The Physiology of the Joints

Churchill Livingstone
Medical Division of Longman Group Limited

Distributed in the United States of America by Churchill Livingstone Inc., 19 West 44th Street, New York, N.Y. 10036, and by associated companies, branches and representatives throughout the world.

1st English edition 1970
reprinted 1974 1975 1976 1977 1978 1980
2nd English edition 1982

ISBN 0 443 02504 5

British Library Cataloguing in Publication Data
Kapandji, I. A.
  The physiology of the joints. — 2nd ed.
  Vol.1: Upper limbs
  1. Joints
  I. Title II. Physiologie articulaire. *English*
  612'.75 QP301 80-42183

The original French edition is entitled *Physiologie Articulaire* and is published by Maloine S.A. Editeur, Paris

Printed in Hong Kong by
Wing King Tong Co Ltd

The Physiology of the Joints

Annotated diagrams of the mechanics of the human joints

I.A. KAPANDJI

Ancien Chef de Clinique Chirurgicale
Assistant des Hôpitaux de Paris
Membre de la Société Française d'Orthopédie et de Traumatologie
Membre du Groupe d'Études de la Main (G.E.M.)

Translated by
L.H. HONORE, B.Sc., M.B., Ch.B., F.R.C.P. (C)

Preface by
Professor F. POILLEUX (Broussais Hôpital, Paris)

Fifth Edition
Completely revised

Volume 1

UPPER LIMB

1 The Shoulder
2 The Elbow
3 Rotation (Pronation and Supination)
4 The Wrist
5 The Hand and the Fingers

With 550 original illustrations by the Author

CHURCHILL LIVINGSTONE
EDINBURGH LONDON MELBOURNE AND NEW YORK 1982

To My Wife

PREFACE TO THE FRENCH EDITION

This book, first of a series of three, has a new and very unusual approach: the author is setting out to give the reader an understanding of the mechanics of the joints with the help of diagrams rather than of a text.

The commentaries are short; the quality, clarity and simplicity of the drawings and diagrams are such that they could be understood without any verbal explanation. Although Dr A. Kapandji first gives us diagrams taken from classical treatises on anatomy, he adds drawings which are very much his own. With his very great knowledge of anatomy and his gift for faithful simplification he can show by these drawings the mechanics of the joint being studied.

Dr A. Kapandji of course intends this book to be helpful to physiotherapists but the student of medicine will find it a necessary and very useful complement to the university course in general physiology of the joints. Surgeons will find ideas of interest for operations which aim to re-establish or re-create normal mechanics in damaged joints.

The drawings are unusually clear: everything which could hinder understanding has been removed and one feels that the author has foreseen the difficulties which the student could encounter. Each time a problem arises it is explained by a diagram which, though simplified, is extremely clear.

The accompanying text which has been included purely for descriptive purposes is short, concise and very well adapted to the author's purpose which is to exploit visual memory to the utmost.

Professor FELIX POILLEUX

FRONTISPIECE OF THE FIFTH EDITION

For the last seventeen years this book, based on the work of Duchenne de Boulogne, the dean of Biomechanics, has undergone only minor changes. The current fifth edition incorporates significant alterations, especially in the chapter devoted to the hand. The rapid developments in hand surgery constantly shed more light on its physiology. Thus the chapter dealing with the thumb and the mechanism of opposition has been rewritten and supplied with new drawings based on recent information. The role of the trapezo-metacarpal joint in the orientation and axial rotation of the thumb is explained mathematically in terms of the mechanics of a universal joint. Emphasis is laid on the role of the metacarpo-phalangeal joint in the locking mechanism essential for the grasping of large objects and of the interphalangeal joint in controlling the degree of thumb opposition with regard to the individual fingers. The infinite variety of static and dynamic grips of the hand is illustrated with new drawings. The different positions of function and immobilization are defined more precisely. Finally, we include a series of test movements which will be more revealing than the systematic analysis of the range of movements at each joint and of the power of each muscle involved. This approach, we feel, is better suited to allow a rapid overview of the full functional capacity of the human hand.

In sum this edition has been significantly updated and expanded.

I.A.K.

CONTENTS

THE SHOULDER

Physiology of the Shoulder	2
Flexion and Extension and Adduction	4
Abduction	6
Axial Rotation of the Arm	8
Movements of the Shoulder Girdle in the Horizontal Plane	8
Horizontal Flexion and Extension	10
The Movement of Circumduction	12
Codman's 'Paradox'	14
Quantitation of Shoulder Movements	16
Movements for Assessing the Overall Function of the Shoulder	18
The Multiarticular Complex of the Shoulder	20
The Articular Surfaces of the Shoulder Joint	22
Instantaneous Centres of Rotation	24
The Capsule and Ligaments of the Shoulder	26
The Intra-articular Course of the Biceps Tendon	28
The Role of the Gleno-Humeral Ligament	30
The Coraco-Humeral Ligament in Flexion and Extension	32
Coaptation of the Articular Surfaces by the Periarticular Muscles	34
The Subdeltoid 'Joint'	36
The Scapulo-Thoracic 'Joint'	38
Movements of the Shoulder Girdle	40
The Real Movements of the Scapulo-Thoracic 'Joint'	42
The Sterno-Clavicular Joint: The Articular Surfaces	44
The Movements	46
The Acromio-Clavicular Joint	48
The Role of the Coraco-Clavicular Ligaments	52
Motor Muscles of the Shoulder Girdle	54
The Supraspinatus and Abduction	56
The Physiology of Abduction	60
The Three Phases of Abduction	64
The Three Phases of Flexion	66
Rotator Muscles of the Arm	68
Adduction and Extension	70

THE ELBOW

Flexion and Extension 72
The Elbow: The Joint Which Allows the Hand to Be Moved Towards
or Away from the Body 74
The Articular Surfaces 76
The Distal End of the Humerus 78
The Ligaments of the Elbow 80
The Head of the Radius 82
The Trochlea Humeri 84
The Limitations of Flexion and Extension 86
Flexor Muscles of the Elbow 88
Extensor Muscles of the Elbow 90
Factors Ensuring Coaptation of the Articular Surfaces 92
The Range of Movements of the Elbow 94
Position of Function and Position of Immobilisation 96

ROTATION (PRONATION AND SUPINATION)

Significance 98
Definitions 100
The Usefulness of Pronation-Supination (Rotation) 102
General Anatomical Relationships 104
Functional Anatomy of the Superior Radio-Ulnar Joint 106
Functional Anatomy of the Inferior Radio-Ulnar Joint 108
Dynamics of the Superior Radio-Ulnar Joint 112
Dynamics of the Inferior Radio-Ulnar Joint 114
Axis of Pronation-Supination 118
The Two Radio-Ulnar Joints Are Co-congruent 122
Muscles of Pronation and Supination 124
Mechanical Disturbances of Pronation-Supination 126
The Position of Function and Compensatory Movements 128

THE WRIST

Significance 130
Movements of the Wrist 132
Range of Movements of the Wrist 134
The Movement of Circumduction 136
The Articular Complex of the Wrist 138
The Articular Surfaces of the Radio-Carpal and Mid-Carpal Joints 140
The ligaments of the Radio-Carpal and Mid-Carpal Joints 142
The Stabilising Function of the Ligaments 144
The Dynamics of the Carpus 148
The Scaphoid-Lunate Couple 152
The Geometrically Variable Carpus 154
Abnormal Movements 156
The Motor Muscles of the Wrist 158
The Actions of the Muscles of the Wrist 160

THE HAND

Its Role	164
Topography of the Hand	166
The Architecture of the Hand	168
The Carpal Bones	172
The Hollowing of the Palm	174
The Metacarpo-Phalangeal Joints	176
The Ligaments of the Metacarpo-Phalangeal Joints	180
The Range of Movements of the Metacarpo-Phalangeal Joints	184
The Interphalangeal Joints	186
The Tunnels and Synovial Sheaths of the Flexor Tendons	190
The Tendons of the Long Flexors of the Fingers	192
The Tendons of the Extensor Muscles of the Fingers	196
The Interosseous and Lumbrical Muscles	198
Extension of the Fingers	200
Abnormal Positions of the Hand and Fingers	204
The Muscles of the Hypothenar Eminence	206
The Thumb	208
The Geometry of Opposition of the Thumb	210
The Trapezo-Metacarpal Joint	212
The Metacarpo-Phalangeal Joint of the Thumb	228
The Interphalangeal Joint of the Thumb	236
The Motor Muscles of the Thumb	238
The Action of the Extrinsic Muscles of the Thumb	242
The Action of the Intrinsic Muscles of the Thumb	244
Opposition of the Thumb	248
Opposition and Counteropposition	254
The Modes of Prehension	256
Percussion — Contact — Gestures	274
Positions of Function and Immobilisation	276
Fictional Hands	278
The Human Hand	280
REFERENCES	282

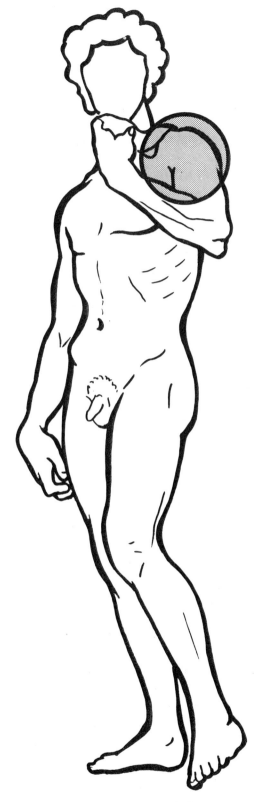

The SHOULDER

THE SHOULDER

Physiology of the Shoulder

The shoulder, the **proximal joint** of the upper limb, is *the most mobile* of all the joints in the human body (Fig. 1, p. 1).

It has **three** degrees of freedom and this permits movement of the upper limb with respect to the *three planes in space and the three major axes* (Fig. 2):

1. **The transverse axis,** lying in a frontal plane, controls the movements of flexion and extension *performed in a sagittal plane* (cf. Fig. 3 and plane A, Fig. 9).

2. **The antero-posterior axis,** lying in a sagittal plane, controls the movements of abduction (the upper limb moves away from the body) and of adduction (the upper limb moves towards the body), which are *performed in a frontal plane* (cf. Fig. 4 and 5 and plane B, Fig. 9).

3. **The vertical axis,** running through the intersection of the sagittal and frontal planes and corresponding to the third axis in space, controls the movements of flexion and extension, which *take place in a horizontal plane* with the arm abducted to 90° (see also Fig. 8 and plane C, Fig. 9.)

About the long axis of the humerus (4) occur two distinct types of lateral and medial rotation of the arm and the upper limb:

— *voluntary rotation*, which depends on the *third degree* of freedom and this can only occur in triaxial-*ball-and-socket-joints*. It is produced by contraction of the rotator muscles.

— *automatic rotation*, which occurs without voluntary movement in biaxial joints or even in triaxial joints when only two of these axes are in use. We will come back to this point when discussing Codman's paradox.

The reference position is obtained when the upper limb hangs vertically at the side of the trunk, so that the long axis of the humerus (4) is continuous with the vertical axis (3) of the limb. The long axis of the humerus also coincides with the transverse axis (1) when the arm is abducted to 90° and with the anteroposterior axis (2) when the arm is flexed to 90°.

Thus the shoulder is a joint with *three main axes* and three degrees of freedom. The long axis of the humerus can coincide with any of these axes or lie in any intermediate position thereby permitting the movement of lateral or medial rotation.

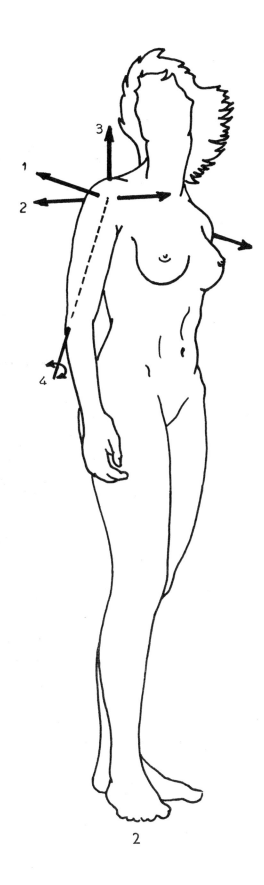

FLEXION AND EXTENSION AND ADDUCTION

Movements of flexion and extension (Fig. 3) performed in a *sagittal plane* (plane A, Fig. 9) and around a *transverse axis* (I, Fig. 2):

(a) extension: movement of small range, up to 45°–50°.

(b) flexion: Movement of great range, up to 180°. Note that the position of flexion at 180° can also be defined as abduction at 180° associated with axial rotation (see Codman's paradox).

Adduction (Fig. 4) in the frontal plane starting from the reference position (i.e. absolute adduction) is mechanically impossible because of the *presence of the trunk*.

Starting from the reference position, adduction is only possible when combined with:

(a) extension: this allows a trace of adduction.

(b) flexion: adduction can reach 30° to 45°.

Starting from any position of abduction, adduction, also called '*relative adduction*', is always possible, in the frontal plane, up to the reference position.

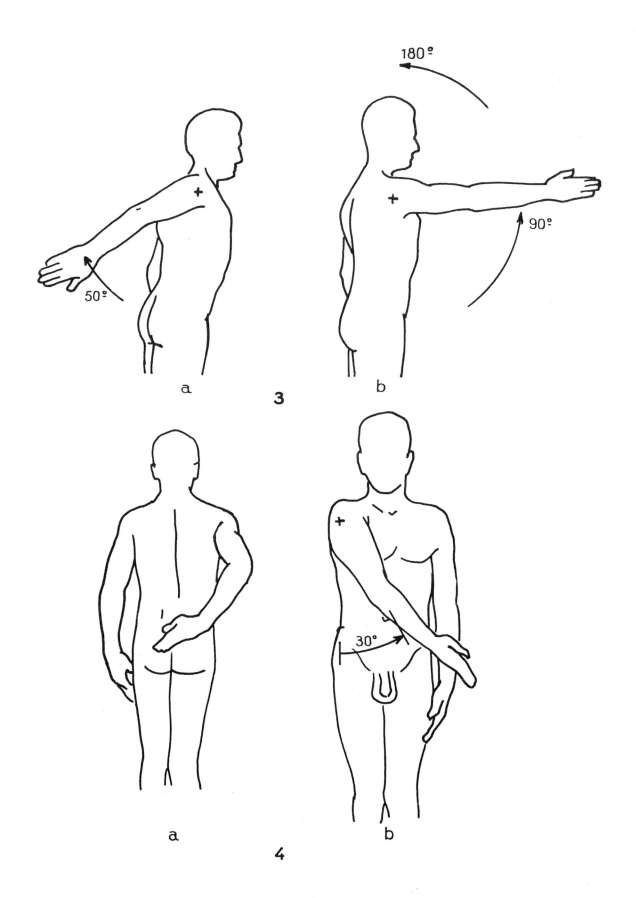

a   **3**   b

a   **4**   b

5

ABDUCTION

Abduction (Fig. 5), the movement of the upper limb away from the trunk, takes place in a *frontal plane* (plane B, Fig. 9) around an *antero-posterior axis* (axis 2, Fig. 2).

When abduction has a full range of 180°, the arm comes to lie vertically above the trunk (d).

Two points deserve attention:

— After the 90° position, the movement of abduction brings the upper limb once more closer to the sagittal plane of the body. The final position of abduction at 180° can also be attained by flexion to 180°.

— As regards the muscles and joint movements involved, abduction, starting from the reference position (a), proceeds through three phases:

(b) abduction from 0° to 60°, taking place only at the shoulder joint.

(c) abduction from 60° to 120°, which requires recruitment of the scapulo-thoracic "joint".

(d) abduction from 120° to 180°, involving movement at the shoulder joint and the scapulo-thoracic "joint" and flexion of the trunk to the opposite side.

Note that pure abduction, occurring exclusively in the frontal plane, is rare. On the contrary, abduction combined with flexion, i.e. elevation of the arm *in the plane of the scapula*, at an angle of 30° in front of the frontal plane, is the most common movement, used particularly to bring the hand to the nape or the mouth.

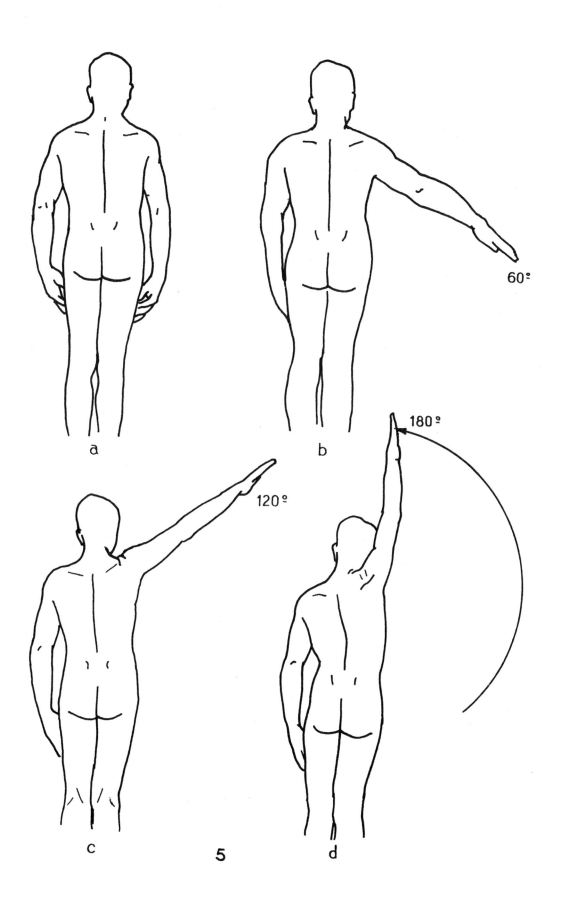

60°

120°

180°

a

b

c

d

5

AXIAL ROTATION OF THE ARM

Rotation of the arm about its long axis (axis 3, Fig. 2) can occur in any position of the shoulder. It is a *voluntary rotation* taking place at joints with three axes and three degrees of freedom. This rotation is usually quantitated starting from the reference position, i.e. with the arm hanging vertically along the body. (Fig. 6, seen from above).

(a) **Reference position**, i.e. the position of null rotation: to measure the range of rotatory movements *the elbow must be flexed to 90°* with the forearm lying within a sagittal plane. If this were not so, the range of such rotatory movements of the arm would be compounded with that of pronation and supination of the forearm.

This reference position, with the forearm lying in a sagittal plane, is purely arbitrary. In practice, the starting position most commonly used, since it corresponds with the point of equilibrium of the rotator muscles, is that of a 30° internal rotation with respect to the true reference position (the hand then lies in front of the trunk). This position can thus be called the *physiological reference position.*

(b) **Lateral rotation:** up to 80° and falling short of 90°. The full range of 80° is rarely used with the arm hanging vertically along the body. On the contrary, the type of lateral rotation most commonly used, and so most important functionally, lies between the physiological reference position (lateral rotation = 30°) and the classic reference position (rotation 0°).

(c) **Medial rotation:** up to 100°–110°. The full range is only achieved *with the forearm passing behind the trunk* and the shoulder slightly extended. This movement must occur freely to allow the hand to reach the back and is *essential for anal toilette.* The first 90° of medial rotation must also be associated with shoulder flexion as long as the hand stays in front of the trunk.

The muscles responsible for rotation will be discussed on page 68. Axial rotation of the arm in positions outside the reference position can only be accurately evaluated *with the use of polar coordinates* (see p. 16). For each position the rotator muscles behave differently, with some losing and others acquiring rotator function. This is another example of the *law of inversion of muscular action* depending on the position of the muscle.

MOVEMENTS OF THE SHOULDER GIRDLE IN THE HORIZONTAL PLANE

These movements (Fig. 7) also involve movements of the *scapula on the thorax.* In the diagram:

(a) **reference position**

(b) **backward movement of the shoulder girdle**

(c) **forward movement of the shoulder girdle**

Note that the range of forward movement is *greater* than that of backward movement.
The muscles involved in these movements are as follows:

Forward movement: pectoralis major, pectoralis minor, serratus anterior.

Backward movement: rhomboids, trapezius (the transverse fibres), latissimus dorsi.

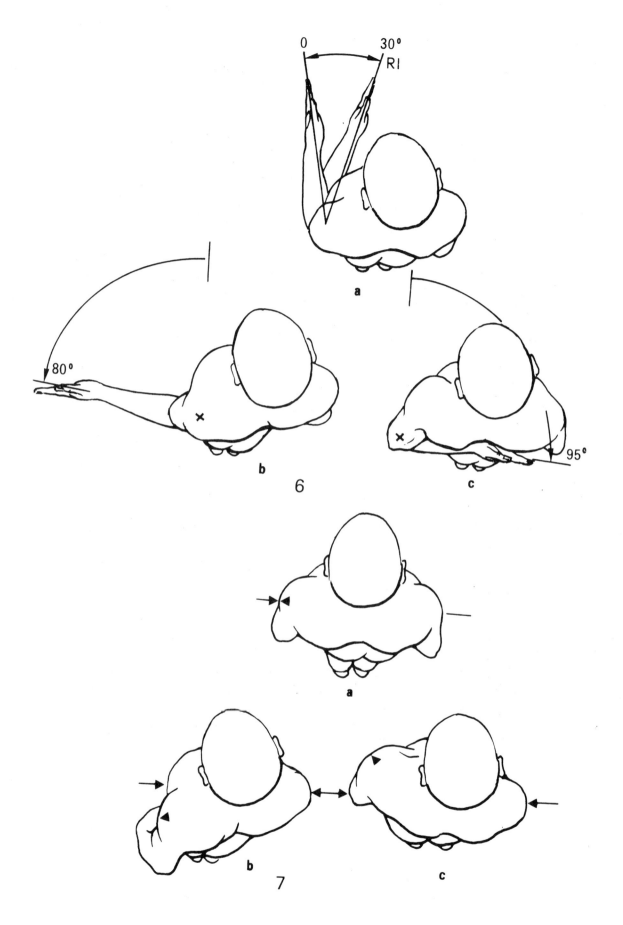

6

7

9

HORIZONTAL FLEXION AND EXTENSION

These movements of the upper limb occur in the horizontal plane (Fig. 8 and plane C, Fig. 9) around a vertical axis or more exactly a series of vertical axes, since they involve both the shoulder joint (axis 4, Fig. 2) and the scapulo-thoracic 'joint' (cf. Fig. 37).

(a) **Reference position:** the upper limb is abducted 90° in the frontal plane, calling into action the following muscles:
Deltoid (acromial fibres: III, Fig. 65).
Supraspinatus.
Trapezius (acromial, clavicular and tubercular fibres).
Serratus anterior.

(b) **Horizontal flexion,** associated with adduction, has a range of 140° and calls into action the following muscles:
Deltoid (anteromedial fibres I and anterolateral fibres II to a variable degree and lateral fibres III).
Subscapularis.
Pectoralis major and pectoralis minor.
Serratus anterior.

(c) **Horizontal extension,** associated with adduction, has a limited range of 30°–40° and calls into action the following muscles:
Deltoid (posterolateral fibres IV and V and posteromedial fibres VI and VII to a variable degree and lateral fibres III)
Supraspinatus
Infraspinatus
Teres major and teres minor
Rhomboids
Trapezius (all fibres including transverse fibres)
Latissimus dorsi, acting as an antagonist-synergist with the deltoid, which cancels its important adductor function

The overall range of this movement of horizontal flexion and extension falls short of 180°. Movement from the extreme position anteriorly to the extreme position posteriorly successively mobilises the various fibres of the deltoid (see p. 60), which is the dominant muscle involved.

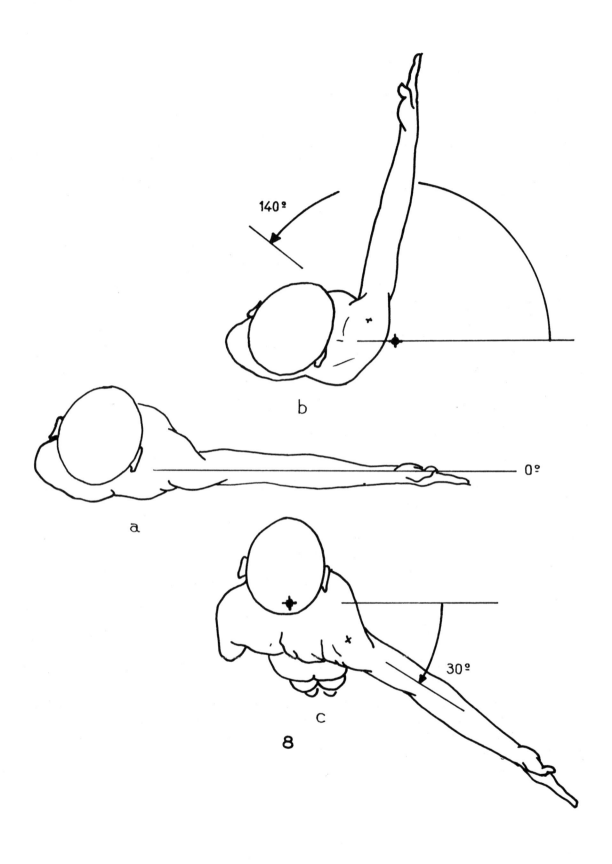

140°

0°

b

a

30°

c

8

11

THE MOVEMENT OF CIRCUMDUCTION

Circumduction combines the elementary movements *about the three cardinal axes* (Fig. 9). When circumduction is taken to its maximum amplitude, the arm describes an irregular cone in space, *the cone of circumduction*. This cone demarcates, within a sphere centred on the shoulder and with a radius equal to the length of the upper limb, a *spherical sector of accessibility*, wherein the hand can grasp objects and bring them to the mouth *without displacement of the trunk*.

In this figure the curve represents the base of the cone of circumduction (the path of the fingertips) crossing the various sectors of space as defined by the planes of reference of the shoulder joint:

A Sagittal plane (flexion — extension)

B Frontal plane (adduction — abduction)

C Horizontal plane (horizontal flexion — extension).

Starting from the reference position, which is marked by a heavy dot, the curve (for the right upper limb) passes successively through the following sectors:

III Below, in front and to the left

II Above, in front and to the left

VI Above, behind and to the right

V Below, behind and to the right

VIII Below, behind and to the left for a very short distance as the combined movement of extension and adduction is very limited (in the diagram sector VIII lies below plane C, behind sector III and to the left of sector V. Sector VII, not seen, lies just above).

The arrow which extends the axis of the arm indicates *the axis of the cone of circumduction* and also corresponds to the axis of the position of function (cf. Fig. 16), with the exception that the elbow is extended in this case. Sector V, which contains the axis of the cone of circumduction, is the *sector of preferential accessibility*. The *forward* orientation of the axis of the cone of circumduction is in line with the need to keep working hands under visual control. Also in line with this need is the partial overlapping of the two sectors of accessibility of the upper limbs anteriorly, which allows the two hands *to work together under visual control*, to cooperate and, if need be, to compensate one for the other. Besides, the full extent of the two spherical sectors of accessibility of the upper limbs is conditioned by the eyes as they move from one extreme position to another with the head fixed in the sagittal plane. Thus the visual fields and the sectors of preferential accessibility of the hands are almost identical.

It must be noted that this congruence has been achieved during phylogeny by the downward migration of the foramen magnum. As a result the face can look forward and *the eyes can glance in a direction perpendicular to the long axis of the body*, whereas in quadrupeds the direction of the gaze coincides with the axis of the body.

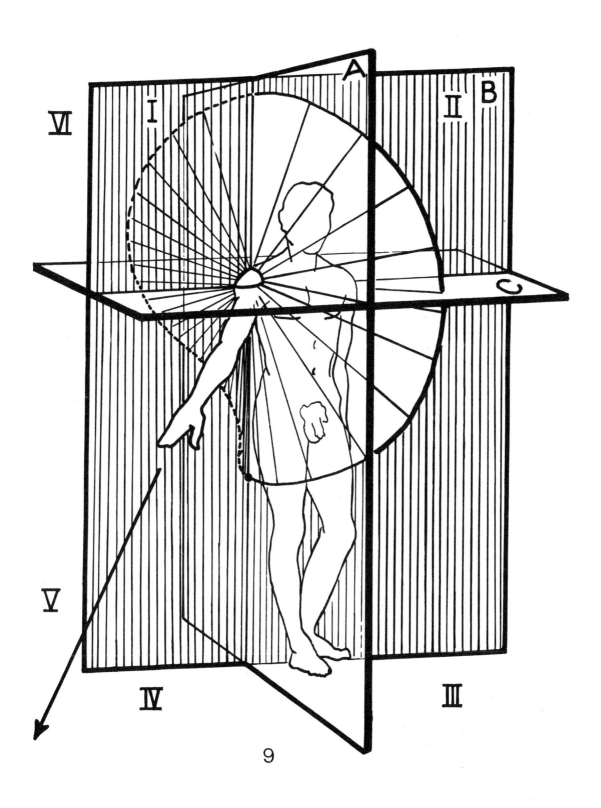

9

CODMAN'S "PARADOX"

Start from the reference position (a and b, Fig. 10), with the upper limb hanging vertically along-side the trunk, the palm of the hand facing medially and the thumb facing *anteriorly* (a), and abduct the limb to 180° in the frontal plane (c) and then extend the limb in the sagittal plane for −180° (d). The limb once more lies vertically alongside the body but with the *palm facing laterally* and the *thumb facing posteriorly* (e).

The movements can also be reversed starting with 180° flexion followed by 180° adduction. The limb is laterally rotated through 180°.

It is easy to note that the orientation of the palm has changed and that the limb has been axially rotated through 180°.

This double movement of abduction followed by extension is **automatically** associated with *medial rotation* of 180°. Thus sequential movements about the two axes of the shoulder bring about a *mechanical* and involuntary movement about the longitudinal axis of the upper limb. This **conjunct rotation** (Mac Conaill) occurs only during *sequential movements*, i.e. movements performed successively about the two axes of a joint with two degrees of freedom. In the present case the shoulder joint, which has three degrees of freedom, is *functioning as a biaxial joint*.

If the limb *is voluntarily and simultaneously* rotated inversely through 180° around the third axis, the hand lies in the same position as at the start with the thumb pointing anteriorly, after completing an *ergonomic cycle*. Such cycles are frequently used by professionals and athletes in the performance of repetitive movements, e.g. in swimming. This voluntary axial rotation, called **adjunct rotation** by Mac Conaill, can only take place in joints with three degrees of freedom and is essential for the completion of an ergonomic cycle. This is well brought out by the following experiment. Start in the reference position after medial rotation so that the palm faces laterally and the thumb points posteriorly. Abduct to 180° but, after 90°, abduction becomes impossible and can only resume after voluntary lateral rotation. Anatomical factors, such as stretching of ligaments and muscles, limit conjoint medial rotation and a voluntary lateral rotation becomes necessary to cancel the conjoint medial rotation and complete the ergonomic cycle. Hence *the need for a triaxial joint at the root of a limb*.

In summary, **two types of axial rotation** can occur at the shoulder joint: voluntary or **adjunct** rotation and automatic or **conjunct** rotation. At every moment these two rotations summate algebraically:

— if *voluntary rotation is nil*, automatic rotation is maximal, giving rise to Codman's (pseudo) paradox.

— if *voluntary rotation occurs in the same direction* as the automatic rotation, the latter is rein-forced.

— if *voluntary rotation takes place in the opposite direction*, it reduces or even cancels automatic rotation, giving rise to the ergonomic cycle.

All these ideas concerning automatic and voluntary rotations and the ergonomic cycle will be further developed and illustrated in volume IV, yet to be published.

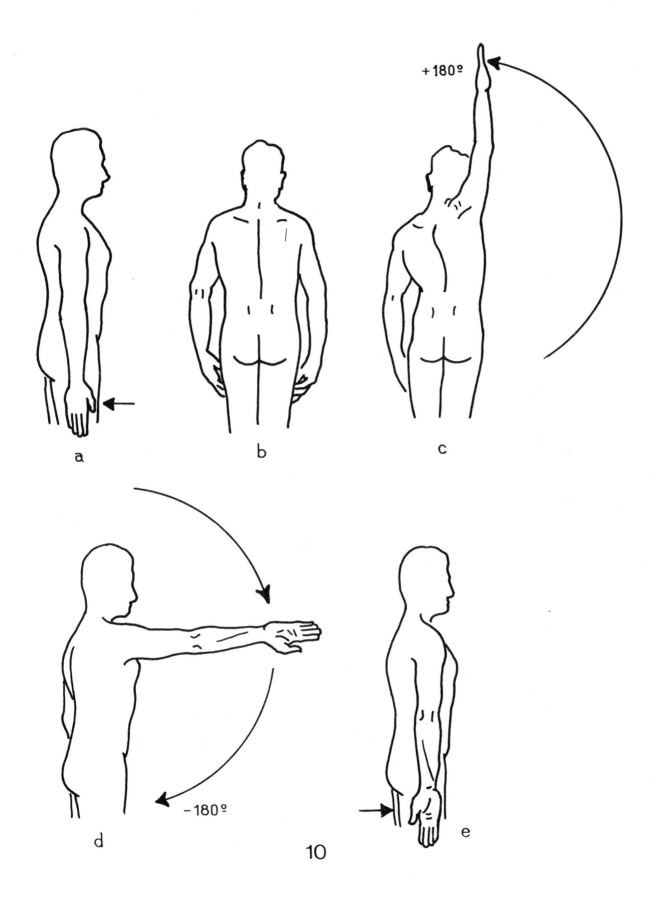

a

b

+180º

c

d

−180º

e

10

QUANTITATION OF SHOULDER MOVEMENTS

The quantitation of movements and positions of joints with three major axes and three degrees of freedom, like the shoulder, is difficult because of basic ambiguities in interpretation. For instance, if *abduction* is broadly defined as a movement of the upper limb away from the sagittal plane of the body, the definition is only valid up to 90°, since past that point the upper limb moves towards the body and yet the term abduction is still used. It is even more difficult to evaluate axial rotation.

While it is fairly easy to quantitate a movement performed in a cardinal plane, frontal or sagittal, though arbitrarily chosen, it is more difficult to do so in intermediate planes. At least *two angular coordinates* are needed, whether a system of rectangular or polar coordinates is used.

Using *rectangular coordinates* (Fig. 11), one measures the angle of projection of the long axis of the arm on two or three reference planes: frontal F, sagittal S and transverse T. The centre of the shoulder lies at the intersection O of these three planes. The projections of the point P on the frontal plane F (M) and on the sagittal plane S (Q) allow one to measure the angle of abduction SÔM and the angle of flexion SÔQ. Note that the position of N, the projection of P on the transverse plane T, is accurately determined when M and Q are known. But in this system of measurements one cannot quantitate rotation along the long axis OP.

Using *polar coordinates* (Fig. 12), one defines the direction of the arm by the position taken by the elbow P on a sphere centred on the shoulder joint O and having a radius OP equal to the length of the humerus. As on the globe, the position of the point P is defined by two lines the longitude and the latitude. The point P lies at the intersection of a large circle passing through the poles and of a small circle parallel to the equatorial plane, which here corresponds to the large circle contained in the sagittal plane S. The line joining the poles corresponds to the intersection of the frontal plane F and the transverse plane T, while the meridian O is represented by the half circle lying within the frontal plane F and below the transverse plane T. *Flexion* is measured as a line of *longitude* reckoned anterior to the body, i.e the angle BÔL (L being the intersection of the meridian running through P and of the equator). *Abduction* is measured as a line of *latitude*, i.e. the angle AÔK or rather its complement BÔK. It is also possible to quantitate the *axial rotation* of the humerus using the line of longitude BPA as reference. The angle of rotation is given as the angle APC.

The latter system of quantitation is thus more precise and complete than the former. It is even the only system that allows the *cone of circumduction* to be represented as a closed loop on the shpere. However it is less often used in practice because of its complexity.

There is also an important difference in the observations obtained by these two methods (Fig. 13). The angle of flexion BÔL is the same but the angle of abduction BÔK is not the same as BÔM (in rectangular coordinates) and this differences widens as flexion approaches 90°. In fact, for a flexion of 90° the point P lies on the horizontal meridian through E. Hence the angle BÔM is always equal to 90° while the angle AÔK can vary from 0° to 90°.

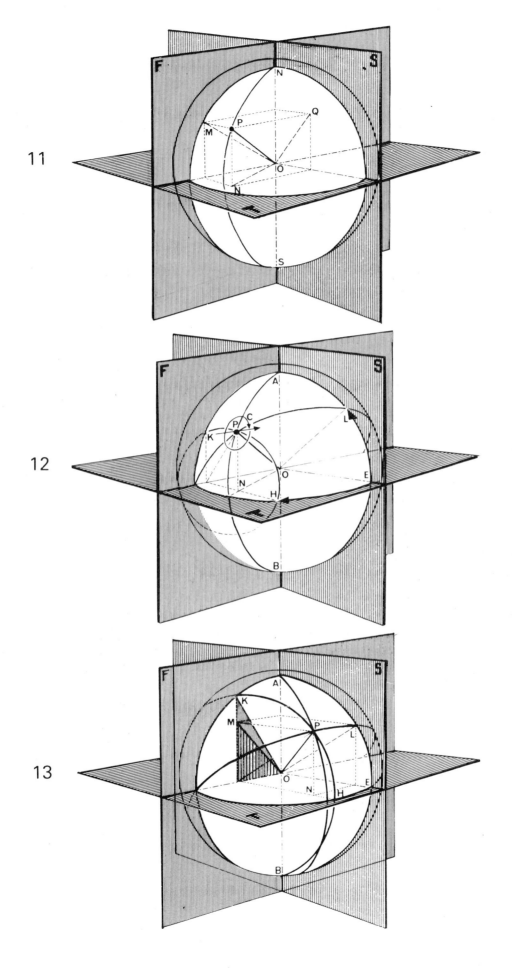

11

12

13

MOVEMENTS FOR ASSESSING THE OVERALL FUNCTION OF THE SHOULDER

The first movement (Fig. 14):

(a) Combing the hair

(b) *Putting the hand behind the neck*.

When this movement is free and of normal range, the hand can reach the opposite ear and the superior aspect of the contralateral scapula. When done with the elbow bent it allows assessment of abduction up to 120° and of lateral rotation up to 90°.

The second movement (Fig. 15):

Putting on a jacket or an overcoat:

— the arm which goes into the first sleeve (left arm in the diagram) is flexed and abducted.

— the arm which makes for the second sleeve is extended and medially rotated (the right arm in the diagram) while the hand reaches the lumbar region.

When this movement is free and of normal range, the hand can reach up to the lower aspect of the contralateral scapula.

The position of function of the shoulder (Fig. 16) is attained when:

The long axis of the arm is flexed at 45° and abducted at 60°, i.e. it lies in a vertical plane forming a solid angle of 45° with the sagittal (or frontal) plane and is *medially rotated* to 30°–40°.

This position corresponds to the *position of equilibrium of the periarticular muscles of the shoulder*. Hence its use when immobilising fractures of the humeral shaft. When this position is adopted, the lower fragment, which is the only one that can be manipulated, is aligned with the upper fragment, which is acted upon by the periarticular muscles.

This position also corresponds to the axis of the cone of circumduction (Fig. 9).

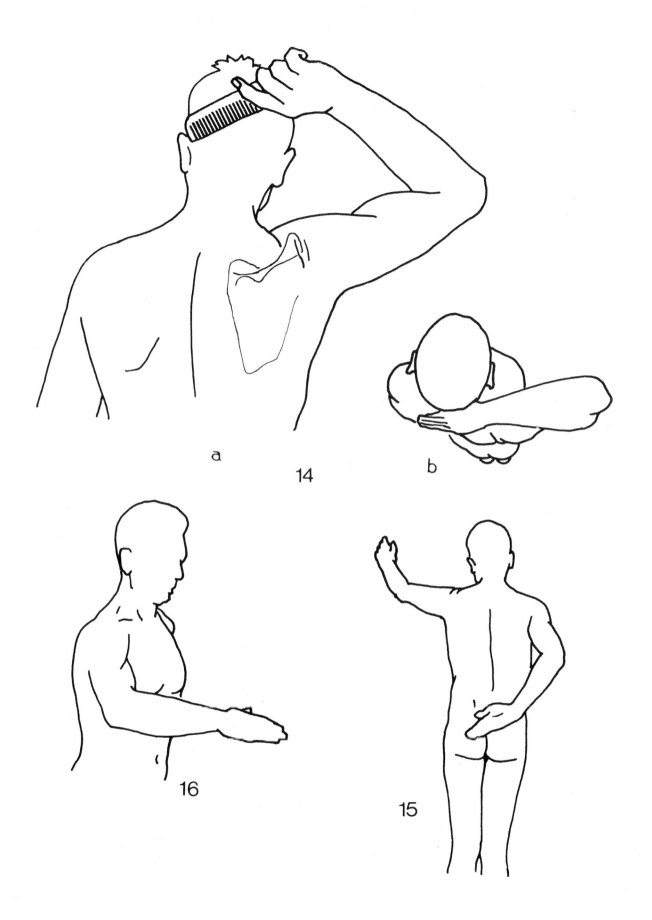

a

14

b

16

15

19

THE MULTIARTICULAR COMPLEX OF THE SHOULDER

The shoulder comprises not one but **five** joints (Fig. 17). We have already described its movement as seen from the upper limb. These five joints fall into two groups:

First group: *two joints:*

1. **The shoulder or scapulo-humeral joint,** which is a true joint anatomically with apposition of two articular surfaces lined by hyaline cartilage. It is the most important joint of this group.

2. **The subdeltoid 'joint'** or 'the second shoulder joint'. This is not an anatomical but a physiological joint, as it consists of two surfaces sliding with respect to each other. The subdeltoid 'joint' is mechanically linked to the shoulder joint because any movement in the latter brings about movement in the former.

Second group: *three joints:*

3. **The scapulo-thoracic 'joint'**

   This is also a physiological and not an anatomical joint. It is the most important joint of this group, although it cannot function without the other two, which are mechanically linked to it.

4. **The acromio-clavicular joint,** a true joint, located at the acromial end of the clavicle.

5. **The sterno-clavicular joint,** a true joint, located at the sternal end of the clavicle.

In sum, the joints of the shoulder can be summarized as follows:

First group: an anatomical main joint — the shoulder joint — mechanically linked to a physiological (false) joint — the subdeltoid 'joint'.

Second group: a physiological (false) main joint — the scapulo-thoracic 'joint' mechanically linked the two anatomical joints — the acromio-clavicular and the sterno-clavicular joints.

In each group the joints are *mechanically linked*, i.e. they must function in concert. In practice both groups also work simultaneously with a variable contribution from each set depending on the type of movement.

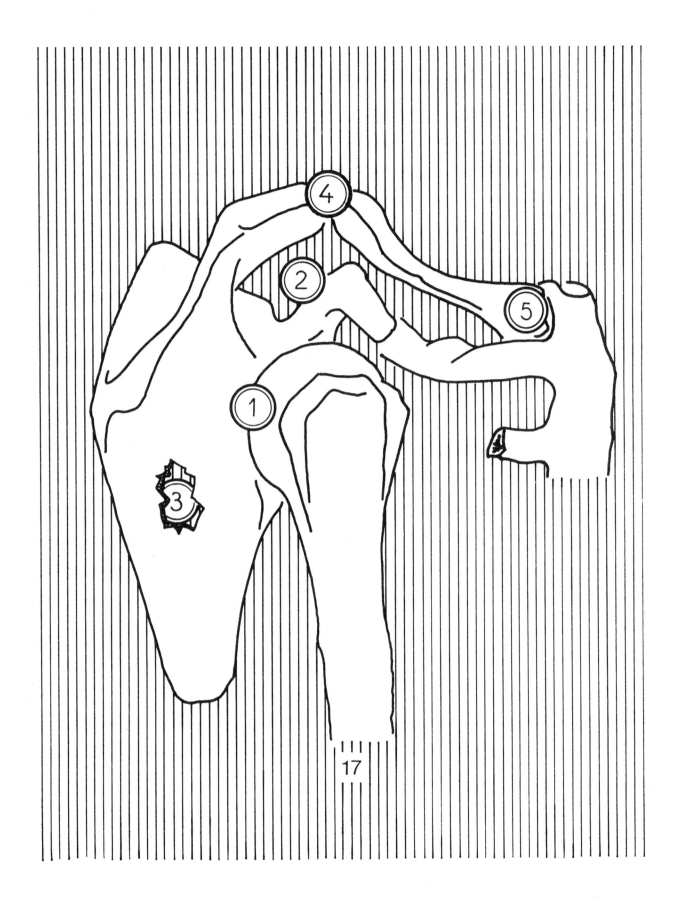

17

THE ARTICULAR SURFACES OF THE SHOULDER JOINT

These are *spherical* surfaces, typical of a ball-and-socket joint, which has *three axes* and *three degrees of freedom*. (Fig. 18).

(a) The head of the humerus

Facing superiorly, medially and *posteriorly* it corresponds to a third of a sphere 3 cm in radius. In effect this sphere is far from regular since its *vertical diameter is 3 to 4 mm greater* than its posterior diameter. Moreover, a vertico-frontal cut (inset) shows that its *radius of curvature decreases slightly in a supero-inferior direction* and that it contains not one centre of curvature but a *series of centres of curvature spirally arranged*. Thus, when the superior portion of the humeral head is in contact with the glenoid cavity, the joint is maximally stable, the more so as the middle and inferior fibres of the gleno-humeral ligament are taut. This position of abduction at 90° corresponds to the **locked** or the close-packed position of Mac Conaill.

Its axis forms with the axis of the shaft an angle of 135° (the neck-shaft angle) and with the frontal plane an angle of 30° (the retrotorsion angle).

It is separated from the rest of the superior epiphysis of the humerus by the *anatomical neck* which makes an angle of 45° with the horizontal plane. It bears two tuberosities, which receive the insertions of the periarticular muscles:

— the lesser tuberosity pointing anteriorly:

— the greater tuberosity pointing laterally.

(b) The glenoid cavity of the scapula

It lies at the supero-lateral angle of the scapula and points laterally, *anteriorly* and slightly superiorly. It is biconcave vertically and transversely but its concavity is *irregular* and less marked than the convexity of the humeral head. Its margin is slightly raised and is grooved anteroposteriorly. The glenoid cavity is *much smaller* than the head of the humerus.

(c) The glenoid labrum

This is a *ring of fibro-cartilage* attached to the margin of the glenoid cavity and bridging the antero-superior groove. It widens the cavity only slightly but deepens it appreciably so as to make the articular surfaces more *congruent*.

It is triangular in section and has three surfaces:

— a basal surface attached to the margin of the glenoid

— an outer (peripheral) surface giving attachment to the capsular ligaments

— an inner (*articular*) surface lined by cartilage continuous with that of the glenoid cavity and in contact with the head of the humerus.

22

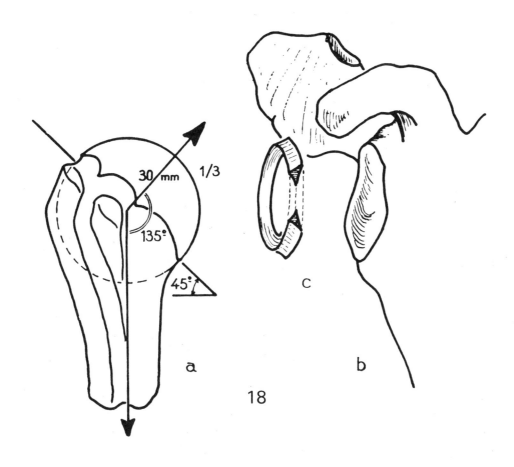

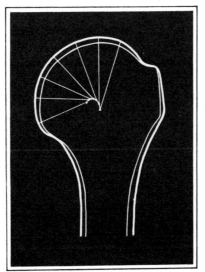

a

b

c

18

23

INSTANTANEOUS CENTRES OF ROTATION

The centre of curvature of an articular surface does not necessarily coincide with the centre of rotation, since other factors, i.e. the shape of the articular surface, mechanical factors within the joint, the tension of ligaments and muscular contractions, influence movements.

In the past the head of the humerus was likened to a portion of a sphere and this led to the belief that it had a fixed and unchangeable centre of rotation. Recent studies by Fischer et al have shown that there exists a series of instantaneous centres of rotation (I.C.R.), corresponding to the centre of a movement occurring between two very close positions. These centres are determined by a computer from a series of radiographs taken in succession.

Thus, during *abduction*, only the component of rotation of the humerus in the frontal plane is considered, and there are two *sets of I.C.R.* (Fig. 19), which for unknown reasons are separated by a distinct gap (3–4). The first set lies within a circular domain C1, located near the inferomedial aspect of the humeral head and having as centre the centre of gravity of the I.C.R.'s and as radius the mean of the distances between the centre of gravity and each I.C.R. The second set lies within a another circular domain C2 located near the upper half of the humeral head. These two domains do not overlap.

During abduction the shoulder joint can thus be broken down into two joints (Fig. 20):

— during abduction to 50°, rotation of the humeral head occurs around a point located *somewhere* within circle C1.

— the end of abduction (from 50° to 90°), the centre of rotation lies within circle C2,

— about 50° abduction, there is a discontinuity in the movement so that the centre of rotation now lies superior and medial to the humeral head.

During *flexion* (Fig. 21, lateral view) a similar analysis fails to disclose any discontinuity in the path of the I.C.R.'s which lie within a *single* circular domain located in the inferior part of the humeral head midway between its two borders.

Finally, during *axial rotation* (Fig. 22, superior view), the circular domain of the I.C.R.'s lies at the junction of the head and shaft midway between the two lateral borders of the humeral head.

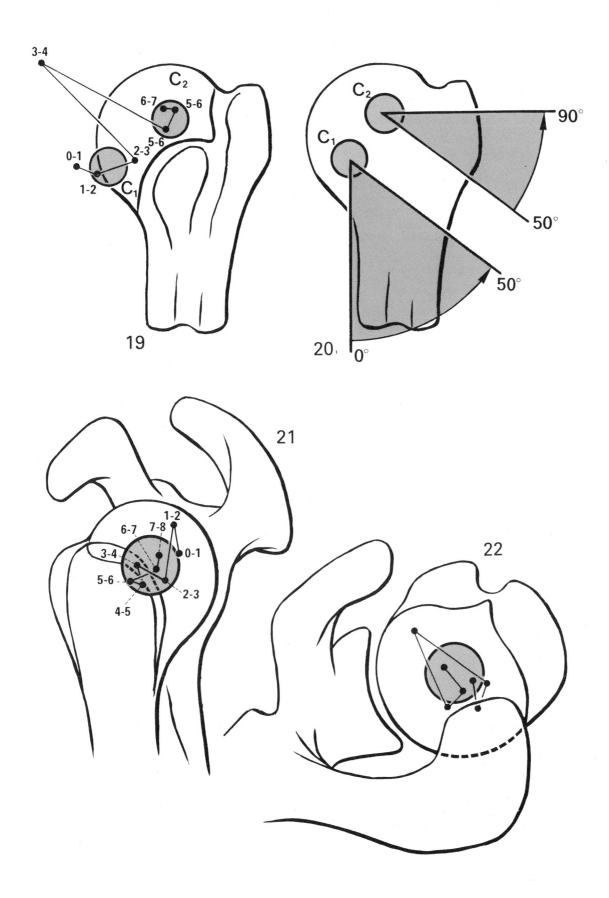

THE CAPSULE AND LIGAMENTS OF THE SHOULDER

The articular surfaces and the capsular cuff (Fig. 23, according to Rouvière)

(a) *The head of the humerus* (medial view)
It is surrounded by a capsule (1) and the diagram shows:
- the inferior synovial folds (2), below the head and raised by the recurrent fibres of the capsule.
- the superior band (3) of the gleno-humeral ligament which strengthens the capsule.

Inside the capsule is the (cut) tendon of the long head of biceps (4).
Outside the capsule is the stump of the subscapularis muscle (5) near its insertion.

(b) *The glenoid cavity* (seen from outside)
The glenoid labrum (1) is shown bridging the groove in the glenoid margin (2). At its upper pole it gives origin to the long tendon of the biceps which is therefore *intracapsular* (3).

Also shown in the diagram are:

The joint capsule (4) and its related ligaments, i.e. coraco-humeral ligament (5) and the three bands of the gleno-humeral ligament: superior (6), middle (7) and inferior (8).

The coracoid process (9), the (cut) spine of the scapula (10), the infraglenoid tubercle (11) which gives origin to the tendon of the long head of triceps *extracapsularly*.

The ligaments of the shoulder (Fig. 24, anterior aspect, according to Rouvière)
- **Coraco-humeral ligament** (1) running from the coracoid process (2) to the greater tuberosity (3), where the supraspinatus tendon (4) is inserted and to the lesser tuberosity (5), where the subscapularis muscle (6) is inserted. The two bands of the ligament diverge above the bicipital groove at the point where the biceps tendon emerges from the joint and proceeds along the groove now *transformed into a tunnel* (7) *by the transverse humeral ligament* (8).
- **Gleno-humeral ligament** with its three bands, the **superior** band (9) running from the upper margin of the glenoid over the humeral head; the **middle** band (10) running from the upper margin of the glenoid in front of the humerus; the **inferior** band (11) running across the anterior edge of the glenoid and below the humeral head.

These three bands form a Z in front of the joint capsule. Between these bands lie two points of weakness:
The foramen of Weitbrecht (12), which is the opening into the subscapularis fossa.
The foramen of Rouvière (13), through which the synovial cavity can communicate with the subcoracoid bursa.
- long head of triceps (14).

Posterior aspect of the shoulder (Fig. 24a, according to Rouvière) An opening has been made in the posterior part of the capsule and the head of the humerus has been resected (1). On a cadaver the **looseness of the capsule** allows the articular surfaces to be parted 3 cm from each other.

Shown in the figure are the following:
- the deep surface of middle (2) and inferior (3) bands of the gleno-humeral ligament.
- the coraco-humeral ligament (4) to which is attached the coraco-glenoid ligament (5) of no mechanical significance.
- the intra-articular portion of the tendon of the long biceps (6),
- the glenoid cavity (7) and the glenoid labrum (8).
- two ligaments with no mechanical function, i.e. the suprascapular ligament (9) and the spino-glenoid ligament (10)
- the insertion of three periarticular muscles: the supraspinatus (11), the infraspinatus (12) and the teres minor (13).

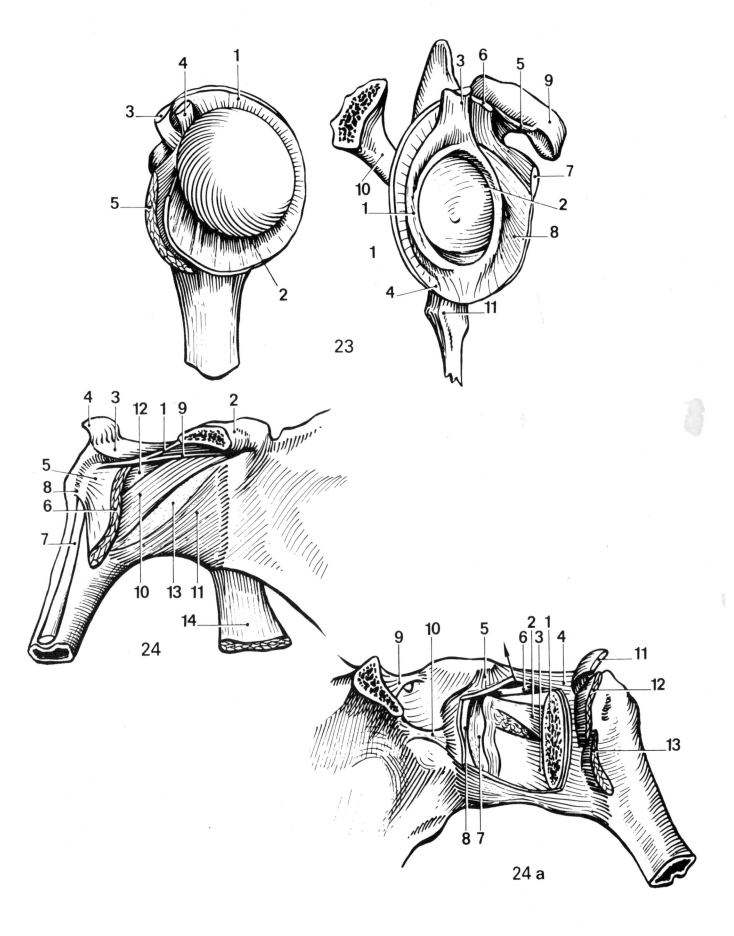

23

24

24 a

27

THE INTRA-ARTICULAR COURSE OF THE BICEPS TENDON

A coronal section through the shoulder (Fig. 25 according to Rouvière) shows:

— The irregularities of the bony glenoid cavity are *smoothed out* by the articular cartilage (1).

— The glenoid labrum (2) deepens the glenoid cavity. However the interlocking of the articular surfaces is only *slight*; hence the *frequent occurrence of dislocations*. In its upper part (3) the glenoid labrum is not completely fixed to the bone and its inner edge lies free in the cavity like a meniscus.

— In the reference position of the joint the upper part of the capsule (4) is taut while the lower part is slack. This 'slack' in the capsule (5) and the unfolding of the synovial folds (6) allow abduction to occur.

— The tendon of the long head of the biceps (7) arises from the supra-glenoid tubercle and the superior margin of the glenoid labrum. As it emerges from the joint cavity in the bicipital groove (8) it passes deep to the capsule (4).

Inset: The section shows the relations of the biceps tendon to the synovium of the joint. Inside the joint cavity the tendon of the long head of the biceps is in contact with the synovium in the following three positions:

1. It is pressed against the deep surface of the capsule (c) by the synovial lining (s).

2. The tendon invaginates the synovium which forms a suspensory sling for it underneath the capsule, i.e. a *meso-tendon*.

3. The tendon now lies free but is completely invested by synovium.

In general, these three positions of the tendon occur successively as it courses away from its origin, but in every case the tendon, though *intracapsular*, remains *extrasynovial*.

It is now known that the biceps tendon plays an important role in the physiology and pathology of the shoulder.

When the biceps contracts to lift a heavy load its two heads are crucial in maintaining the *coaptation of the articular surfaces of the shoulder*. The short head, resting on the coracoid process, lifts the humerus relative to the scapula and, along with the other longitudinal muscles (triceps, coracobrachialis and deltoid), prevents its downward dislocation. At the same time the long head of the biceps presses the humeral head against the glenoid, especially during abduction (Fig. 26), since *the long head of the biceps is also an abductor*. Following its rupture there is a 20 per cent drop in the strength of abduction.

The initial degree of tension of the biceps depends on the length of its horizontal intra-articular path (Fig. 27, seen from above), which is maximal when the humerus is in an intermediate position of flexion-extension (A) and in lateral rotation (B). In these positions the efficiency of the long head is at its greatest. When the humerus is medially rotated (C), the intra-articular path of the biceps, and hence its efficiency, are minimal.

It is clear therefore that the biceps, bent as it is at the level of the bicipital groove without an associated sesamoid bone, is subject to severe mechanical stress, which can only be tolerated when the muscle is in good condition. If the collagen fibres degenerate with age, the intra-articular tendon may snap as a result of the slightest effort, giving rise to a typical clinical picture associated with periarthritis of the shoulder.

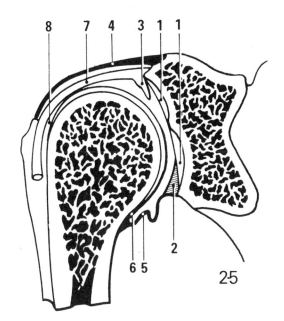

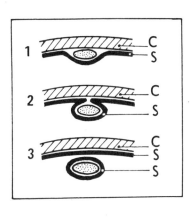

25

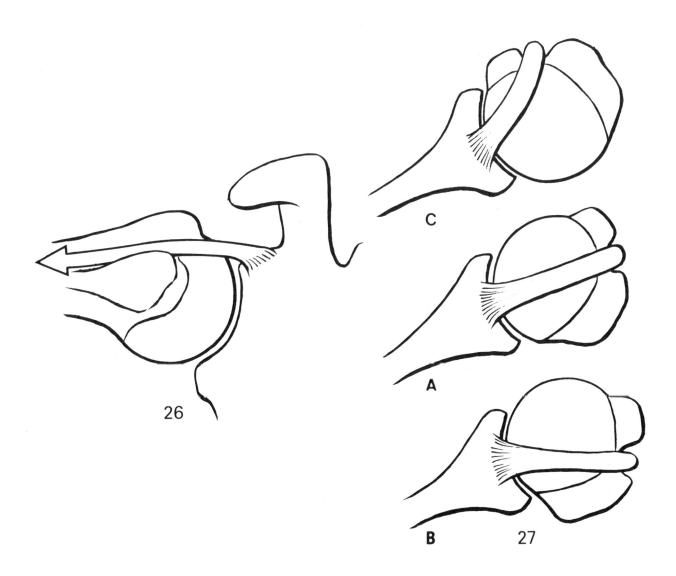

26

C

A

B

27

THE ROLE OF THE GLENO-HUMERAL LIGAMENT

During abduction (Fig. 28):

    (a) reference position (the hatchings show the middle and inferior bands of the ligament)

    (b) The middle and inferior bands of the gleno-humeral ligament become taut while the superior band and the coraco-humeral ligament (not shown here) relax. Thus in abduction the ligaments are maximally stretched and the articular surfaces achieve maximal contact because the radius of curvature of the humeral head is greater superiorly than inferiorly. Hence abduction is the locked or *close-packed position of the shoulder* (Mac Conaill).

Abduction is also checked when the greater tuberosity comes into contact with the upper part of the glenoid and the glenoid labrum. This contact is delayed by lateral rotation, which pulls back the greater tuberosity near the end of abduction, brings the bicipital groove to face the acromio-coracoid arch and slackens slightly the inferior fibres of the gleno-humeral ligament. As a result abduction reaches 90°

When abduction is combined with a 30° flexion in the plane of the scapula, the tightening of the gleno-humeral ligament occurs more slowly and abduction can reach up to 110°.

During rotation (Fig. 29)

    (a) Lateral rotation tenses up all three bands of the gleno-humeral ligament.

    (b) Medial rotation relaxes them.

30

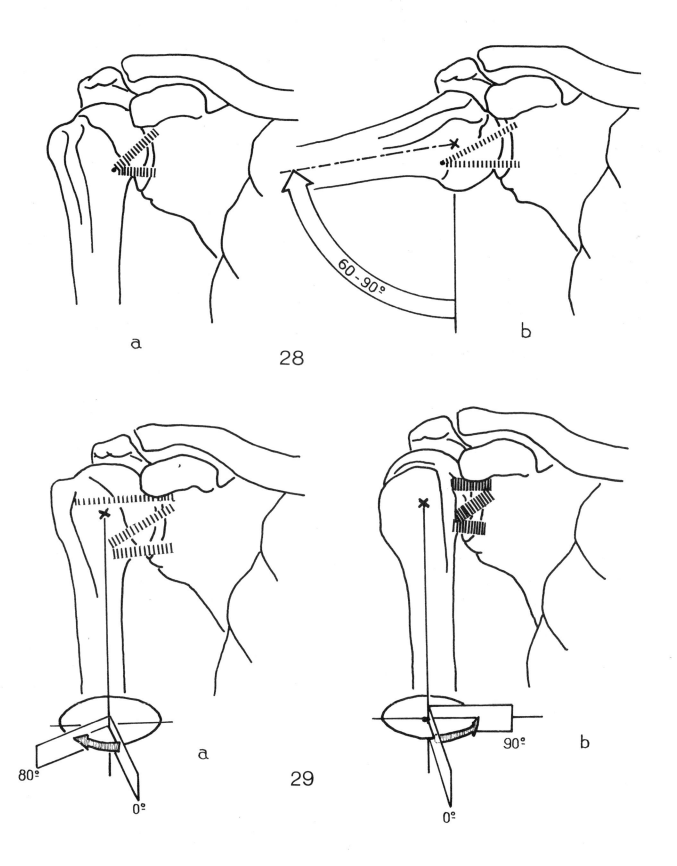

a   b

28

a   29   b

31

THE CORACO-HUMERAL LIGAMENT IN FLEXION AND EXTENSION

The differential development of tension in the two bands of the coraco-humeral ligament is shown in Fig. 30 (the shoulder seen from outside):

(a) Reference position showing the coraco-humeral ligament with its two bands (the posterior inserted into the greater tuberosity and the anterior into the lesser tuberosity).

(b) Tension develops mainly in the anterior band during *extension*.

(c) Tension develops mainly in the posterior band during *flexion*. Medial rotation of the humerus occurring at the end of flexion slackens the coraco- and gleno-humeral ligaments, thus increasing the range of movement.

30

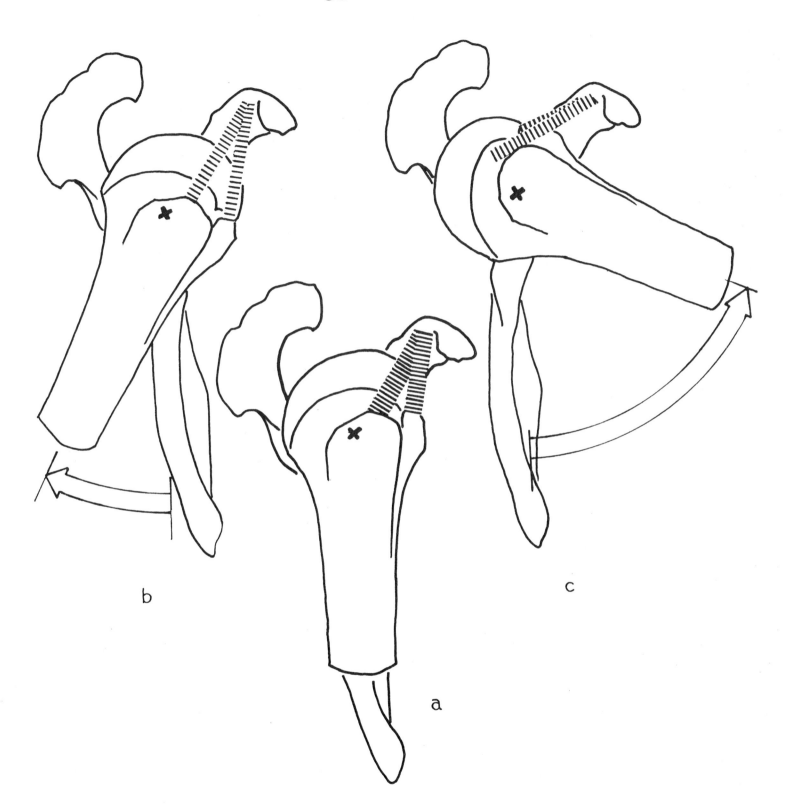

b

a

c

33

COAPTATION OF THE ARTICULAR SURFACES BY THE PERIARTICULAR MUSCLES

These muscles, *running transversely* across the joint, act as active ligaments and *keep the head of the humerus pressed against the glenoid cavity* (Fig. 31):

  (a) Seen from behind

  (b) Seen from the front

  (c) Seen from above.

In these figures the following muscles are seen:

  1. Supraspinatus

  2. Subscapularis

  3. Infraspinatus

  4. Teres minor

  5. Tendon of the long head of the biceps. When this muscle contracts, the tendon, attached to the supra-glenoid tubercle, forces the humeral head medially.

According to some authors the articular surfaces are also kept together by atmospheric pressure, acting not in the glenoid cavity but beneath the periarticular muscular cuff. (see also Fig. 33 and 34).

The *long muscles* of the arm and of the shoulder girdle (Fig. 32) are *tonically* active and prevent *infraglenoid dislocation* of the head of the humerus as a result of a weight carried in the hand or of the sheer weight of the upper limb itself. This inferior dislocation is seen in the syndrome of 'the swinging arm', when, for some reason, the muscles of the shoulder and of the arm are paralysed.

Recent electromyographic studies, however, have shown that these muscles are only active when heavy weights are being carried. Otherwise the head of the humerus is essentially supported far less by the coraco-humeral ligament, as formerly believed, than by the inferior fibres of the capsule, as shown by the recent studies of Fischer et al. By contrast, superior dislocation, brought about by an excessively strong contraction of the long muscles, is prevented and checked by the presence of the coraco-acromial arch, and the contraction of supraspinatus. If the supraspinatus is out of action, the humeral head hits directly the inferior aspect of the acromion and of the acromio-coracoid ligament, causing pain as in the syndrome of periarthritis of the shoulder associated with damage of the muscles of the rotator cuff.

  (a) Seen from the back

  (b) Seen from the front

In these diagrams the following muscles can be seen:

  5. Short head of biceps

  6. Coraco-brachialis

  7. Long head of triceps

  8. and (8') Deltoid muscle (the clavicular and scapular fibres)

  9. Clavicular head of pectoralis major.

(The black arrow indicates a downward pull.)

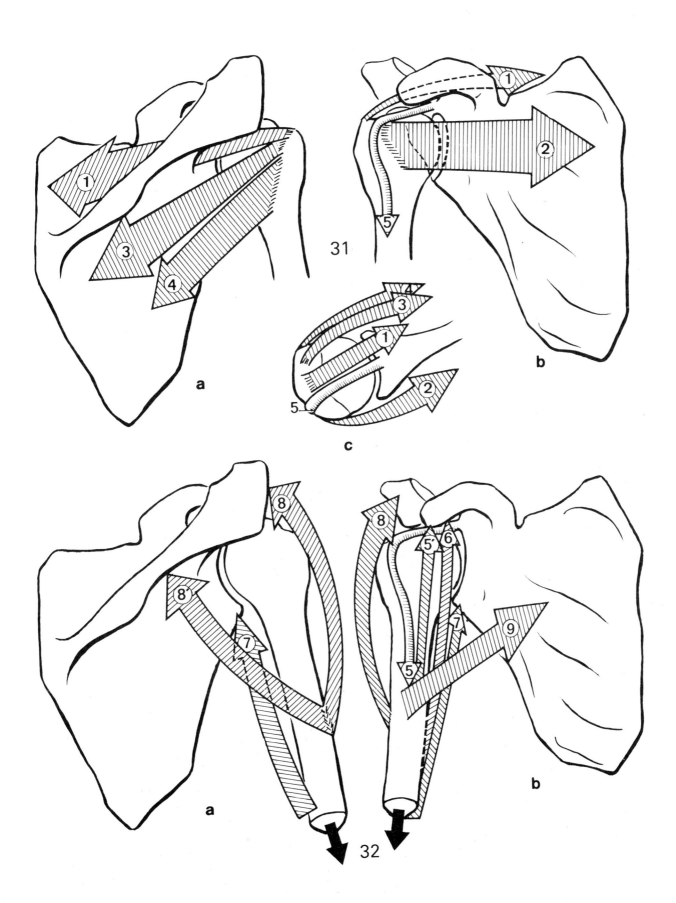

31

a

b

c

32

a

b

35

THE SUBDELTOID "JOINT"

The deltoid has been horizontally sectioned and retracted (1), revealing the "articular" surfaces of this false (physiological) "joint". The deep surface (Fig. 33, according to Rouvière) consists of:

— The upper extremity of the humerus (2);

— the periarticular cuff of muscles, i.e. supraspinatus (3), infraspinatus (4), teres minor (5).

The subscapularis muscle is not seen in the diagram, but the tendon of the long head of the biceps (6) is clearly seen as it emerges from the bicipital groove.

Between the surface just described and the deep surface of the deltoid the fibroadipose plane of cleavage contains the *subdeltoid bursa* (shown opened) (7).

Other muscles seen in the diagram are: teres major (8), long head of triceps (9), brachialis (10), coraco-brachialis (11), short head of biceps (12), pectoralis minor (13) and pectoralis major (14).

Coronal section of the shoulder girdle (Fig. 34) shows:

(a) The arm is hanging **vertically** beside the body and the following structures are seen:

The supraspinatus (1), traversing deep to the acromio-clavicular joint (2) before its insertion into the greater tuberosity (3).

The deltoid (4) lying superficial to the subdeltoid bursa (5).

(b) During **abduction:** The greater tuberosity (3) is pulled superiorly and medially by the supraspinatus (1), so that the superior recess of the subdeltoid bursa is pulled underneath the acromio-clavicular joint (2); the deep wall of the bursa glides medially on the superficial wall (6), which wrinkles, thus allowing the head of the humerus to slip deep to the acromio-deltoid vault.

On the other hand, the inferior recess of the shoulder joint (7) unpleats and becomes taut. The long head of the triceps (8) is also seen.

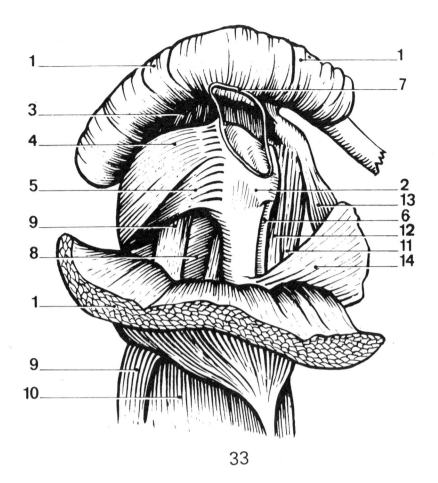

33

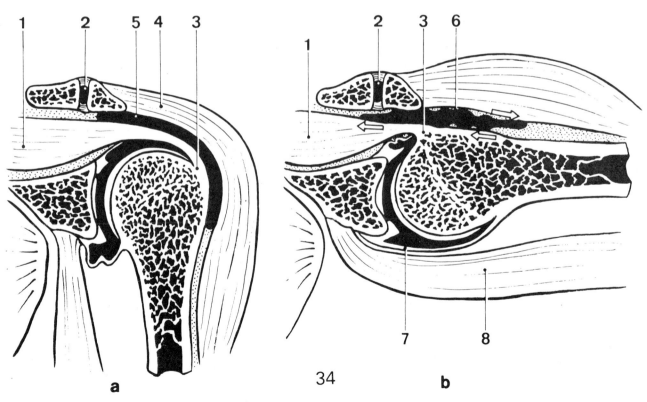

a   34   b

THE SCAPULO-THORACIC 'JOINT'

A horizontal section of the thorax helps to understand the function of the scapulo-thoracic 'joint' (Fig. 35).

In the *left half of the section* (showing the anatomical arrangement) the *two 'spaces'* of this false joint can be seen.

1. **The 'space' between the scapula and the serratus muscle** is bounded as follows:

   — posteriorly and laterally, by the scapula (shown in black), covered by the subscapularis muscle.

   — anteriorly and medially, by the serratus anterior muscle arising from the medial border of the scapula and inserted into the antero-lateral border of the thorax.

2. **The 'space' between the thoracic wall and the serratus muscle** is bounded as follows:

   — medially and anteriorly, by the thoracic wall (ribs and intercostal muscles).

   — posteriorly and laterally, by the serratus anterior.

The *right half of the section*, which is a functional diagram of the shoulder girdle, shows that:

— the scapula does not lie in a frontal plane but runs *obliquely*, medio-laterally and postero-anteriorly, forming with the frontal plane a solid angle of 30° open antero-laterally.

— The clavicle runs obliquely in a postero-lateral direction and forms with the scapula an angle of 60°.

A posterior view of the thorax shows (Fig. 36):

The scapula in its normal position stretches from the second to the seventh rib. Relative to the vertebral spines (median line): its supero-medial angle corresponds to the first thoracic vertebra; its inferior angle corresponds to the seventh or eighth thoracic spine; the medial extremity of the spine of the scapula (i.e. the angle formed by the two segments of the medial border) corresponds to the third thoracic spine.

The medial or spinal border of the scapula lies 5 to 6 cm lateral to the thoracic spines.

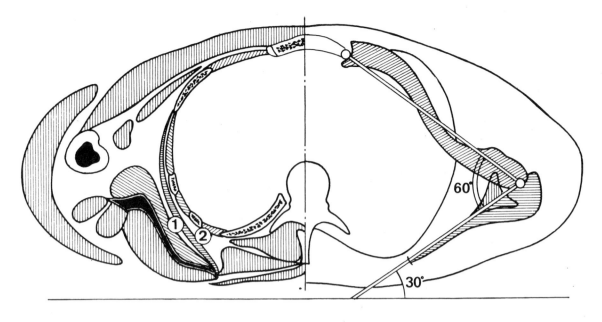

35

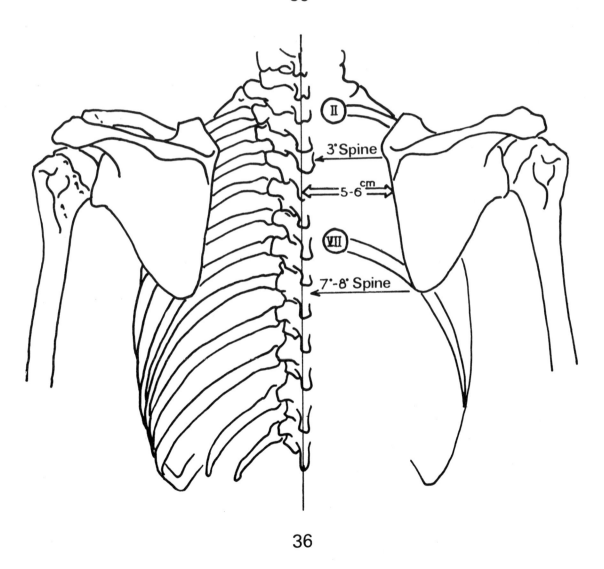

36

39

MOVEMENTS OF THE SHOULDER GIRDLE

Medial and lateral movements of the scapula on the thorax (Fig. 37: schematic horizontal section)

(1) *Right side of section.* When the scapula moves medially it comes to lie more and more *in a frontal plane;* the glenoid cavity faces more directly *laterally;* the lateral extremity of the clavicle moves medially and posteriorly; the angle between scapula and clavicle tends to *open out.*

(2) *Left. side of section.* When the scapula moves laterally it comes to lie more and more *in a sagittal plane*; the glenoid cavity faces more directly anteriorly; the lateral extremity of the clavicle moves laterally and anteriorly and its long axis tends to lie in a frontal plane. At this point the transverse diameter of the shoulders is at its greatest. The angle between clavicle and scapula tends *to close.*

These two extreme positions of the scapula form a solid angle of 40° to 45° and this corresponds to the total range of movement of the glenoid cavity in a horizontal plane, i.e. about an imaginary vertical axis.

Medial and lateral movements of the scapula round the chest wall (Fig. 38, seen from behind)

Right side: Medial displacement (N.B. slight tilting).

Left side: Lateral displacement.

The total range of this movement is 15 cm.

Elevation and depression of the scapula (Fig. 39):

Right side: Depression.

Left side: Elevation.

Total range of movement; 10 to 12 cm
These vertical movements are necessarily associated with *some tilting.*

'Tilting' or rotation of the scapula (Fig. 40):

Rotation of the scapula occurs on an *axis perpendicular* to the plane of the scapula and situated a little below the spine, *not far from the supero-lateral angle.*

Right side: *'Downward'* rotation (clockwise for the right scapula); the inferior angle moves medially, the supero-lateral angle moves inferiorly and the glenoid tends to face downwards.

Left side: *'Upward'* rotation: this is the opposite movement in which the glenoid comes to face more directly superiorly and the supero-lateral angle moves superiorly.

Total range of movement: 60°.

Displacement of the inferior angle is 10 to 12 cm and that of the supero-lateral angle is 5 to 6 cm.

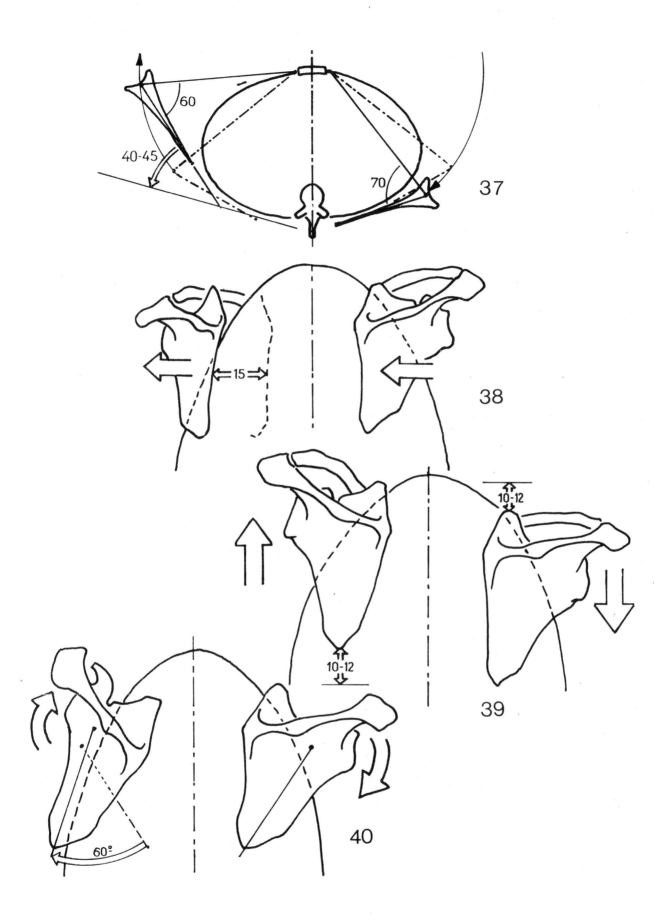

37

38

39

40

41

THE REAL MOVEMENTS OF THE SCAPULO-THORACIC 'JOINT'

The elementary movements of the scapulo-thoracic 'joint' have been described but it is now known that during abduction or flexion of the upper limb these elementary movements are variably combined. By comparing radiographs of the scapula taken during abduction (Fig. 41) with radiographs of the dried bone taken in various positions, J.Y. de la Caffinière has been able to determine the real movements of the scapula. Views of the acromion (Fig. 42) and of the coracoid and glenoid cavity (Fig. 43) taken in perspective show that, during active abduction, the scapula is subjected to four movements:

— *elevation* of 8–10 cm without any associated forward displacement, as usually believed.

— *angular rotation* of 38°, increasing almost linearly as abduction increases from 0° to 145°. From 120° abduction onwards the degree of angular rotation is the same in the shoulder joint and in the scapulo-thoracic 'joint'.

— *tilting* around a transverse axis running obliquely medio-laterally and posteroanteriorly, so that the tip of the scapula moves forwards and upwards while its upper part moves backwards and downwards. This movement recalls that of a man bending over backwards to look at the top of a skyscraper. The range of tilting is 23° during abduction from 0° to 145°.

— *swivelling* around a vertical axis with a biphasic pattern:

  • initially, during abduction from 0° to 90°, the glenoid cavity paradoxically moves over an angle of 10° to face posteriorly.

  • as abduction exceeds 90°, the glenoid cavity moves over an angle of 6° to face anteriorly and thus does not quite resume its initial position in the anteroposterior plane.

During abduction, the glenoid cavity undergoes a complex series of displacements, being elevated and displaced medially so that the greater tuberosity of the humerus just 'misses' the acromion anteriorly and slides under the acromio-coracoid ligament.

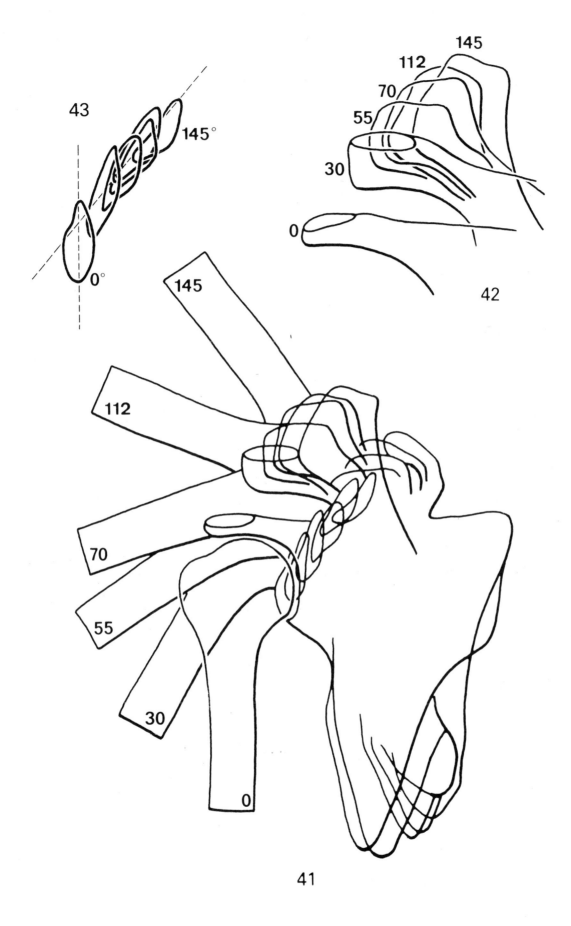

43

THE STERNO-CLAVICULAR JOINT: THE ARTICULAR SURFACES

The two surfaces, (Fig. 44), shown here separated from each other, are *saddle-shaped* (cf. the trapezo-metacarpal joint) and are reciprocally concavo-convex. The axis of the concave surface is *perpendicular in space* to that of the convex surface and these two axes lie on either side of the saddle. The smaller surface (1) is clavicular and the larger (2) is sterno-costal. In fact, the clavicular surface (1), greater horizontally than vertically, overlaps the sterno-costal surface anteriorly and particularly posteriorly.

The clavicular surface (Fig. 45) fits snugly on to the sterno-costal surface, even as the rider sits on the saddle and the saddle fits on to the back of the horse. The concavity of the former fits the convexity of the latter and vice versa. The two axes of each surface coincide so closely that the system has only two axes perpendicular to each other in space, as shown in the diagram.

— axis 1 corresponds to the concavity of the clavicular surface and allows movements of the clavicle in the horizontal plane;

— axis 2 corresponds to the concavity of the sterno-costal surface and allows movements of the clavicle in the vertical plane.

This joint has two axes and two degrees of freedom, corresponding mechanically to a **universal joint.** However, there also occurs at this joint some *axial rotation* (see p. 54)

The right sterno-clavicular joint is seen opened anteriorly (Fig. 46).

The medial end of the clavicle (1) with its articular surface (2) has been tilted after section of the superior ligament (3), the anterior ligament (4) and the most powerful costo-clavicular ligament (5). Only the posterior ligament is intact (6). The sterno-costal surface (7) is clearly visible with its two curvatures: concave vertically and convex antero-posteriorly.

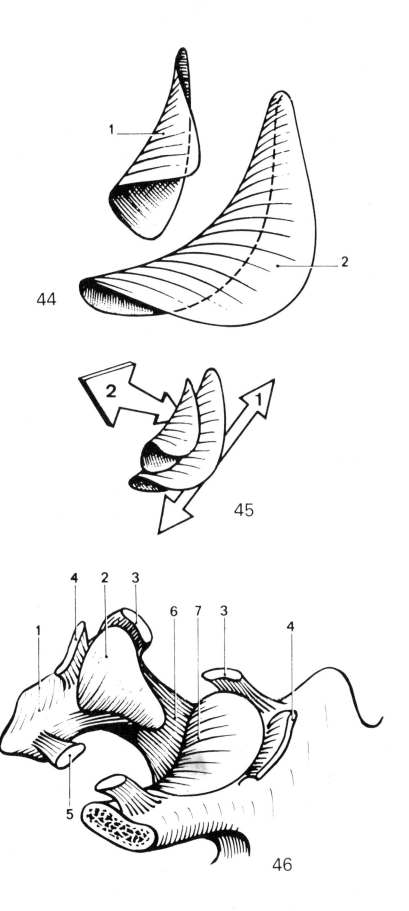

44

45

46

THE STERNO-CLAVICULAR JOINT: THE MOVEMENTS

A composite view of the sterno-clavicular joint (Fig. 47, according to Rouvière) brings out:

Right half: **Coronal section** showing the following:

— The costo-clavicular ligament (1) inserted into the superior aspect of the first rib and running superiorly and laterally towards the inferior aspect of the clavicle.

— Very often the two articular surfaces do not have reciprocally similar radii of curvature and congruence of the surfaces is provided by a *meniscus* (3), like the saddle between rider and horse. This meniscus subdivides the joint into two secondary cavities, which may or may not communicate with each other according to whether the meniscus is centrally perforated or not.

— The sterno-clavicular ligament (4), lining the superior aspect of the joint, is strengthened superiorly by the interclavicular ligament (5)

Left half: **Anterior aspect** of the joint, showing the following:

— The costo-clavicular ligament (1) and the subclavius muscle (2).

— The axis X, horizontal and slightly oblique anteriorly and laterally corresponds to the movements of the clavicle in the vertical plane with range: superiorly 10 cm and inferiorly 3 cm.

— The axis Y, lying in a vertical plane obliquely, inferiorly and slightly laterally, traverses the middle part of the costo-clavicular ligament and corresponds, according to traditional teaching, to the movements of the clavicle in the horizontal plane. The range of these movements is as follows: the lateral extremity of the clavicle can move 10 cm anteriorly and 3 cm posteriorly. From a strictly mechanical point of view the real axis (Y') is parallel to the axis (Y), but situated inside the joint (cf. axis 1, Fig. 45).

There is also a third type of movement occurring at this joint, viz. a 30° axial rotation of the clavicle. It is only possible because of the *'slack'* of the joint due to the laxity of the ligaments. As the sterno-clavicular joint is biaxial, there is also an automatic (conjoint) rotation occurring during voluntary rotation around its two axes. This is borne out by the practical observation that this automatic rotation of the clavicle is always associated with voluntary movements at the joint.

Movements of the clavicle in the horizontal plane (Fig. 48, superior view).

In bold outline is shown the position of the clavicle at rest.

The movements occur about the point Y'.

The two crosses represent the extreme positions of the clavicular insertion of the costo-clavicular ligament.

Inset: A section taken at the level of the costo-clavicular ligament to show the tension developed in the ligament in the extreme positions.

Movement anteriorly is checked by the tension of the costo-clavicular ligament and of the anterior capsular ligament (1).

Movement posteriorly is limited by the tension of the costo-clavicular ligament and the posterior capsular ligament (2).

Movements of the clavicle in the frontal plane (Fig. 49, anterior view)

The cross corresponds to axis X of movement. When the lateral extremity of the clavicle is raised (shown in bold outline), the medial extremity slides inferiorly and laterally (white arrow). The movement is limited by *the tension of the costo-clavicular ligament* (striped band) and by the tone of the subclavius muscle (large striped arrow).

When the clavicle is lowered its medial extremity rises. This movement is limited by the tension of the superior capsular ligament and by *contact* between the clavicle and the superior surface of the first rib.

46

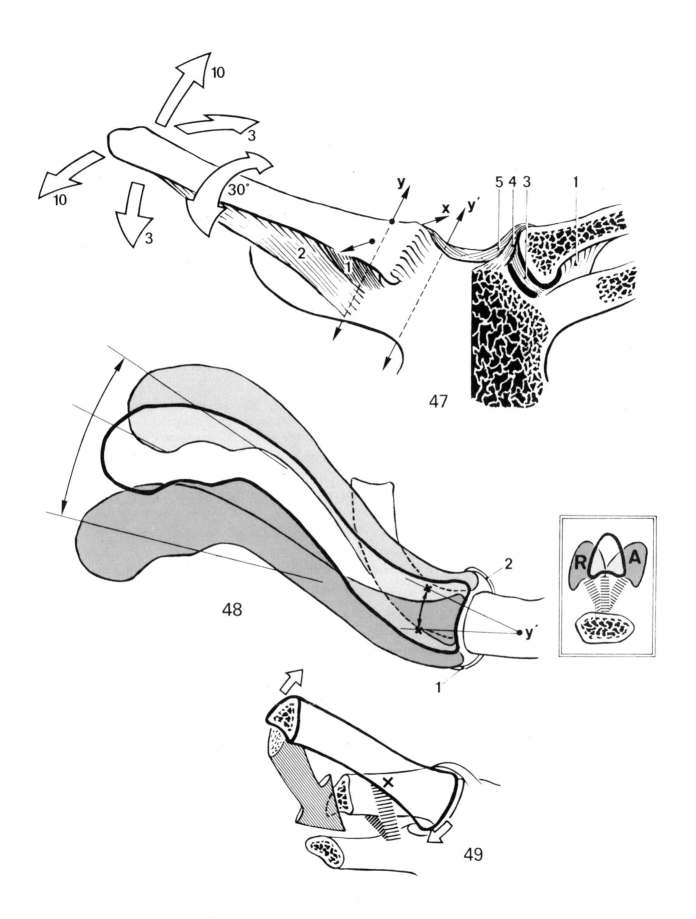

47

48

49

THE ACROMIO-CLAVICULAR JOINT

In the diagram (Fig. 50: postero-lateral aspect of the joint) the scapula and clavicle have been *separated* from each other. The following structures can be seen:

— the spine of the scapula (1), continuous laterally with the acromion (2), which bears on its
— antero-medial border an articular surface (3) which is flat or slightly convex. This joint is of the **plane** variety and faces anteriorly, medially and superiorly.

— the lateral extremity of the clavicle (4) with its inferior aspect thinned by a sloping articular surface (5). This surface is flat or slightly convex and faces *inferiorly*, posteriorly and laterally.

— two powerful ligaments arising from the base of the coracoid process (6):

(a) the *conoid ligament* (7), which is inserted into the inferior surface of the clavicle on the conoid tubercle near its posterior edge;

(b) the *trapezoid ligament* (8) which runs obliquely superiorly and laterally towards the trapezoid ridge of the clavicle; this is a roughened patch, triangular in shape, running from the conoid tubercle anteriorly and laterally on the inferior surface of the clavicle.

— the supraspinatus fossa (9) and the glenoid cavity (10).

The vertical plane P cuts the acromio-clavicular joint through its middle. This section is shown in the inset and contains the different structures already described and in addition the following features can be observed:

— the capsule is strengthened superiorly by the *powerful* acromio-clavicular ligament (15)

— an *intra-articular fibro-cartilaginous plate* (seen in one-third of cases) which makes the articular surfaces congruent (11). Only exceptionally does this plate form a proper meniscus.

— the *obliquity of the plane of the joint:* the clavicle is, as it were, 'placed' on the acromion.

An anterior view of the right coracoid process (Fig. 51) shows:

— **The conoid ligament** (C) is fan-shaped with its apex lying inferiorly; it is inserted into the tip of the 'elbow' of the coracoid process and lies in a *frontal plane*.

— **The trapezoid ligament** (T), inserted into the medial border of the upper surface of the coracoid process, runs superiorly and laterally. It is a thin quadrilateral sheet obliquely set so that its antero-medial aspect points medially, anteriorly and superiorly and its postero-lateral aspect points posteriorly, laterally and inferiorly.

The posterior edge of the trapezoid ligament is in contact with the conoid ligament, most frequently at its lateral edge. These two ligaments lie in two planes more or less at right angles to each other and they form a solid angle facing anteriorly and medially.

48

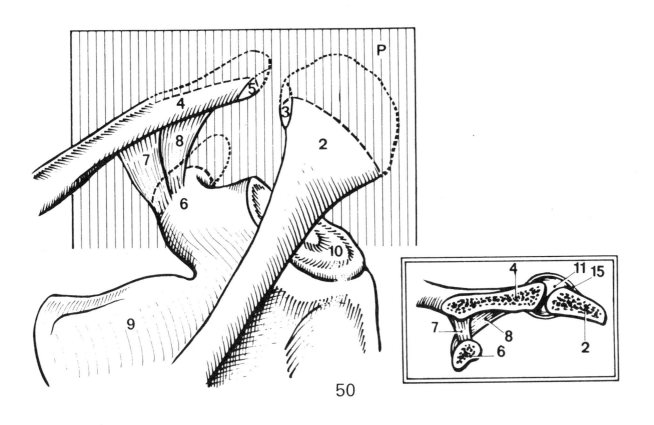

50

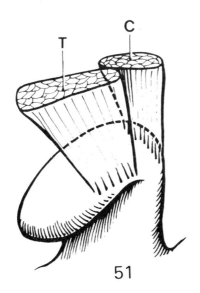

51

49

THE ACROMIO CLAVICULAR JOINT (continued)

In Fig. 52 (supero-lateral aspect, according to Rouvière) can be seen:

— the superficial portion of the acromio-clavicular ligament (11), cut to show its deep aspect which strengthens the capsule.

— the conoid (7), trapezoid (8) and medial coraco-clavicular ligaments (12); the coraco-acromial ligament (13), which plays no part in joint control and helps to form the supraspinatus sulcus (cf. Fig. 49).

— superficially (not shown in the diagram) the interwoven fibres of the deltoid and trapezius, which play a crucial role in keeping the articular surfaces of the acromio-clavicular joint together and curtailing its tendency to subluxation.

In Fig. 53 (infero-medial aspect, according to Rouvière):

The clavicle is shown 'running away' from its medial extremity. The structures already described can be seen as well as the suprascapular ligament (14), which bridges across the suprascapular notch and plays no mechanical role.

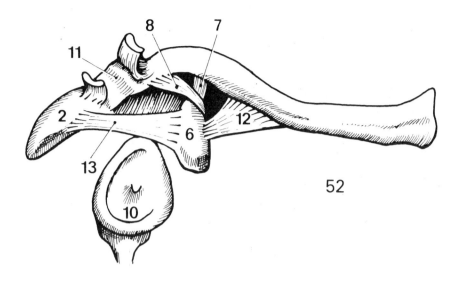

52

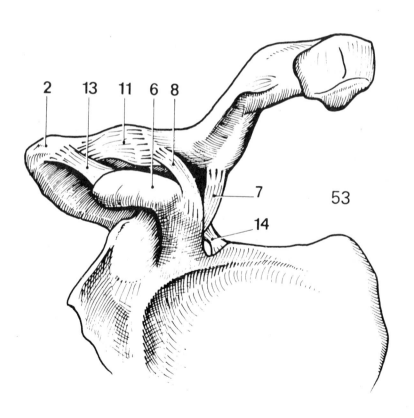

53

THE ROLE OF THE CORACO-CLAVICULAR LIGAMENTS

A diagrammatic view of the acromio-clavicular joint (Fig. 54: seen from above) shows the importance of the conoid ligament:

— The scapula (dotted) seen from above.

— The broken line shows the contours of the clavicle in its resting position.

— The heavy continuous line shows the final position of the clavicle.

This shows how, when the solid angle between clavicle and scapula *is opened out*, the conoid ligament *is stretched and checks the movement* (the two stippled lines represent the two successive positions of the conoid ligament).

Figure 55 (seen from above) shows the role of the trapezoid ligament.

When the angle between the clavicle and the scapula is *closed* the trapezoid ligament *is stretched and limits the movement*.

Axial rotation at the acromio-clavicular joint is well illustrated in Fig. 56 (antero-medial aspect.):

— The cross marks the centre of rotation of the joint.

— The heavy line shows the initial position of the scapula (the lower half has been cut).

— The striped surface shows the final position of the scapula after it has rotated at the acromio-clavicular joint, like the swingle of a flail on the handle.

The tension developed in the conoid ligament (hatched band) and the trapezoid ligament (stippled) is also seen. This 30° rotation is added to the 30° rotation at the sterno-clavicular joint to allow a 60° rotation of the scapula.

A recent photographic study by Fischer et al has brought to light the complexity of the movements taking place at the poorly interlocked acromio-clavicular joint.

During *abduction* (with reference to the scapula):

— the medial end of the clavicle is raised by 10°.
— the angle between the scapula and the clavicle is widened to 70°.
— the clavicle is rotated posteriorly up to 45°.

During *flexion*, the elementary movements are similar, though less pronounced as regards the widening of the scapulo-clavicular angle.

During *extension*, the scapulo-clavicular angle is narrowed to 10°.

During *medial rotation*, the only movement is an opening of the scapulo-clavicular angle up to 13°.

52

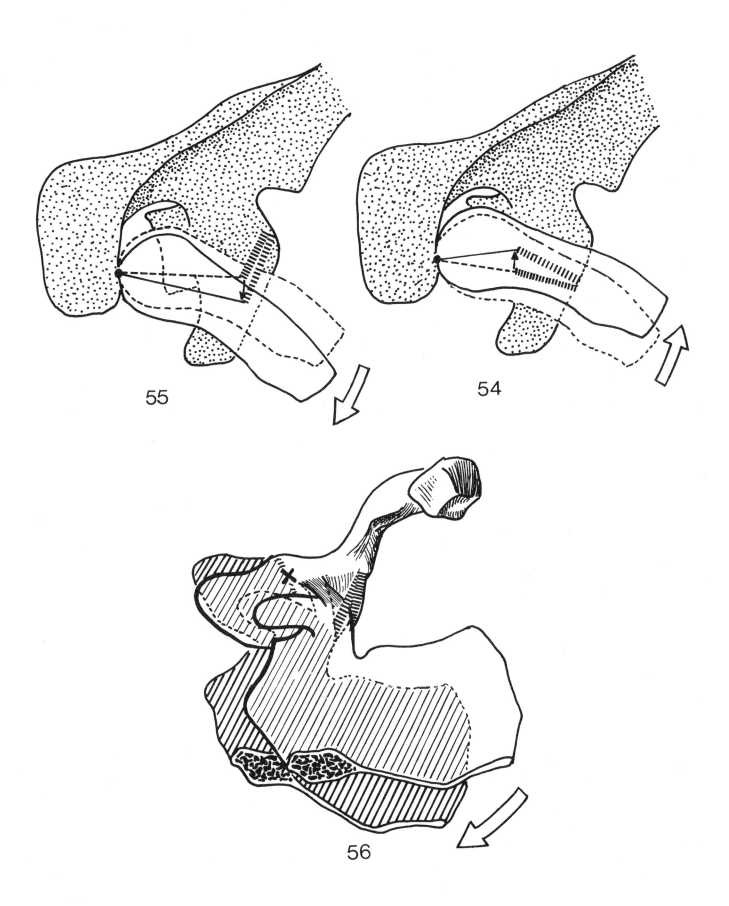

55

54

56

MOTOR MUSCLES OF THE SHOULDER GIRDLE

Figure 57 (thorax shown diagrammatically):

Right half (posterior aspect)

1. **Trapezius**, consisting of three parts with different actions:

   Upper acromio-clavicular fibres (1). They raise the shoulder girdle and prevent it from sagging under the weight of a load; they hyperextend the neck and turn the head to the other side when the shoulder is stationary.

   Intermediate transverse fibres (1'). They bring the medial edge of the scapula 2 to 3 cm nearer the vertebral spines and press the scapula against the thorax; they move the shoulder posteriorly.

   Lower fibres (1″), running obliquely inferiorly and medially.

   They pull the scapula inferiorly and medially.

   Simultaneous contraction of the three bands draws the scapula medially and posteriorly; rotates the scapula superiorly (20°), playing a minor part in abduction but a major part in the carrying of heavy loads; prevents the arm from sagging and the scapula from leaving the thoracic wall.

2. **Rhomboid muscles,** running obliquely, superiorly and medially. They draw the inferior angle superomedially and so elevate the scapula and rotate it inferiorly with the glenoid cavity facing inferiorly; they fix the inferior angle of the scapula against the ribs and paralysis of the rhomboids is followed by separation of the scapulae from the thoracic wall.

3. **Levator scapulae,** sloping obliquely, superiorly and medially. Like the rhomboids, it draws the superior angle superiorly and medially by 2 or 3 cm (as in shrugging the shoulders). It is active during the carrying of a load. Its paralysis is followed by the sagging of the shoulder girdle.

   It rotates the scapula slightly so that the glenoid points inferiorly.

4. **Serratus anterior** (cf. Fig. 58)

Left half (anterior aspect, Fig. 57).

5. **Pectoralis minor,** running obliquely, inferiorly, anteriorly and medially. It depresses the shoulder girdle so that the glenoid cavity faces inferiorly (e.g. during movements on parallel bars); it pulls the scapula laterally and anteriorly so that its posterior edge leaves the thoracic wall.

6. **Subclavius,** running obliquely, inferiorly and medially, almost parallel to the clavicle. It lowers the clavicle and so the shoulder girdle; it presses the medial extremity of the clavicle against the manubrium sterni and so *brings into apposition the articular surfaces of the sterno-clavicular joint.*

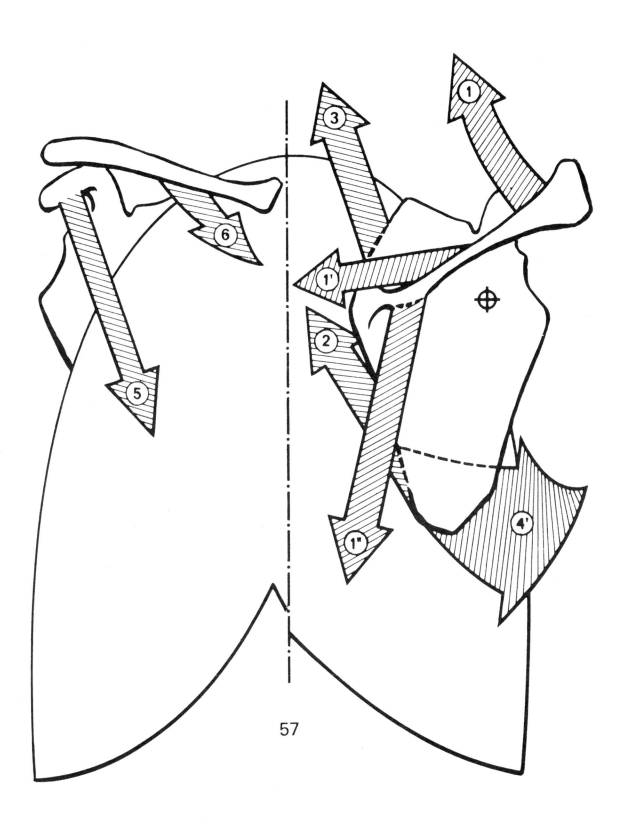

57

55

MOTOR MUSCLES OF THE SHOULDER GIRDLE (continued)

The diagrammatic profile of the thorax shows the **serratus anterior** with its two parts (Fig. 58):

— *Upper part*, running horizontally and anteriorly. It draws the scapula 12 to 15 cm anteriorly and laterally and stops it from moving back when a heavy object is being pushed forwards. If it is paralysed this action causes the medial edge of the scapula to leave the thoracic wall (used as a clinical test).

— *Lower part*, running obliquely, anteriorly and inferiorly. It rotates the scapula upwards so that the glenoid faces superiorly; it is active during flexion and abduction of the arm and in the carrying of loads, only when the arm is already abducted at a minimum of 30° (e.g. carrying a bucket of water).

In Figure 59 (horizontal section):

Left side shows the action of the trapezius (middle fibres), levator scapulae and rhomboids. They adduct the scapula by moving it nearer to the midline. As a group (excepting the lower fibres of the trapezius) they elevate the scapula.

Right side shows the action of serratus anterior and pectoralis minor, which abduct the scapula, i.e. they move it away from the midline. In addition, pectoralis minor and subclavius depress the shoulder girdle.

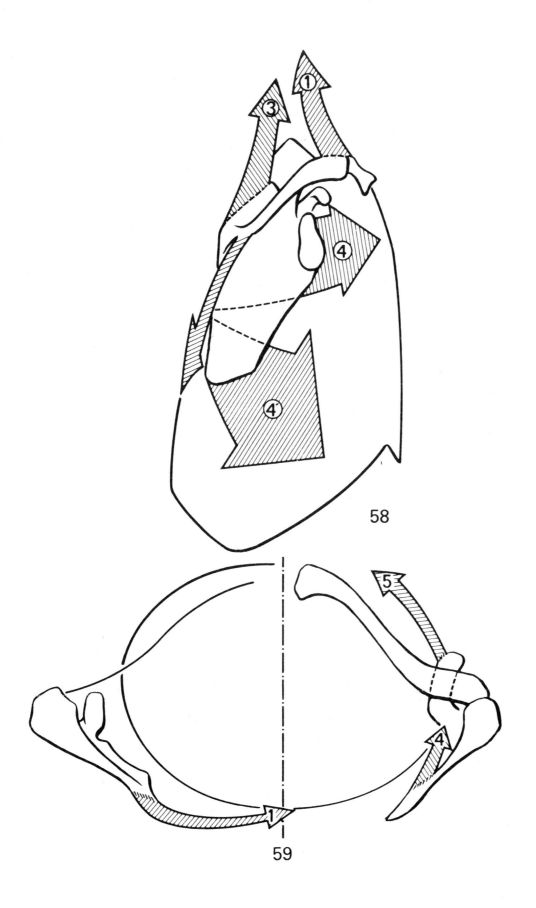

58

59

THE SUPRASPINATUS AND ABDUCTION

Figure 60 (superior aspect of scapula)

The supraspinatus canal (starred), which connects the supraspinatus fossa with the subdeltoid region, is bounded:

posteriorly, by the spine of the scapula and the acromion;

anteriorly, by the coracoid process;

superiorly, by the coraco-acromial ligament.

The acromion, the ligament and the coracoid process together form a fibro-osseous arch called *the coraco-acromial arch*.

The supraspinatus canal forms a rigid and inextensible ring; if the muscle increases in size as a result of a scar or of an inflammatory process, it cannot glide through the canal without sticking. If, however, the nodular swelling manages to glide through eventually, abduction can proceed after a jump; this is known as the 'jumping shoulder'.

When the rotator cuff is damaged the degenerate and ruptured supraspinatus tendon no longer lies between the humeral head and the coraco-acromial arch. Direct contact between these two structures is responsible, according to modern authors, for the pain associated with abduction in the syndrome of 'rotator cuff rupture'.

Figure 61 (the scapula seen from in front and from above) shows how the supraspinatus, attached to the supraspinatus fossa and the greater tuberosity, passes beneath the coraco-acromial ligament.

Figure 62 (posterior aspect of the scapula and humerus) shows: the four muscles of abduction are shown schematically:

(1) Deltoid

(2) Supraspinatus

These two muscles form a *couple* which initiates abduction at the shoulder

(3) Serratus anterior

(4) Trapezius

These two muscles form a *couple* which initiates abduction at the scapulo-thoracic 'joint'.

The subscapularis, infraspinatus and teres minor (not shown in the diagram) are now considered to play a role in abduction. They pull the humeral head inferiorly and medially, thus forming with the deltoid a second functional couple at the level of the shoulder joint.

Finally the biceps tendon also participates in abduction since its rupture causes a 20 per cent drop in the strength of abduction.

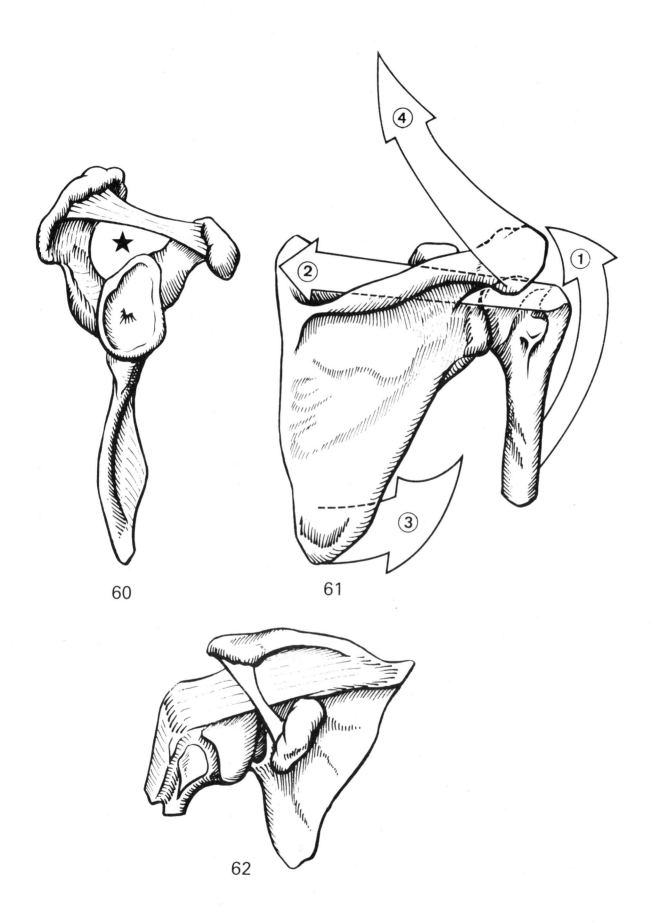

60

61

62

59

THE PHYSIOLOGY OF ABDUCTION

Though at first sight abduction is a simple process involving two muscles, the deltoid and the supraspinatus, there is controversy regarding their respective contributions. Recent electromyographic studies (J.-J. Comtet & Y. Auffray 1970) have shed new light on the problem.

Role of the deltoid

According to Fick (1911), the deltoid is made up of seven *functional* components (Fig. 65: horizontal cut through the inferior part of the muscle):

— the anterior (*clavicular*) band contains 2 components: I and II
— the middle (*acromial*) band contains one: III
— the posterior (*spinal*) band contains four: IV, V, VI, and VII.

When the position of each component is considered with regard to the axis of pure abduction AA' (Fig. 63: seen from in front and Fig. 64: seen from behind), it is evident that some components, i.e. the acromial band (III), the most lateral portion of component II of the clavicular band and component IV of the spinal band lie lateral to the abduction axis and thus *from the start produce abduction* (Fig. 65). The other components (I, V, VI, VII) on the contrary act as *adductors* when the upper limb hangs vertically alongside the body. Thus the latter components of the deltoid are *antagonists* to the former and they only start to abduct when during abduction they are progressively displaced lateral to the abduction axis AA'. Hence their *action is inverted* depending on the site of initiation of abduction. Note that some components (VI and VII) are always adductors regardless of the degree of abduction.

Strasser (1917) by and large agrees with this view but notes that when abduction takes place *in the plane of the scapula*, i.e. with an associated 30° flexion and around an axis BB' (Fig. 65) perpendicular to the plane of the scapula, nearly the whole of the clavicular band is abductor from the start.

Electromyographic investigations have shown that *different portions of the muscle are recruited successively* during abduction and that the more powerfully adductor the fibres are at the start the later they are recruited. Thus the abductor components are not opposed by the antagonistic adductor components. This is an example of *reciprocal innervation* (Sherrington).

During **pure abduction** the order of recruitment is as follows:

— acromial band III;
— parts of IV and V almost immediately following;
— finally II after 20°–30° abduction.

During **abduction associated with 30° flexion**:

— III and II are called into action from the start.
— IV, V and I are recruited later progressively.

During **lateral rotation of the humerus associated with abduction**:

— II contracts from the start.
— IV and V are not called into action even at the end of abduction.

During **medial rotation of the humerus combined with abduction**:

— the order of recruitment is reversed.

In sum, the deltoid, active from the very start of abduction, can *by itself complete the full range of abduction*. It achieves maximal efficiency at about 90° abduction, when it generates a force equivalent to 8.2 times the weight of the upper limb (Inman).

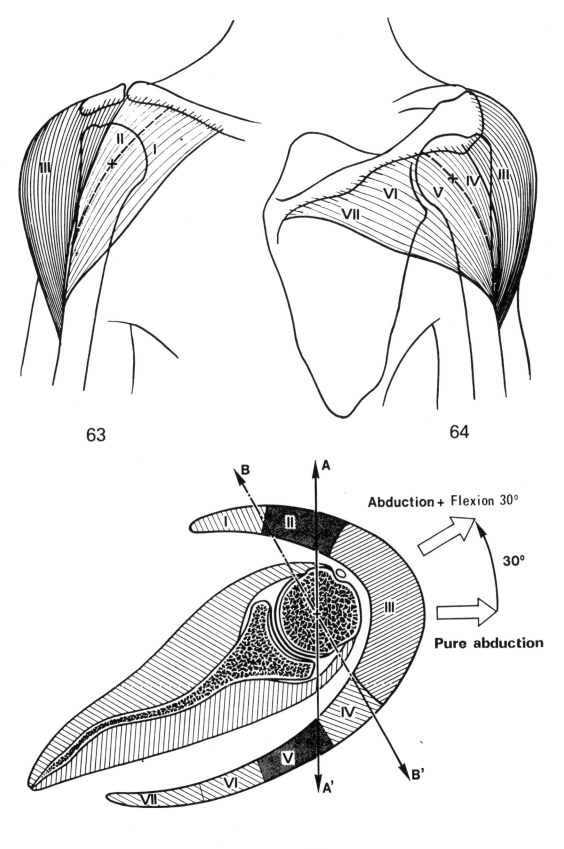

63

64

Abduction + Flexion 30°

30°

Pure abduction

65

61

THE PHYSIOLOGY OF ABDUCTION (continued)

The role of the rotator muscles

It is now evident that the other muscles of the rotator cuff not only play a vital role in the deltoid-supraspinatus synergism but also are essential for the efficiency of the deltoid (Inman).

During abduction (Fig. 66) the force exerted by the deltoid D can be resolved into a longitudinal component Dr, which will be applied to the humeral head as a force R after subtraction of the longitudinal component Pr of the weight of the upper limb P (acting through its centre of gravity). This force R can also be resolved into a force Rc which presses the humeral head against the glenoid cavity and a stronger force Ri which tends to dislocate the head superiorly and laterally. If the rotator muscles (infraspinatus, subscapularis and teres minor) contract at this point, their overall force Rm directly opposes the dislocating force Ri, preventing dislocation of the humeral head superiorly and laterally (inset). Thus the force Rm, which tends to lower the upper limb, and the elevating component of the deltoid Dt 'act as a functional couple leading to abduction. The force generated by the rotator muscles is maximal at 60° abduction. This has been confirmed electromyographically for the infraspinatus (Inman).

The role of the supraspinatus

The supraspinatus has long been viewed as the "abduction-starter". Recent studies (B. Van Linge and J. D. Mulder), producing paralysis of the muscle by anaesthetizing the suprascapular nerve, have shown that it is *not essential for abduction even at the start*. The deltoid by itself is enough to produce complete abduction.

But the *supraspinatus can by itself produce a range of abduction equal to that produced by the deltoid*, as shown by Duchenne de Boulogne's electrical experiments and clinical observations following isolated paralysis of the deltoid.

Electromyography reveals that the supraspinatus contracts during the full duration of abduction and *achieves peak activity at 90° of abduction*, just like the deltoid.

At the start of abduction (Fig. 67), its tangential component of force Et is greater than that of the deltoid Dt but it has a shorter leverage. Its radial component Er presses the humeral head strongly against the glenoid cavity and thus significantly opposes superior dislocation of the head provoked by the radial component of force of the deltoid Dr. Thus it reinforces the *action of the rotator muscles in keeping together the articular surfaces* of the shoulder. Likewise it tenses the superior fibres of the capsule and opposes inferior subluxation of the humeral head (Dautry and Gosset).

The supraspinatus is thus a *synergist of the other muscles of the cuff*, i.e. the rotators. It is a powerful helper of deltoid, which on its own tires rapidly.

In sum, its action is important *qualitatively* in helping to keep articular surfaces together and *quantitatively* in improving the endurance and power of abduction. Its mode of action is simple compared with that of the deltoid. Though it cannot any more be viewed as the abduction starter, it is clearly useful and effective particularly *at the start of abduction*.

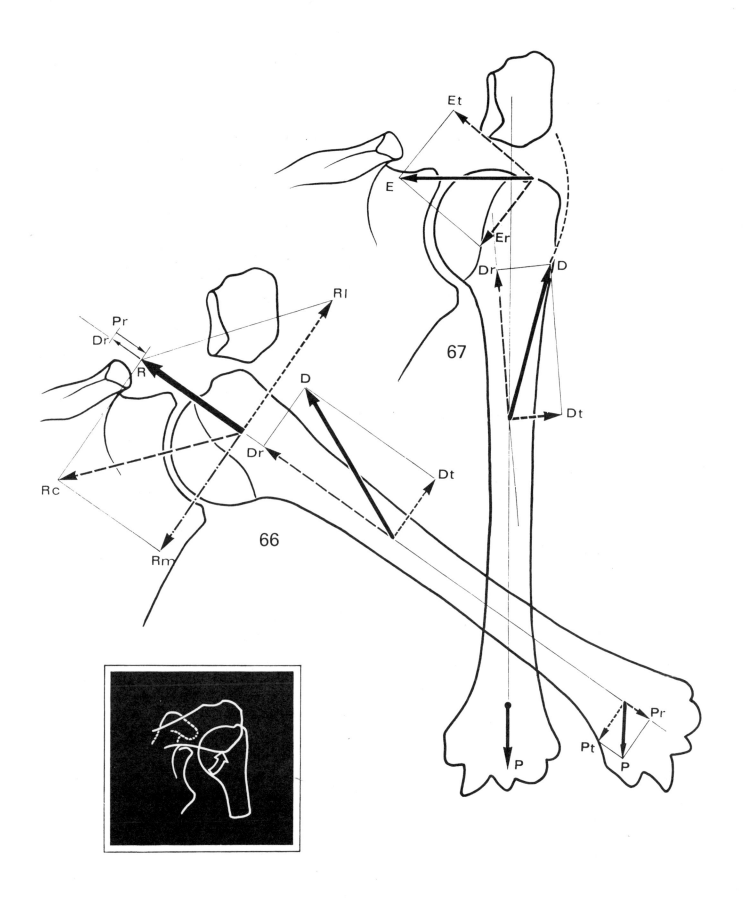

67

66

63

THE THREE PHASES OF ABDUCTION

First phase of abduction (Fig. 68): 0° to 90°.

The muscles involved are essentially the deltoid (1) and the supraspinatus (2), which form a couple at the level of the shoulder joint. It is in this joint that the movement of abduction starts. This first phase ends at 90° when the shoulder 'locks' as a result of the greater tuberosity hitting the superior margin of the glenoid. Lateral rotation of the humerus, by displacing the greater tuberosity posteriorly, delays this mechanical locking. Thus abduction combined with 30° flexion and taking place in the plane of the scapula, is the true *physiological* movement of abduction (Steindler).

Second phase of abduction (Fig. 69): 90° to 150°.

The shoulder is locked and abduction can only proceed with *participation of the shoulder girdle*. These movements are:

A 'swing' of the scapula with anticlockwise rotation (for the right scapula) which makes the glenoid cavity face superiorly. The range of this movement is 60°.

Axial rotation at the sterno-clavicular and acromio-clavicular joints, each joint contributing a movement of 30°.

The muscles involved in this second phase are: trapezius (3 and 4), and serratus anterior (5) which constitute the couple acting at the level of the scapulo-thoracic 'joint'.

This movement is checked at about 150° (90° + 60° produced by the rotation of the scapula) by resistance of the stretched adductor muscles i.e. latissimus dorsi and pectoralis major.

The third phase of abduction (Fig. 70); 150° to 180°

To allow the hand to reach the vertical position once more, *movement of the spinal column becomes necessary*. If only one arm is in abduction, *lateral displacement* of the spinal column produced by the contralateral spinal muscles (6) is adequate. If both arms are in abduction, they can only come to lie parallel vertically by being maximally flexed. For the vertical position to be attained *exaggeration of the lumbar lordosis* becomes necessary, and this is achieved by action of the spinal muscles.

This division of abduction into three phases is, of course, artificial; in fact these various movements *run into one another*. Thus it is easy to note that the scapula begins to swing before the arm has reached 90° abduction; likewise, the spinal column begins to bend before 150° abduction is reached. At the end of abduction, all the muscles are in contraction.

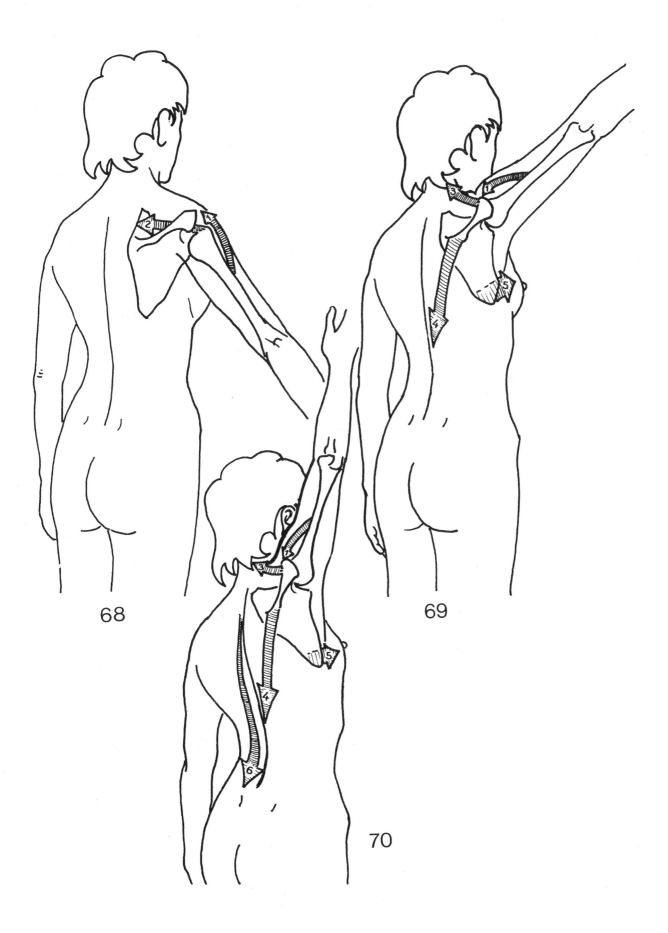

68

69

70

THE THREE PHASES OF FLEXION

First phase of flexion (Fig. 71): 0° to 50°–60°.

The muscles involved are:

— the anterior fibres of the deltoid (1)

— coraco-brachialis (2);

— the clavicular fibres of pectoralis major (3).

This *movement of flexion at the shoulder* is limited by two factors:

— Tension of the coraco-humeral ligament (cf. Fig. 30c).

— Resistance offered by teres minor, teres major and infraspinatus.

Second phase of flexion (Fig. 72); 60° to 120°

The shoulder girdle participates as follows:

— Sixty degrees rotation of the scapula, so that the glenoid cavity faces superiorly and anteriorly.

— Axial rotation at the sterno-clavicular and acromio-clavicular joints, each joint contributing 30°.

The muscles involved are the same as in abduction: trapezius (4 and 5); serratus anterior (6).

Flexion at the scapulo-thoracic 'joint' is limited by the resistance of latissimus dorsi and the costo-sternal fibres of pectoralis major.

Third phase of flexion (Fig. 73): 120° to 180°

When flexion is checked at the shoulder and at the scapulothoracic 'joint', *movement of the spinal column becomes necessary*. If one arm is being flexed, it is possible to complete the movement by passing into the position of maximal abduction and then bending the spinal column to one side. If both arms are flexed, the terminal phase of the movement is identical with that of abduction, i.e. exaggeration of the lumbar lordosis by the lumbar muscles (7).

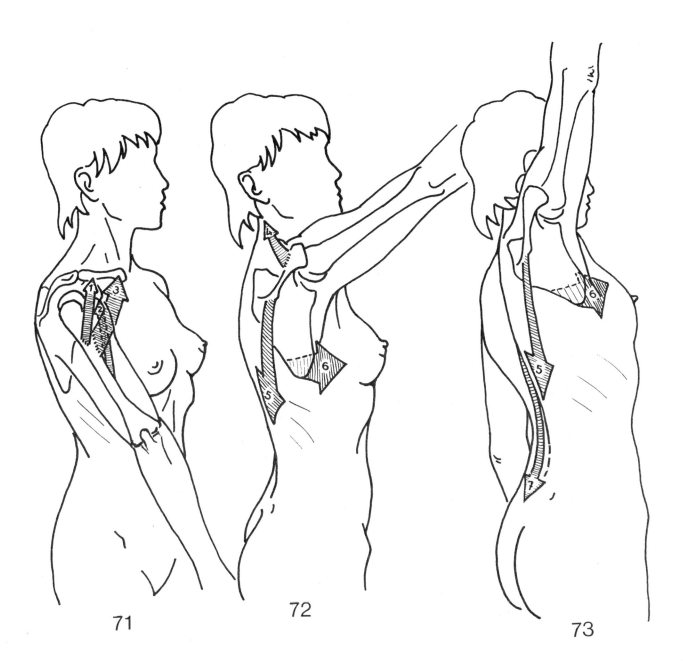

71

72

73

ROTATOR MUSCLES OF THE ARM

A superior view of the shoulder shows the rotator muscles (Fig. 74a):

(b) **Medial rotators** (diagrammatically shown):

    1. Latissimus dorsi

    2. Teres major

    3. Suprascapularis

    4. Pectoralis major

(c) **Lateral rotators** (diagrammatically shown):

    5. Infraspinatus

    6. Teres minor

In comparison with the numerous and powerful medial rotators, the lateral rotators are *weak*. They are nevertheless indispensable for the proper function of the upper limb because by themselves they can *act on the hand as it lies in front of the trunk and move it anteriorly and laterally*. This medio-lateral movement of the right hand is *essential for writing*.

It should be noted that, though these muscles have a separate nerve supply (suprascapular nerve for infraspinatus, circumflex nerve for teres minor), these two nerves *come from the same root* (C5) of the brachial plexus. So these muscles can be paralysed simultaneously as a result of traction injuries of the brachial plexus during a fall on to the shoulder (motor-cycle accident).

But rotation at the shoulder does not account for the whole range of rotation of the upper limb. There are in addition changes in the direction of the scapula (and so of the glenoid) as it moves round on the chest wall (cf. Fig. 37); this 40° to 45° change in direction of the scapula produces a corresponding increase in the range of the movement of rotation. The muscles involved are:

— for lateral rotation (adduction of scapula), rhomboids and trapezius;

— for medial rotation (abduction of scapula), serratus anterior and pectoralis minor.

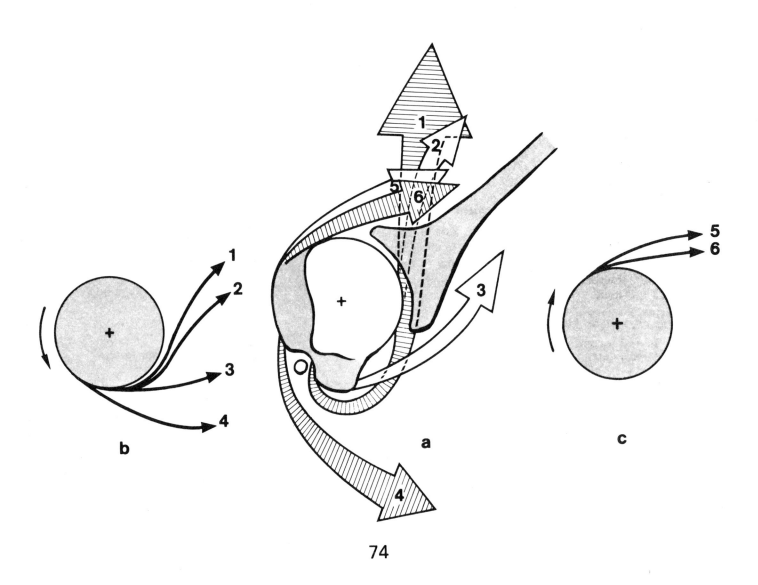

b

a

c

74

69

ADDUCTION AND EXTENSION

The adductor muscles (Fig. 75: anterior aspect and Fig. 76: postero-lateral aspect):

1. Teres major

2. Latissimus dorsi

3. Pectoralis major

4. Rhomboids.

Inset: diagrammatic representation of the action of the two muscular couples producing adduction.

(a) *Couple formed by the rhomboids* (1) and *teres major* (2):

Synergism of these two muscles is indispensable for adduction; in fact, if teres major alone contracts and the upper limb resists adduction, there follows upward rotation of the scapula about its axis (marked with a cross). Contraction of the rhomboids prevents this scapular rotation and allows teres major to adduct the arm.

(b) *Couple formed by long head of triceps* (4) and *latissimus dorsi* (3):

Contraction of latissimus dorsi, which is a powerful adductor, tends to displace the head of the humerus inferiorly (black arrow).

The long head of triceps, which is a weak adductor, opposes this inferior displacement by contracting simultaneously and lifting the head of the humerus (white arrow).

The extensor muscles (Fig. 77: postero-lateral aspect) are:

— *for extension at the shoulder joint:*

Teres major (1)

Teres minor (5)

Posterior fibres of the deltoid (6)

Latissimus dorsi (2)

— for *extension at the scapulo-thoracic 'joint'*, by adduction of the scapula:

Rhomboids (4)

Middle transverse fibres of the trapezius (7)

Latissimus dorsi (2).

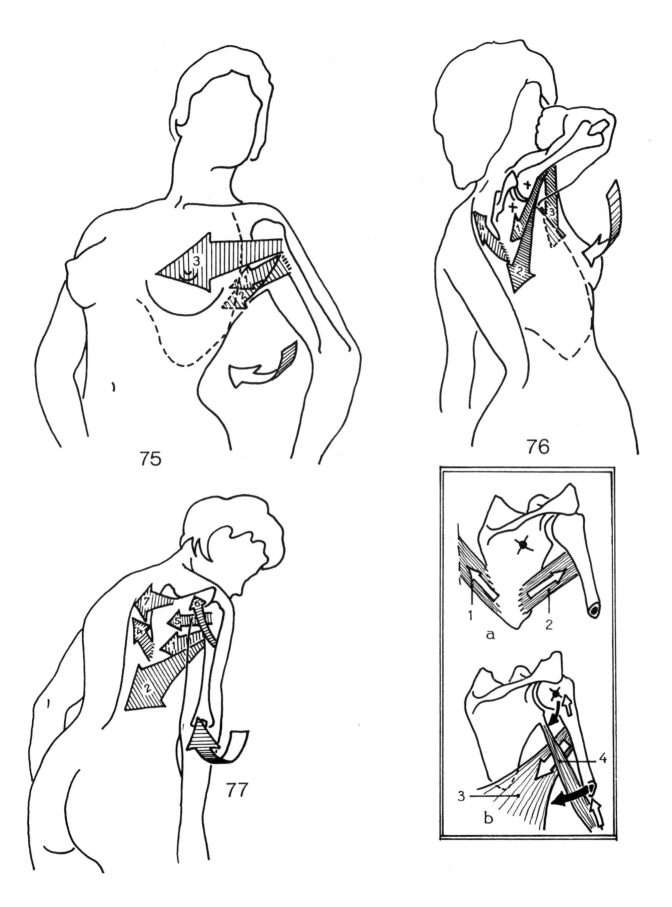

75

76

77

a

b

1   2

3   4

71

THE ELBOW:

FLEXION AND EXTENSION

Anatomically the elbow consists of a single joint with *only one joint cavity:*

Physiologically, however, it has *two distinct functions:*

— **pronation-supination** (axial rotation), involving the superior radio-ulnar joint.

— **flexion-extension,** involving the true elbow joint.

In this chapter only **flexion and extension** will be studied.

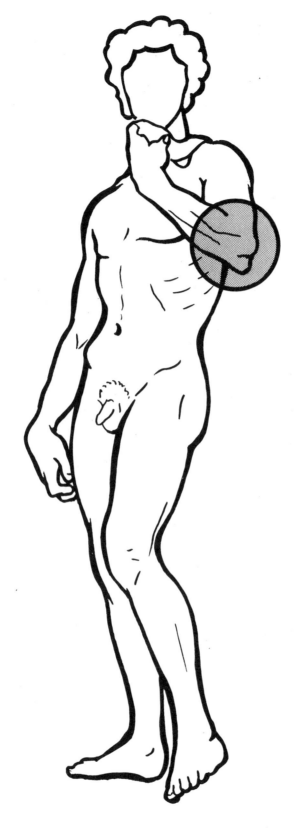

The ELBOW

73

THE ELBOW: THE JOINT WHICH ALLOWS THE HAND TO BE MOVED TOWARDS OR AWAY FROM THE BODY

The elbow is the **intermediate joint** of the upper limb constituting the mechanical link between the first segment — the upper arm — and the second segment — the forearm — of the upper limb. It allows the forearm, which can assume any position in space as a result of movements at the shoulder, to place its functional extremity (the hand) at any distance from the body.

Flexion at the elbow underlies man's ability to carry food to his mouth. Thus the extended and pronated forearm (Fig. 1) takes hold of food and carries it to the mouth as a result of flexion and supination. In this respect the biceps can be called *the feeding muscle*.

The elbow, the upper arm and the forearm form *a pair of compasses* (Fig. 2a), which allows the wrist almost to touch the shoulder S (with first intervening). As a result the hand easily reaches the shoulder and the mouth. In the telescoping model (Fig. 2b), it is clear that the hand cannot reach the mouth, since the shortest distance possible between hand and mouth is the sum of the length of the segment L and the length of the encasing (e) needed to maintain the rigidity of the system. Thus as regards the elbow, the 'compasses' provide a more logical and better solution than the 'telescope', even if the latter were possible.

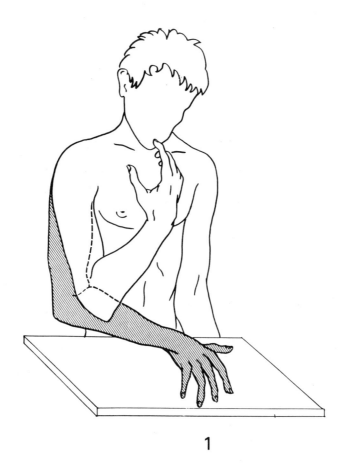

1

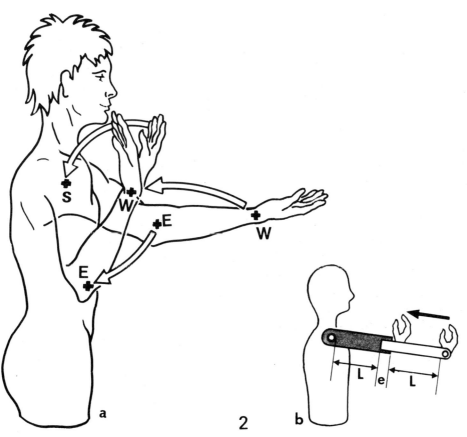

a

2

b

75

THE ARTICULAR SURFACES

(the numbers have the same meaning in all diagrams)

The distal end of the humerus has two articular surfaces (Fig. 3, according to Rouvière):

— The **trochlea** (2), (Fig. 4a) pulley-shaped with a central groove (1) lying in a sagittal plane and bounded by two convex lips (2).

— The **capitulum**, a spherical surface (3) lying lateral to the trochlea.

The complex formed by the trochlea and capitulum (Fig. 4) is like *a ball and spool threaded on to the same axis*. This axis constitutes, to a first approximation, *the axis of flexion and extension of the elbow*.

The following two points must be made:

The capitulum is not a complete sphere but a *hemisphere* (the anterior half of the sphere), placed, as it were, 'in front' of the lower end of the humerus. Therefore the capitulum, unlike the trochlea, does not extend posteriorly and stops short at the lower end of the humerus.

The *capitulo-trochlear groove* (Fig. 3) has the shape of a segment of a cone (4) with its wider base resting on the lateral lip of the trochlea. The usefulness of this capitulo-trochlear groove will emerge later.

The proximal ends of the two bones of the forearm have *two* surfaces corresponding to those of the humerus:

— The **trochlear notch of the ulna** (Fig. 3), which articulates with the trochlea and *has the corresponding shape*. It consists of a longitudinal rounded ridge (10) extending from the *olecranon process* (11) superiorly to the *coronoid process* (12) anteriorly and inferiorly. On either side of this ridge, which corresponds to the trochlear groove, is a concave surface (13) corresponding to the lips of the trochlea. The articular surface is shaped like one unit of a *corrugated iron sheet* (white arrow), formed by a ridge (10) and two gutters (11) (Fig. 4b).

— The **cupped proximal surface of the head of the radius** (Fig. 3) with a *concavity (14) corresponding to the convexity of the capitulum humeri (3)*. It is bounded by a rim which articulates with the capitulo-trochlear groove (cf. p. 83).

These two surfaces constitute in effect one articular surface owing to the annular ligament (16).

Figures 5 and 6 show **apposition of the articular surfaces**. Figure 5, seen from the front (*right side*), shows the olecranon fossa (5) above the trochlea and the radial fossa (6), the medial epicondyle (7) and the lateral epicondyle (8). Figure 6, seen from the back (*left side*), shows also the olecranon fossa (17) which receives the olecranon process (20).

A coronal section taken through the joint (Fig. 7, according to Testut) shows that the capsule (17) invests a single anatomical joint cavity with two functional joints: the true elbow joint (Fig. 7, 18 & 19, and Fig. 8: vertical stripes) and the superior radio-ulnar joint (Fig. 8: horizontal stripes), essential for pronatoin-supination. The olecranon process is also seen (11), lying inside the olecranon fossa during extension.

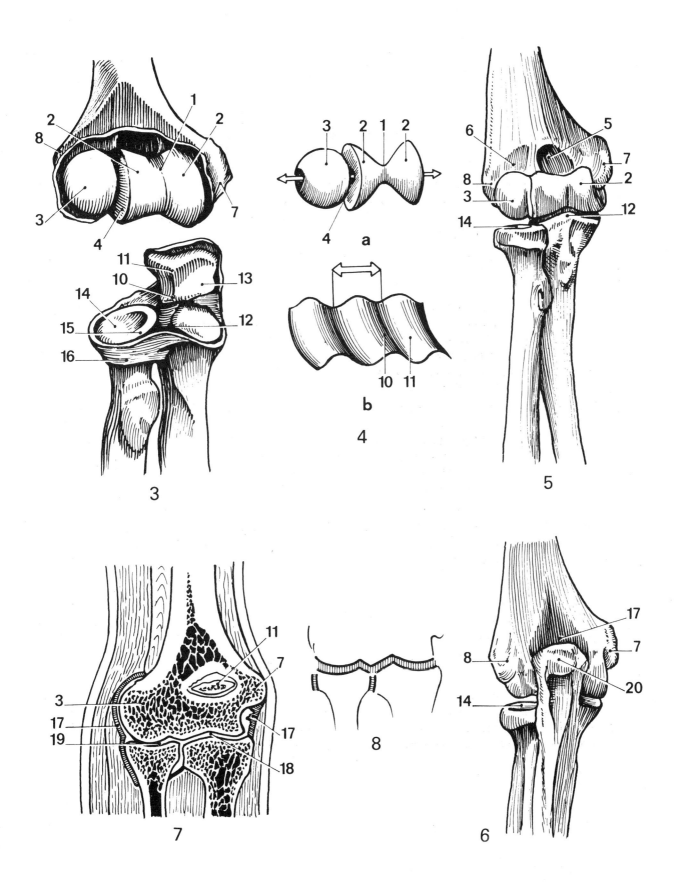

a

b

3

4

5

7

8

6

THE DISTAL END OF THE HUMERUS

This has the shape of an artist's palette (Fig. 12: anterior view, and Fig. 13: posterior view) and is *flattened antero-posteriorly*. On its distal aspect it bears the two articular surfaces — the trochlea and the capitulum. It is important to know the structure and shape of this segment of the humerus in order to understand the physiology of the elbow.

1. The distal end of the humerus **resembles a fork** which holds between its two prongs the axis of the articular surfaces (Fig. 14).

Immediately above the articular surfaces two concavities are present: viz. anteriorly, the *coronoid fossa* which receives the coronoid process of the ulna during flexion (Fig. 11); and posteriorly the *olecranon fossa* which receives the olecranon process during extension (Fig. 9). These fossae increase the range of flexion and extension at the elbow by delaying the moment of impact of the coronoid and olecranon processes on the shaft of the humerus. They also allow the trochlear notch of the ulna, which has a range of movement of 180°, to glide over the trochlear for an appreciable distance on either side of the neutral position (Fig. 10).

These two fossae are occasionally so deep that the intervening thin plate of bone is *perforated* and so they communicate with each other. The compact portions of the distal end of the humerus lie on either side of these fossae forming two divergent pillars, the one ending on the medial epicondyle, the other on the lateral epicondyle (Fig. 13); between these the capitulo-trochlear articular complex lies supported. This fork-like structure explains why it is so difficult to reduce and especially to control fractures of the distal end of the humerus.

2. The distal end of the humerus (Fig. 15a) bulges anteriorly at an angle of 45° to the shaft so that the *trochlea lies in front of the axis of the shaft;* this is important in the mechanics of the joint.

In the same way, the *trochlear notch of the ulna* projects anteriorly and superiorly at an angle of 45° to the ulnar shaft and so *lies in front of the axis of the ulna* (a and b).

This anterior projection of the articular surfaces and their inclination at 45° *promote flexion* in the following two ways:

1. Contact of the coronoid process with the humerus occurs only when the two bones are almost parallel, i.e. theoretically flexed to 180°.

2. Even during full flexion the two bones are separated by a space (double arrow), which lodges the muscles.

In the absence of these two mechanical factors (f), flexion would clearly be limited to 90° by the impact of the coronoid process (g) on the humerus; and during full flexion there would be no space left for the muscles (h), assuming that the bones could come into contact with each other as a result of, say, communication between the coronoid and the olecranon fossae.

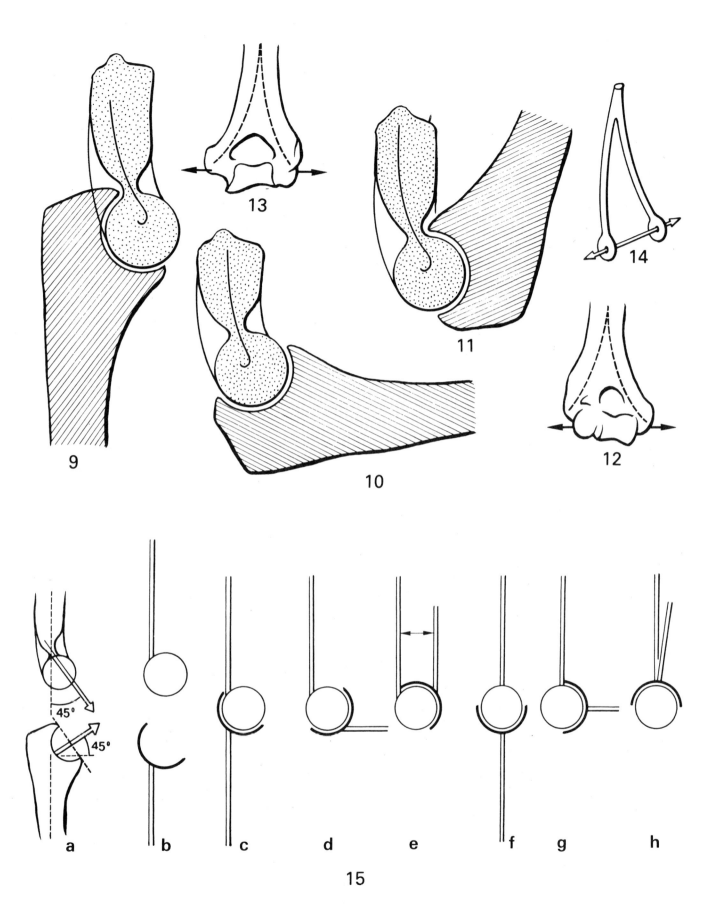

9

13

10

11

14

12

a   b   c   d   e   f   g   h

45°

45°

15

THE LIGAMENTS OF THE ELBOW

(The numbers have the same meaning in all diagrams)

The function of these ligaments is *to keep the articular surfaces in apposition*. They act as two *stays* located on either side of the joint — the medial ligament (Fig. 16, according to Rouvière) and the lateral ligament (Fig. 17, according to Rouvière).

These *fan-shaped* ligaments are inserted proximally on the epicondyles roughly at the level of the transverse axis xx' of the joint and distally round the edge of the trochlear notch (Fig. 18, according to Rouvière).

The **mechanical model of the elbow** is shown in Figure 19: (above) the fork of the distal end of the humerus supporting the articular pulley; (below) a half-ring (the trochlear notch of the ulna) continuous with the ulnar shaft and fitting into the pulley; the ligaments in the shape of two stays continuous with the humerus and inserted at the two ends of the axis of the pulley.

These two *lateral stays* have a *double function* (Fig. 20a): to keep the half-ring fitted on to the pulley (coaptation of articular surfaces); to prevent all sideways movements.

If one of the ligaments gives way (Fig. 20b), for example the medial ligament (white arrow), movement takes place towards the opposite side with loss of contact of the articular surfaces. This is the *mechanism commonly encountered in dislocation of the elbow*, which is, in its first stages, a severe sprain (i.e. rupture of the medial ligament).

The **medial ligament** consists of three parts (Fig. 16):

— The **anterior fibres** (1), some of which strengthen the annular ligament (2).

— The **intermediate fibres**, being the most powerful (3).

— The **posterior fibres** (4) or the ligament of Bardinet, strengthened by the transverse fibres of Cooper's ligament (5).

This diagram also shows the medial epicondyle (6), from which arises the fan-shaped medial ligament; the olecranon (7); the oblique cord (8); the tendon of the biceps (9) inserted into the radial tuberosity.

The **lateral ligament** also consists of three parts (Fig. 17):

— The *anterior fibres* (10) which strengthen the annular ligament posteriorly.

— The *intermediate fibres* (11) which strengthen the annular ligament posteriorly.

— The *posterior fibres* (12).

The lateral epicondyle (13) is also shown.

The **capsule** is strengthened anteriorly by the anterior ligament (14) and the oblique anterior ligament (15) and posteriorly by the fibres of the posterior ligament, which run transversely across the humerus and obliquely from humerus to olecranon.

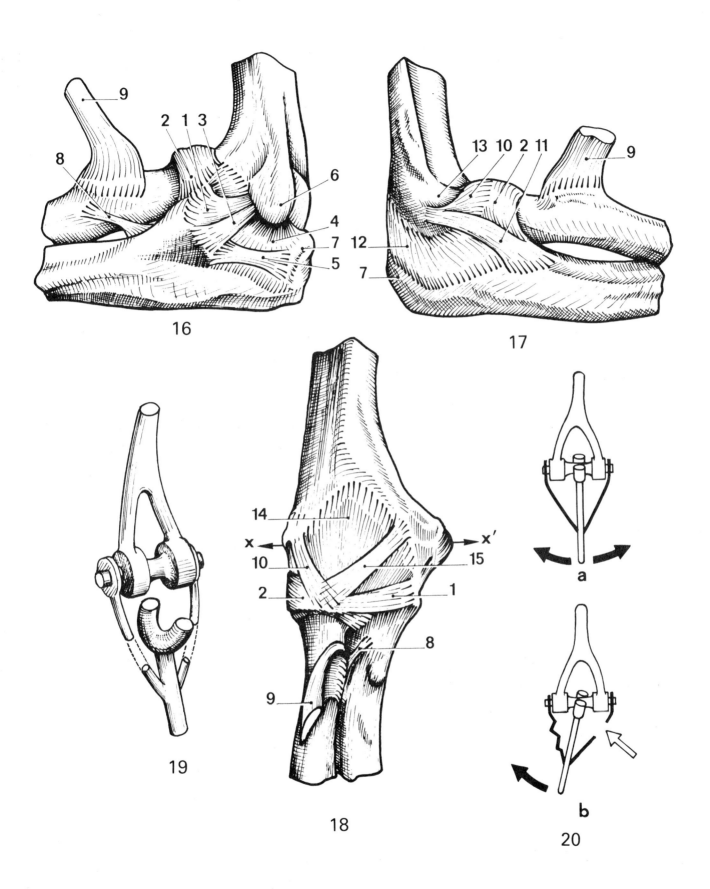

16

17

19

18

20

a

b

x   x'

81

THE HEAD OF THE RADIUS

The shape of the head of the radius is *determined entirely by its articular function:*

— For axial rotation of the radius the head is *cylindrical.*

— For flexion and extension of the elbow about the intercondylar axis xx':

The head of the radius (Fig. 21) must first correspond to the spheroidal capitulum humeri (A). Hence its *upper surface is concave* and **cup-shaped** (B). It is as if there had been removed from the bone a half-sphere (C) with a radius of curvature equal to that of the capitulum. During pronation-supination the radial head can rotate on the humeral condyle regardless of the degree of flexion or extension of the elbow.

But the capitulum has a medial border (Fig. 22) in the shape of a truncated cone (A) (i.e. *the capitulo-trochlear groove*) so that for congruence during flexion and extension a *wedge must be removed* (C) from the medial aspect of the head of the radius. This could be achieved by removing a wedge from the radial head along a plane tangential (B) to that of the trunk of the cone.

Finally, the radial head not only glides on the capitulum and the capitulo-trochlear groove which turning on its axis xx' but can also **simultaneously** rotate about its vertical axis yy' during pronation and supination (B). So, the smooth crescent cut along the edge of the head of the radius (C) extends for some distance along its circumference, as if a *shaving* had been removed by a razor during rotation of the head (Fig. 23).

The articular relations of the head of the radius in extreme positions (Fig. 24):

— In *full extension* (a) only the anterior half of the proximal surface of the radial head articulates with the capitulum; in fact the articular cartilage of the capitulum stretches as far as the inferior end of the humerus without extending posteriorly.

— In *full flexion* (b) the rim of the radial head reaches beyond the capitulum and enters *the radial fossa*, which is much less deep than the coronoid fossa (cf. Fig. 5).

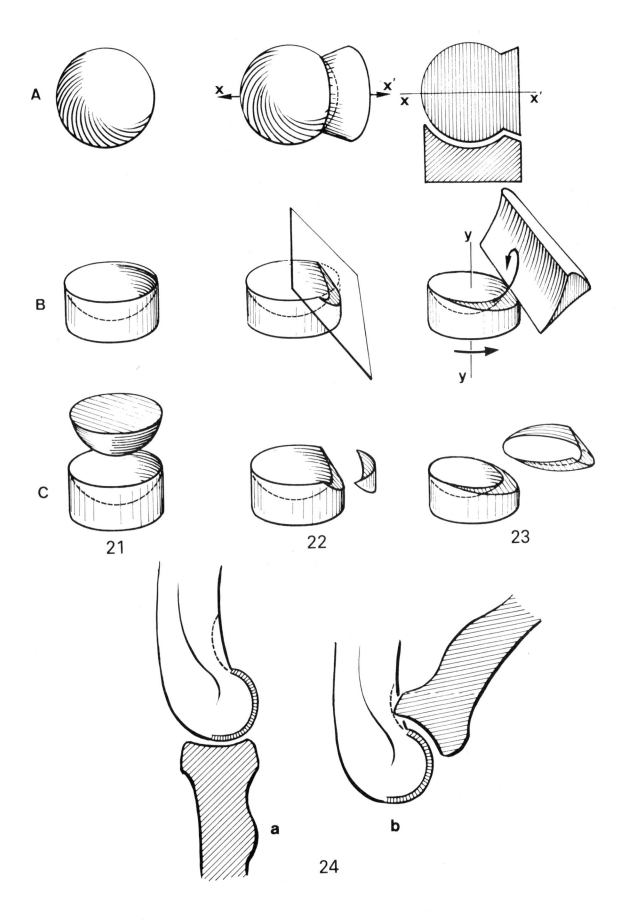

A

B

C

21

22

23

a

b

24

THE TROCHLEA HUMERI

(anatomical variations)

To a first approximation the trochlear groove was said (p. 76) to lie in the sagittal plane but in fact it is *oblique and not vertical*. Its obliquity shows individual variations which are summarised in Figure 25, along with their physiological consequences:

Type I, the most frequent (uppermost row, Fig. 25).

Anteriorly (a) the groove looks *vertical*, but posteriorly (b) it *runs obliquely distally and laterally*. As a whole (c) it runs in a *spiral* around the axis of the bone. The functional consequences are the following:

During extension (d) (according to Roud) the posterior aspect of the groove makes contact with the trochlear notch of the ulna and its obliquity is matched by a similar obliquity of the forearm. As a result the forearm has a slight obliquity inferiorly and laterally and its axis, out of line with that of the arm, forms *an obtuse angle with that of the latter*. This angle, known as *the carrying angle of the arm*, is more marked in women (Fig. 26).

During flexion, the anterior part of the groove is responsible for the direction imparted to the forearm and, as it lies in the vertical plane, the forearm comes to rest anteriorly *in the same plane as the upper arm* (e).

Type II: less common (middle row, Fig. 25)

The trochlear groove runs obliquely *proximally and laterally anteriorly* (a) and *distally and laterally posteriorly* (b). As a whole it runs in a *true spiral* round the axis of the bone.

During extension (d) the forearm runs obliquely distally and laterally with a similar carrying angle of the arm as in Type I.

During flexion (e) the outward obliquity of the anterior aspect of the groove influences the direction of movement of the forearm so that it *comes to rest slightly lateral to the arm*.

Type III: very rare (bottom row, Fig. 25)

The trochlear groove runs *obliquely and medially anteriorly* (a) and *distally and laterally posteriorly* (b). As a whole (c) the groove forms in space either a circle which lies in a plane running obliquely distally and laterally or a very closed spiral pointing medially. The functional effects are the following:

During extension (d), the carrying angle of the arm is normal.

During flexion (e), the *forearm comes to rest medial to the arm*.

Another consequence of this spiral configuration of the trochlear groove is that the groove has in effect a *series of instantaneous axes* lying between the two extreme positions, as shown (Fig. 27):

— An *axis during flexion* (continuous line) which is perpendicular to that of the flexed forearm (this most common variation is shown here, cf. Type I).

— An *axis during extension* (broken line) which is perpendicular to that of the extended forearm.

In fact, the direction of the axis of flexion and extension *changes progressively between the two extreme positions* of flexion and extension (see Fig. 28, where the humerus is shown).

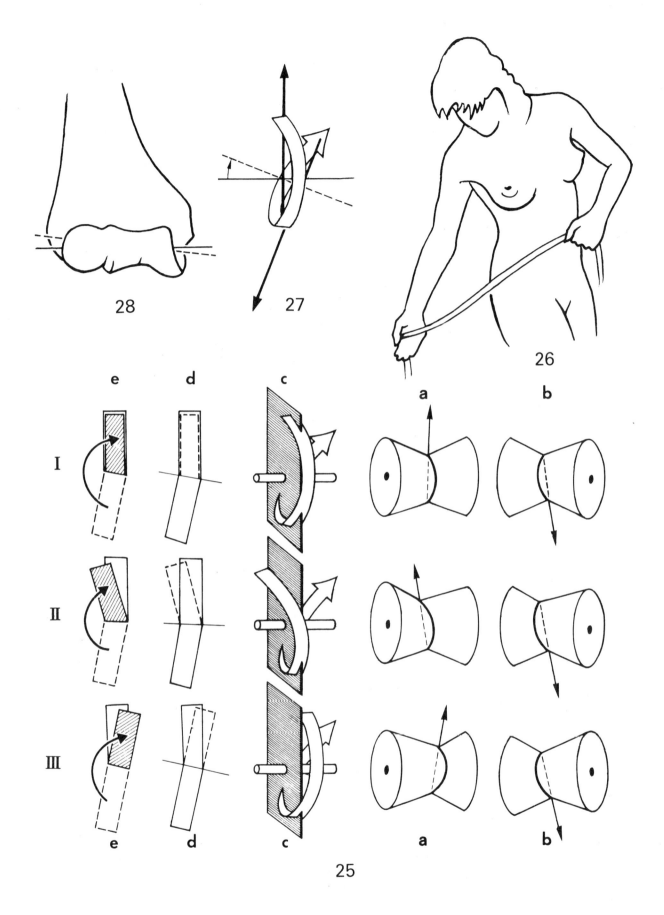

28

27

26

e   d   c   a   b

I

II

III

e   d   c   a   b

25

85

LIMITATIONS OF FLEXION AND EXTENSION

Extension is checked (Fig. 29) by three factors:

1. The impact of the olecranon process on the olecranon fossa
2. The tension of the anterior ligament of the joint
3. The resistance of the flexor muscles (biceps, brachialis, supinator).

If extension proceeds any further, *rupture of one of these limiting structures must occur:*

— The olecranon is fractured (Fig. 30) and the capsule is torn (2).

— The olecranon (Fig. 31) is not fractured but the capsule (2) and the ligaments are torn with posterior dislocation of the elbow (3).

— The muscles are usually unaffected but the brachial artery can be torn or at least bruised.

Limitation of flexion depends upon whether flexion is **active** or **passive**.

Active flexion (Fig. 32):

The first and foremost limiting factor is the apposition of the anterior muscles of the arm and forearm (1), *hardened by contraction*, which prevents active flexion beyond 145°. This effect is more prominent the more sinewy the subject is.

The other factors, i.e. impact of the corresponding bony surfaces (2) and tension of the capsular ligament (3), are insignificant.

Passive flexion (Fig. 33), secondary to an external force (black arrow) tending to 'close' the joint:

— The relaxed muscles (1) can be *flattened against each other* allowing flexion to reach beyond 145°; at this stage the other limiting factors become more important, i.e. impact of the head of the radius against the radial fossa and of the coronoid process against the coronoid fossa (2); tension of the posterior capsular ligament (3); tension developed passively in the triceps (4). Flexion can then reach 160°.

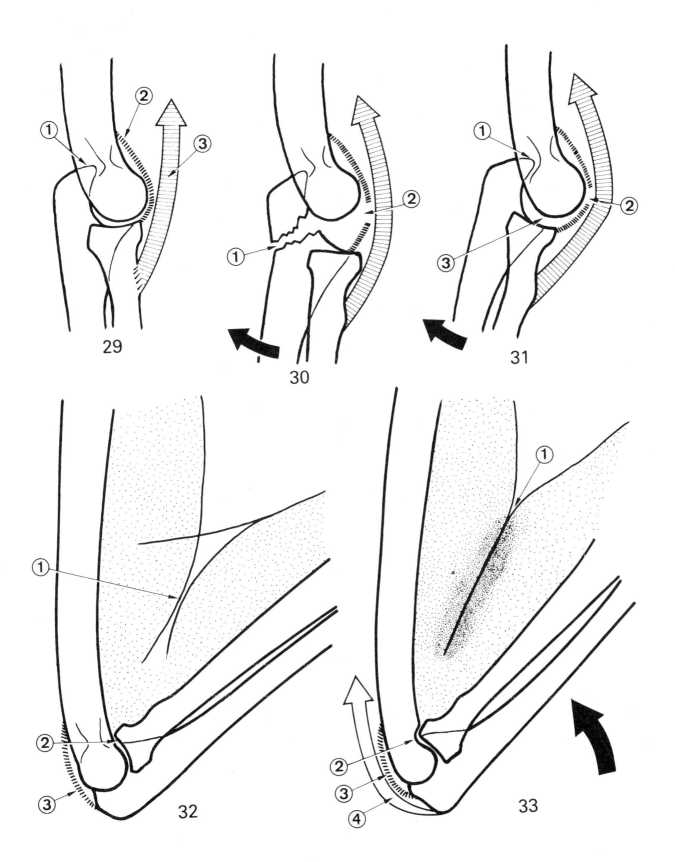

29

30

31

32

33

FLEXOR MUSCLES OF THE ELBOW

There are *three* primary flexor muscles:

— **Brachialis** (1), with its origin from the anterior aspect of the lower half of the humerus and its insertion into the tuberosity of the ulna (Fig. 34); acts *exclusively* as a flexor of the elbow. It is one of the rare muscles of the body with a single function.

— **Brachio-radialis** (2), running from the lateral supracondylar ridge of the humerus (Fig. 34) to the styloid process of the radius, acts *essentially* as a flexor of the elbow and becomes a supinator *only in extreme pronation,* and a pronator in extreme supination.

— **Biceps brachii** (3) is the *main flexor of the elbow* (Fig. 35). It is inserted mostly into the radial tuberosity and it arises not from the humerus (and therefore is a biarticular muscle) but from the scapula as follows:

— *the long head* (3') arises from the supraglenoid tubercle and traverses the upper part of the shoulder (cf. Chapter I: The Shoulder);

— *the short head* (3") arises from the coracoid process.

By virtue of its origin from the scapula the biceps *keeps the articular surfaces of the shoulder in apposition* but its *main action is flexion of the elbow.* It also plays an important, though secondary, role in *supination.* When the elbow is flexed it tends to produce dislocation of the radius (p. 92).

The flexor muscles *work at their best advantage when the elbow is flexed at 90°.*

In fact, during extension (Fig. 36), the direction of the forces exerted by the muscles is nearly parallel (white arrow) to the axis of the arm of the lever. The centripetal component C acting in the direction of the centre of the joint is the more powerful but of little mechanical importance, while the weak transverse component T is the only effective force in flexion.

On the other hand, when the elbow is in mid-flexion (Fig. 37), the muscular pull is *perpendicular* to the arm of the lever (white arrow: biceps; black arrow: brachioradialis) so that the centripetal component is zero and the tangential component is the same as the muscular pull, which is therefore fully utilised for flexion.

This *flexion angle of maximum efficiency* lies between 80° and 90° for the biceps and for the brachioradialis between 100° and 110°, i.e. *at a greater angle of flexion than for the biceps.*

The action of the flexor muscles follows the physical laws applying to levers of the third type and so favours range and speed of movement at the expense of power.

Accessory flexor muscles:

Extensor carpi radialis longus (R_1): lying deep to the brachioradialis (Fig. 37);

Pronator teres: its fibrous retraction (Volkmann's contracture) prevents complete elbow extension.

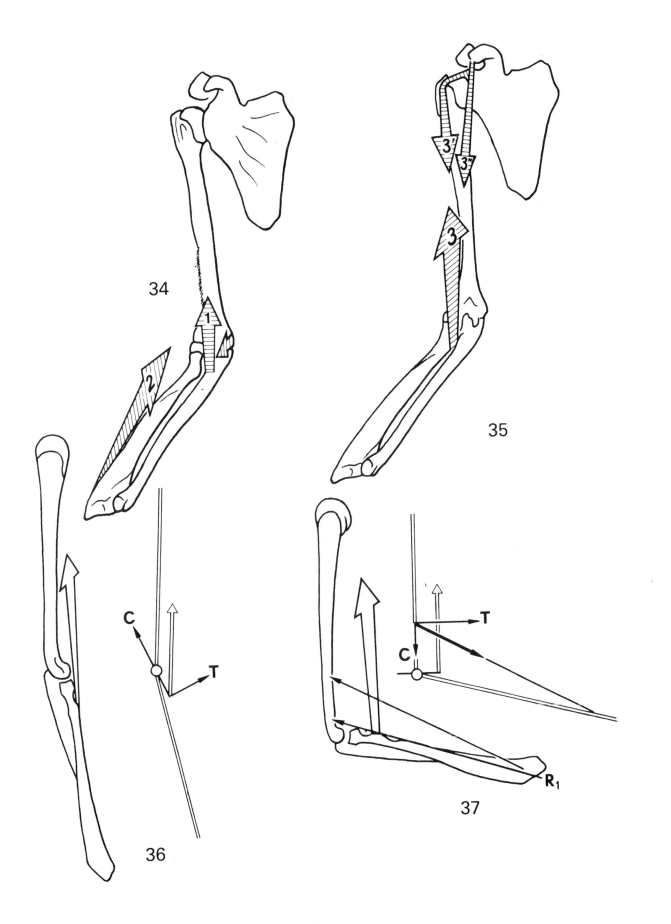

34

35

36

37

EXTENSOR MUSCLES OF THE ELBOW

Extension of the elbow depends on *one muscle*, i.e. the triceps brachii (Fig. 38), as the anconeus (A) exerts a negligible action, (although Duchenne de Boulogne thinks differently).

The **triceps** consists of three separate fleshy heads converging on to a *common tendon* which is inserted into the olecranon process:
- The *medial head* (1) arises from the entire posterior surface of the humerus below the level of the spiral groove for the radial nerve.
- The *lateral head* (2) arises chiefly from the lateral border of the humerus above the spiral groove (these two heads are therefore monoarticular).
- *The long head* (3) arises from the infraglenoid tubercle of the scapula and so is biarticular.

The **efficiency of the triceps** varies according to the state of flexion of the elbow:
- In full extension (Fig. 39) the muscular force can be resolved into two components, i.e. the centrifugal component C which tends to dislocate the ulna posteriorly and the more powerful normal (tangential) component T, which is the only active force in extension.
- When the elbow is slightly flexed to 20° to 30° (Fig. 40) the radial component (centrifugal in the preceding example) becomes zero and the effective tangential component T is the same as the muscular pull. Hence in this position the triceps is *maximally efficient*.
- Subsequently, when the elbow is flexed further (Fig. 41), the effective tangential component T decreases as the centripetal component C increases.
- In full flexion (Fig. 42), the triceps tendon is reflected on the superior surface of the olecranon process *as on a pulley* and this tends to make up for its loss of efficiency. Moreover, its fibres are *maximally stretched* and so its force of contraction is maximal; this further compensates for its loss of efficiency.

The efficiency of the long head of the triceps and so of the whole muscle also depends on the *position of the shoulder* because it is a biarticular muscle (Fig. 43).

It is clear that the distance between its origin and insertion is greater when the shoulder is flexed at 90° than when the arm hangs down vertically (with the elbow in the same position). In fact, the arcs of a circle described by the humerus (1) and the long head of triceps (2) do not coincide. If the length of the triceps did not change, its insertion would reach 0′ but, as the olecranon is now at 0_2, the muscle must be passively stretched from 0′ to 0_2.

Therefore the triceps is more powerful *when the shoulder is in flexion*. Then some of the force generated by the flexor muscles of the shoulder (the clavicular fibres of the pectoralis major and the deltoid) is diverted by the long head of the triceps to enhance the power of extension. This exemplifies one of the functions of biarticular muscles. The triceps is also at its most powerful *when the elbow and shoulder are simultaneously extended* (starting from the position of 90° shoulder flexion), e.g. as when a woodcutter strikes with an axe.

On the other hand, the triceps is at its weakest when the elbow is extended at the same time as the shoulder is flexed, as when a blow is struck forwards. In this case the long head of the triceps is 'caught' between two antagonistic movements, i.e. lengthening due to shoulder flexion and contraction due to extension of the elbow.

Note that the triceps and the latissimus dorsi form a functional couple producing adduction at the shoulder (see p. 70).

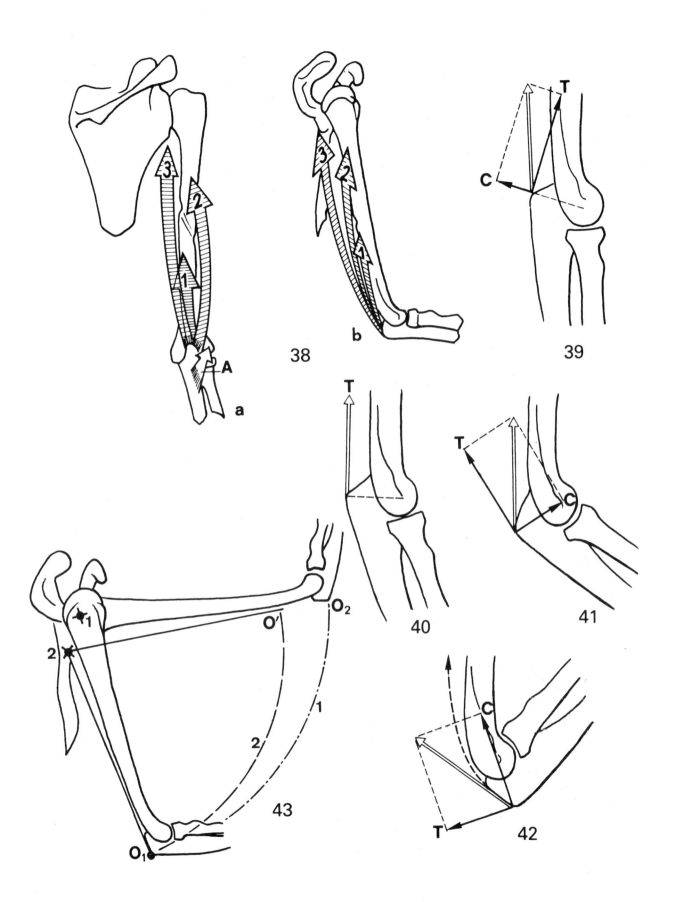

38

a

A

b

39

T

C

40

T

41

T

C

42

C

T

43

O_1

O_2

O'

1

2

1

2

91

FACTORS ENSURING COAPTATION OF THE ARTICULAR SURFACES

Coaptation of the articular surfaces in the long axis of the joint precludes dislocation in extension:

— either when a force is applied *downwards* (Fig. 44: lateral view and Fig. 45: medial view), as when one carries a bucket of water,

— or when a force is exerted *upwards* (Fig. 47 and 48), as when one falls on one's hands with the elbows fully extended.

1. Resistance to longitudinal traction

Because the trochlear notch of the ulna covers an arc of less than 180° it fails to grip the trochlea of the humerus in the absence of the soft tissues. The apposition of the articular surfaces is achieved by the ligaments, i.e. the medial (1) and lateral (2) ligaments; the muscular cuff consisting of the muscles of the arm, i.e. triceps (3), biceps (4), brachialis (5) and also of those of the forearm, i.e. brachioradialis (6) and the muscles arising from the lateral (7) and medial (8) epicondyles.

During full extension the tip of the olecranon hooks over the trochlea in the olecranon fossa, thus imparting some mechanical resistance to the elbow joint in its long axis.

Note that the lateral half of the elbow joint is *structurally unsuited to withstand excessive traction* and the head of the radius tends to dislocate distally through the annular ligament. This mechanism is thought to operate in the condition of 'pulled elbow' in the child.

The only anatomic structure preventing "descent" of the radius relative to the ulna is the interosseous membrane.

2. Resistance to impacting forces

This is provided exclusively by the bones involved:

— In the radius, pressure is transmitted to the head, which is liable to fracture (Fig. 47)

— In the ulna, the coronoid process absorbs the pressure and can be fractured, leading to an irreducible posterior dislocation of the elbow (Fig. 48).

Coaptation during flexion (Fig. 46)

When the elbow is flexed to 90° the ulna is *perfectly stable* (a), because the trochlear notch is surrounded by the powerful musculo-tendinous insertions of the triceps (3) and the brachialis (5) which secure coaptation of the joint surfaces.

The radius, on the other hand, is *liable to proximal and anterior dislocation* (b) under the action of the biceps (4). This dislocation is prevented solely by the annular ligament. When this ligament is torn the radius is dislocated proximally and anteriorly by the slightest flexion of the arm produced by the biceps.

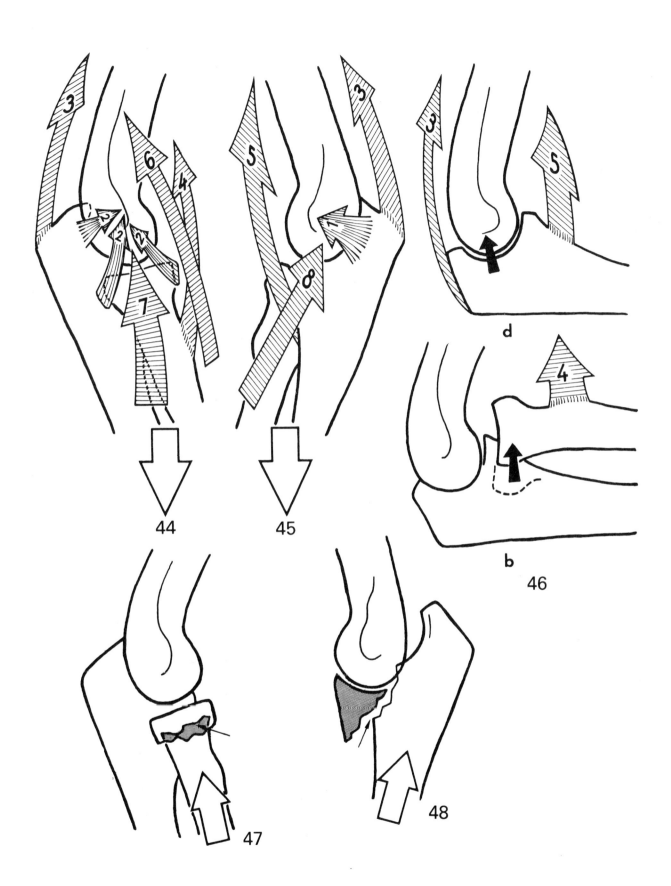

44

45

d

b
46

47

48

93

THE RANGE OF MOVEMENTS OF THE ELBOW

The **reference position** (Fig. 49) is defined as the position achieved *when the axes of the arm and forearm are in a straight line.*

Extension is the movement of the forearm *posteriorly.* Since the position of reference corresponds to complete extension (Fig. 49) the range of extension of the elbow is zero *by definition*, except in subjects (e.g. women and children) in whom great laxity of the ligaments allows hyperextension of 5° to 10° (z, Fig. 50).

By contrast, *relative* extension is always possible from any position of flexion.

When extension is incomplete it is quantitated *negatively*. Thus an extension of −40° corresponds to an extension falling short of 40°, i.e. the elbow remains flexed at 40° when complete extension is the object.

In the diagram (Fig. 50) the shortfall in extension is −y and flexion is +x (Df is the shortfall in flexion). Thus the useful range of flexion-extension is x − y.

Flexion is movement of the forearm *anteriorly* (Fig. 50) with approximation of the forearm to the anterior aspect of the arm.

Active flexion has a range of 145° (Fig. 51)

Passive flexion has a range of 160°, with the fist width separating the wrist from the shoulder, i.e. the wrist never touches the shoulder.

SURFACE MARKINGS OF THE ELBOW

The three *visible and palpable markings* are:

The **olecranon** (2), projecting from the midline of the elbow joint

The **medial epicondyle** (1), medially

The **lateral epicondyle** (3), laterally.

In extension (Fig. 52) these three landmarks lie in a *horizontal* line. Between the olecranon (2) and the medial epicondyle (1) runs the *ulnar nerve* (stippled arrow), so that any injury to the nerve in this position causes an electric shock felt in the territory of supply of the nerve (medial border of the hand). Laterally below the epicondyle can be felt the head of the radius as it rotates during pronation and supination.

In flexion (Fig. 53), the three landmarks now constitute an *equilateral triangle* (b) lying in a coronal plane tangential to the posterior aspect of the arm (a).

During dislocation this relationship is disturbed:

— In extension the olecranon *reaches above* the interepicondylar line (posterior dislocation).

— In flexion the olecranon *extends posteriorly* beyond the frontal plane of the arm (posterior dislocation).

94

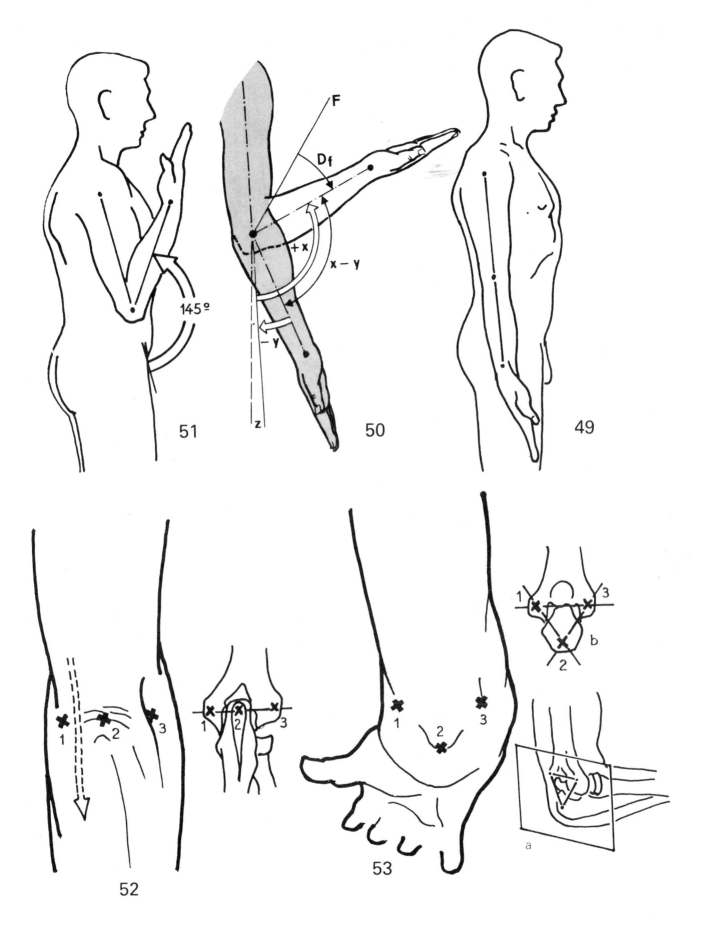

51

F

D_f

+ x

x − y

y

z

145°

50

49

52

1

2

3

1

2

3

53

1

2

3

1

3

2

b

a

POSITION OF FUNCTION AND POSITION OF IMMOBILISATION

Both positions are defined by the same criteria (Fig. 54); flexion at 90°; neutral rotation so that the hand lies in the vertical plane (cf. Chapter III).

EFFICIENCY OF THE FLEXOR AND EXTENSOR MUSCLES

As a whole, the flexors are slightly more powerful than the extensors so that in the relaxed position of the arm hanging loosely beside the body *the elbow is slightly flexed* and this degree of flexion is directly proportional to the muscularity of the subject.

The power of the flexors *varies with rotation of the forearm*, being greater when the forearm is pronated. The biceps is more stretched when the forearm is in pronation and its flexor action is consequently more efficient. Its flexor efficiency ratio for pronation/supination is 5:3.

The power of the muscle groups varies with the position of the shoulder (as shown diagrammatically in the comprehensive Figure 55):

1. **The arm is stretched vertically above the shoulder** (H):

   The force exerted during extension (e.g. lifting dumb-bells) is equivalent to 43 kg (arrow 1).

   The force exerted during flexion (e.g. while pulling oneself up) is equivalent to 83 kg (arrow 2).

2. **The arm is flexed at 90°** (AV):

   — The force produced during extension (e.g. while pushing a heavy load forwards) is equivalent to 37 kg (arrow 3).

   — The force produced during flexion (e.g. while rowing) is equivalent to 66 kg (arrow 4).

3. **The arm is hanging down beside the body** (B):

   — The force during flexion (e.g. while lifting a heavy load) is equivalent to 52 kg (arrow 5)..

   — The force during extension (e.g. lifting oneself up on parallel bars) is equivalent to 51 kg (arrow 6).

Therefore there are *preferential positions* where the muscle groups achieve maximum efficiency:

— for extension: when the arm is pointing downwards (arrow 6).

— for flexion: when the arm is pointing upwards. (arrow 2).

Thus the muscles of the upper limb are adapted for **climbing** (Fig. 56).

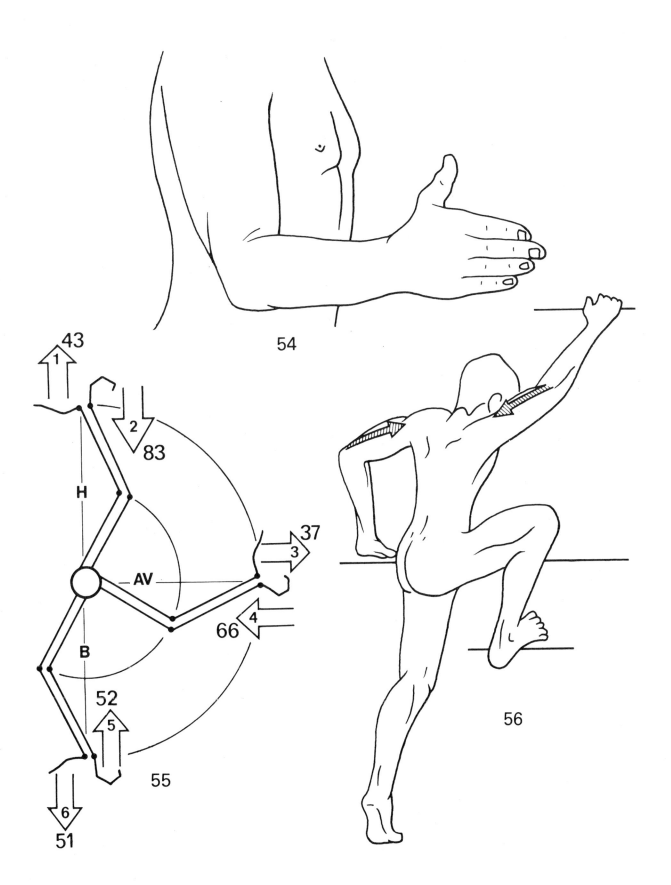

54

43
1

2
83

H

AV

37
3

66
4

B

52
5

55

6
51

56

97

ROTATION (PRONATION-SUPINATION)

SIGNIFICANCE

Rotation (pronation-supination) is *the movement of the forearm about its longitudinal axis*.

It involves **two joints which are mechanically linked** (Fig. 1):

— the *superior radio-ulnar* (SRU) joint, which anatomically belongs to the elbow

— the *inferior radio-ulnar* (IRU) joint, which is anatomically separate from the wrist.

This longitudinal rotation of the forearm introduces **a third degree of freedom** in the articular complex of the wrist. Thus the hand, the effector extremity of the upper limb, can be placed in any position to grasp or support an object. Note that the presence of a synovial joint with three degrees of freedom at the wrist would have created many mechanical problems. Thus it would have been necessary to supply the mobile extremity, i.e. carpus, with bony projections to provide leverage for the rotator muscles. Also it would have been mechanically impossible for the tendons of the forearm muscles to cross the wrist, since the latter would have been free to twist on itself during longitudinal rotation. Hence the hand would have had to contain all the extrinsic muscles, at the expense of muscle efficiency and hand size.

Longitudinal rotation of the forearm itself is at once the logical and elegant solution, even if the skeleton of the forearm is complicated by the presence of a *second bone*, the radius, which not only by itself supports the hand but also rotates around the first bone, the ulna, at the level of two radio-ulnar joints.

This architectural design of the forearm appeared 400 million years ago when certain fishes left the sea to colonise the land and transform into tetrapod amphibians.

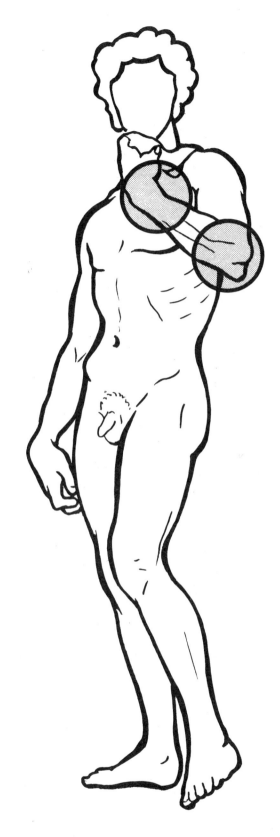

PRONATION-SUPINATION

99

DEFINITIONS

Rotation can only be studied with *the elbow flexed at 90° and resting against the trunk*. If the elbow is extended, the forearm is in line with the arm and *axial rotation* of the former is compounded with that of the latter owing to rotation of the shoulder.

With the elbow flexed at 90°:

— The **position of supination** is achieved (Fig. 2) with the *palm facing superiorly* and the *thumb pointing laterally*.

— The **position of pronation** is achieved (Fig. 3) with the *palm facing inferiorly* and *the thumb pointing medially*.

— The **position of neutral rotation** (Fig. 4), attained when the palm faces medially and the thumb points superiorly, is neither in pronation nor supination. It serves as a *reference position from which is measured the range of pronation and supination*.

When one looks at the arm 'end-on', i.e. along its long axis, the hand in neutral rotation (Fig. 5) lies in a vertical plane parallel to the plane of symmetry of the body (the sagittal plane); the hand in supination (Fig. 6) lies in a horizontal plane and so *the range of the movement of supination is 90°*; the hand in pronation (Fig. 7) fails to reach the horizontal plane and so *the range of the movement of pronation is only 85°*.

As a whole, the range of true rotation of the forearm, i.e. without associated rotation of the arm, is about 180°.

When the movements of rotation of the shoulder are also included, i.e. with the elbow completely extended, the range of rotation attains:

— 360° when the upper limb hangs vertically down beside the trunk;

— 360° when the upper limb is abducted to 90°

— 270° when the shoulder is flexed at 90° or extended at 90°.

— just over 180° when the upper limb lies vertically in abduction at 180°; in this position, therefore, axial rotation of the shoulder is negligible.

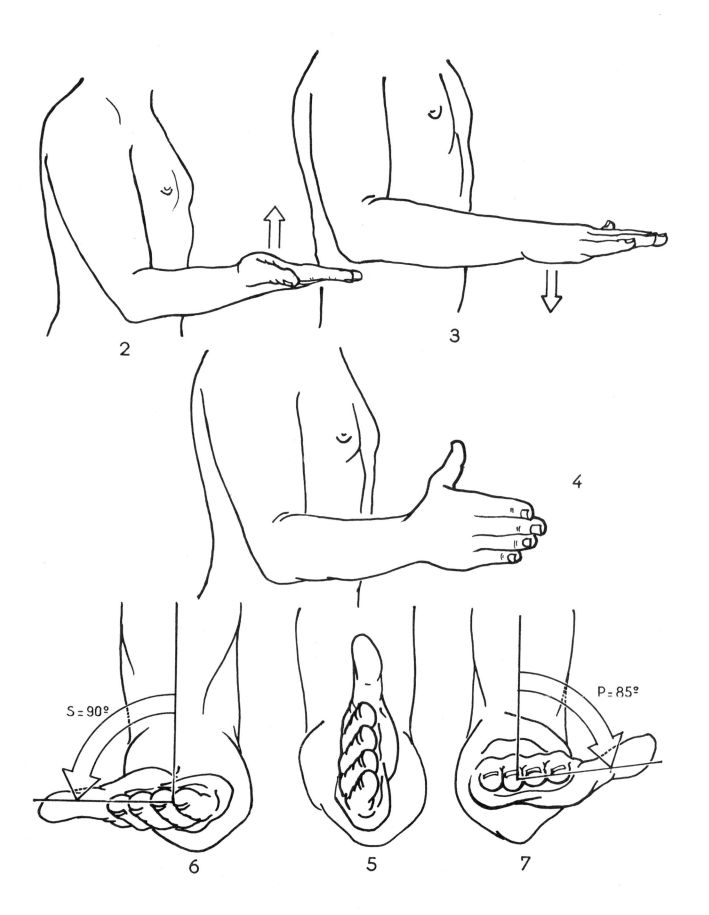

2

3

4

S = 90°

6

5

P = 85°

7

101

THE USEFULNESS OF PRONATION-SUPINATION (ROTATION)

Of the seven degrees of freedom inherent in the joint complexes of the upper limb from shoulder to hand, pronation-supination (rotation) is one of the most important since it is essential for *the control of hand orientation*. It allows the hand to assume the optimum position for grasping an object lying within a spherical sector of space (centred on the shoulder) and for carrying it to the mouth (the feeding function). It also allows the hand to reach any point of the body for protection or cleaning (the cleaning function). It also plays an essential role in all actions of the hand e.g. during work.

As a consequence of pronation-supination, the hand (Fig. 8) can *support* a tray or an object (supination) or compress an object downwards or lean on it (pronation).

Pronation-supination also allows a rotatory movement to be imparted to an object grasped with the centre of the palm and the fingers, as holding a screw-driver (Fig. 9), when the axis of the tool coincides with that of pronation-supination. Since a *handle is grasped obliquely by the whole hand* (Fig. 10) pronation-supination *alters the orientation of the tool* as a result of *conical rotation*. The asymmetry of the hand allows the handle of the tool to lie anywhere in space along the segment of a cone centred on the axis of pronation-supination. Hence the hammer can hit the nail at a controlled angle.

This observation exemplifies one aspect of the *functional coupling of pronation-supination and wrist action*, another aspect being the dependence of abduction-adduction of the wrist on pronation-supination. In pronation or in the intermediate position the hand is usually *tilted towards the ulna in an attempt to bring the dynamic tripod of prehension* (the thumb, index and middle fingers) *into line with the axis of pronation-supination*. In supination the hand is tilted towards the radius favouring a *supportive grip* e.g. carrying a tray.

This functional coupling makes it imperative to integrate the physiology of the inferior radio-ulnar joint with that of the wrist, though mechanically the former is linked to that of the superior radio-ulnar joint.

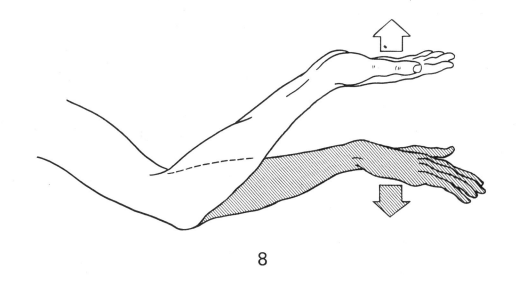

8

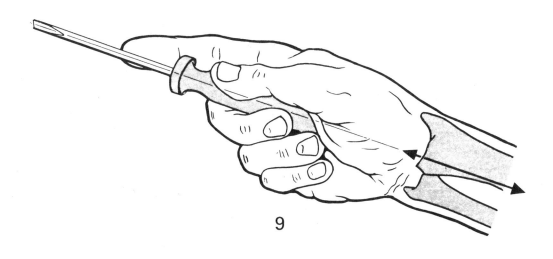

9

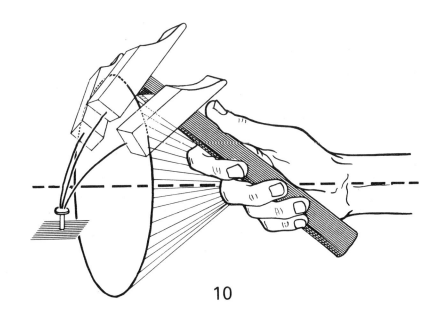

10

GENERAL ANATOMICAL RELATIONSHIPS

In supination (Figs. 11, 12, 13 and diagrams a, b of Fig. 17):

The radius and the ulna lie side by side with the ulna on the medial side. Their axes are parallel (a, Fig. 14). This is illustrated in Fig. 11 (*anterior view*), which also contains:

— The *interosseous membrane,* with its anterior fibres (1) running obliquely distally and medially and its posterior fibres (2) running proximally and laterally, *plays a vital role in binding radius and ulna together* and stopping the distal slippage of the radius.
(The radius is prevented from 'escaping' proximally by the humeral condyle). On its own it can keep these two bones together even after the ligaments of both radio-ulnar joints have been cut.

— the oblique cord (3)

— the anterior ligament of the inferior radio-ulnar joint (4).

N.B. *These three structures become taut during supination and check it.*

— the annular ligament (5) strengthened by

— the anterior fibres of the lateral ligament of the elbow (6)

— the anterior fibres of the medial ligament of the elbow (7)

— the triangular ligament (8), seen in cross-section.

Figure 12 (*seen from behind*) shows: the interosseous membrane with its anterior and posterior fibres (1); the posterior ligament of the inferior radio-ulnar joint (2); the annular ligament strengthened by the intermediate fibres of the lateral ligament of the elbow (4).

Figure 13 (*seen from the side*) shows the radius partially obscuring the ulna. The slight concavity of the anterior aspect of the radius is also apparent and this is also shown in the diagram b on Figure 17 (slightly exaggerated).

In pronation (Figs. 14, 15, 16 and diagrams c and d of Fig. 17):

The radius and the ulna are no longer parallel but *cross each other*, as seen in the anterior view (Fig. 14) and in the posterior view (Fig. 15) and in the diagram of Figure 17. In pronation (Fig. 17d) the radius is lateral to the ulna proximally and medial to it distally.

In Figure 16 (seen from the side) the radius is seen to lie anterior to the ulna and its concavity now facing posteriorly allows it to 'override' the ulna (Fig. 17c).

Clearly pronation can only have a range of just under 90° *because of the curvature of the radius in the sagittal plane.* Thus the flexors, which during supination lie in front of the bones (Fig. 18a), come to lie between the radius and the ulna during pronation (Fig. 18b) and eventually form a 'mattress' that softens the contact between the two bones (Fig. 18c). At the same time, the interosseous membrane wraps itself round the ulna and, helped by the muscular mattress, it displaces the ulna posteriorly with respect to the radius, thus *favouring the posterior subluxation of the ulnar head at the end of pronation.*

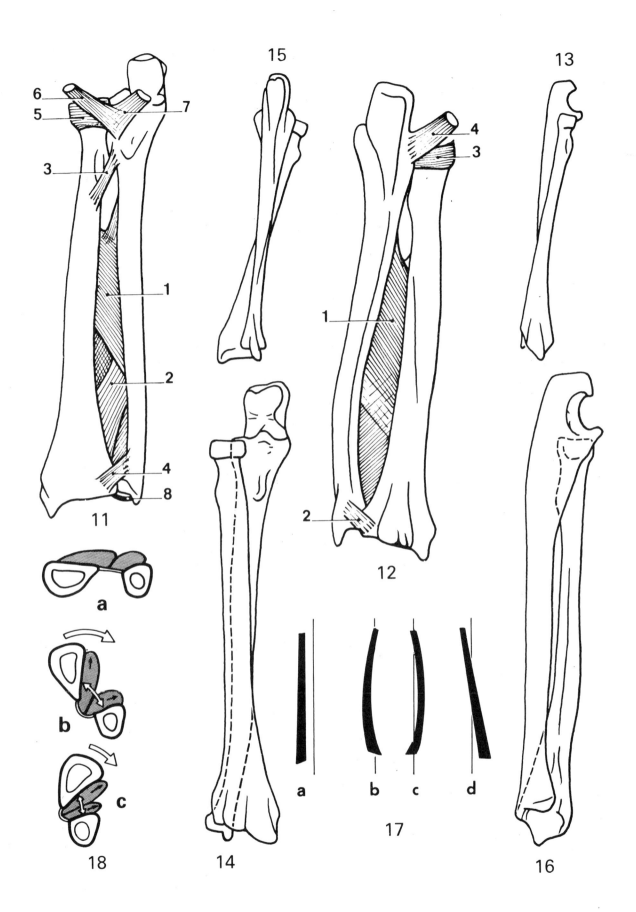

FUNCTIONAL ANATOMY OF THE SUPERIOR RADIO-ULNAR JOINT

(the numbers have the same meaning in all the figures)

The superior radio-ulnar joint is a **trochoid** with cylindrical surfaces and *one degree of freedom*: i.e. rotation about the axis of the two cylinders in contact. It can therefore be compared mechanically to a *system of ball-bearings* (Fig. 20).

It consists of the following *two* cylindrical surfaces:

— **The head of the radius** (Fig. 21) with its cylindrical rim (1) covered by articular cartilage and corresponding to the proximal component (1) of the ball-bearing system. Note also that the cupped surface of the head (2) articulates (Fig. 25, sagittal section) with the capitulum of the humerus. Since the latter does not extend posteriorly, only the anterior half of the head of the radius is in contact with it during extension. The bevelled aspect (3) of the head of the radius is also illustrated (cf. p. 83).

— **A fibro-osseous ring** (shown in Fig. 19 with the radial head removed) corresponds to the distal component of the ball-bearing system (Fig. 20, 5 and 6). It consists of the following:

— the **radial notch of the ulna** (6) covered by articular cartilage, concave antero-posteriorly and separated by a blunt ridge (7) from the trochlear notch (8, Fig. 21).

— the **annular ligament** (5) (shown intact in Fig. 19 and cut in Fig. 21), which consists of a strong fibrous band attached by its ends to the anterior and posterior margins of the radial notch of the ulna and lined internally by cartilage continuous with that lining the radial notch. Therefore it serves *as a ligament*, by surrounding the head of the radius and binding it to the radial notch, and also *as an articular surface* in contact with the head of the radius. Unlike the radial notch of the ulna, it is *flexible*.

Another ligament related to the joint is the **quadrate ligament** (4), which is shown cut in Figure 21, intact in Figure 22 (with the annular ligament cut and the radius displaced laterally) and in Figure 23 (seen from above with the olecranon and annular ligament sectioned). It consists of a fibrous band attached to the inferior border of the radial notch and to the neck of the radius (Fig. 24, frontal section). Its two borders (Figs. 21 and 22) are strengthened by the fibres of the upper border of the annular ligament. It acts the reinforce the inferior aspect of the capsule. The rest of the capsule (10) encloses all the joints at the elbow within one anatomical cavity.

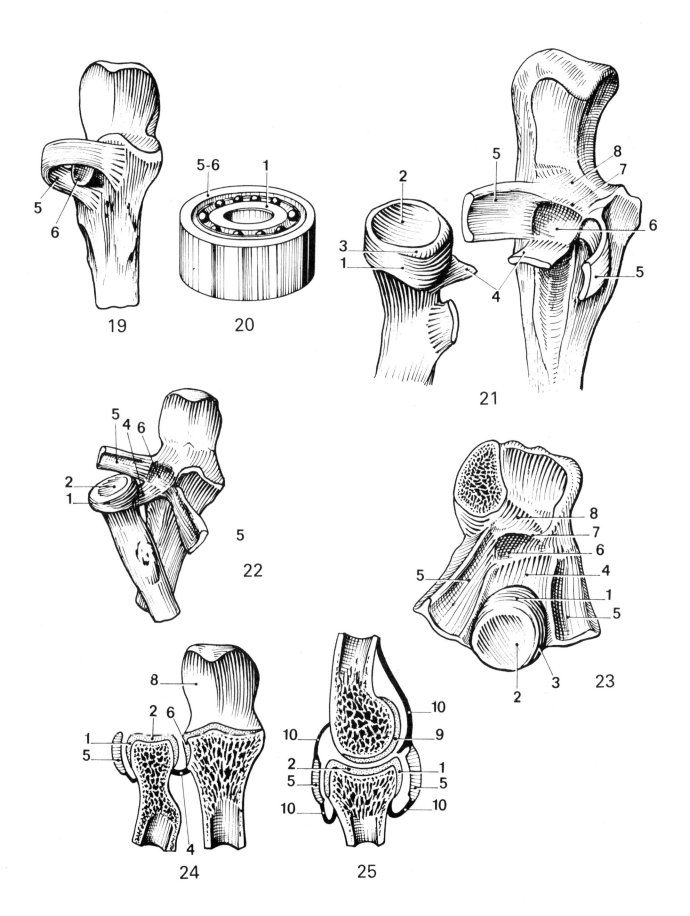

19 20

21

22 5

23

24 25

THE FUNCTIONAL ANATOMY OF THE INFERIOR RADIO-ULNAR JOINT

(architecture and mechanical construction of the inferior end of the ulna)

Like its homologue, the superior radio-ulnar joint, the inferior radio-ulnar joint is a **trochoid** (pivot) joint with cylindrical articular surfaces and *only one degree of freedom*, i.e. rotation about the axes of its interlocked cylindrical surfaces.

The **first of these cylindrical surfaces** (Fig. 26) is supported by the *head of the ulna*. It is possible to consider the distal end of the ulna (a) as formed by the telescoping of a diaphyseal cylinder (1) into an epiphyseal cone (2), so that the axis of the cone is out of line with that of the cylinder. From this composite structure (b) a conical segment (c) is cut along a horizontal plane (3) and the distal surface of the ulna is thus produced (4). Next (d) a solid crescent (6) is shaved off by a second cutting cylinder (5) so that the head of the ulna takes on a cylindrical shape (7). Note that the cutting cylinder (5) is not concentric with the diaphyseal cylinder (1) or with the epiphyseal cone (2). Hence the shape of the articular surface, which resembles a *crescent* wrapped over a cylinder with its anterior and posterior horns abutting on the styloid process (8), displaced to the postero-medial aspect of the epiphysis. In reality, this surface is not quite cylindrical (Fig. 27), because it was originally fashioned from a surface convex outwards. Hence it has the shape of a *keg* slightly bent downwards and inwards, so that it can be inscribed on an inverted cone, whose axis is parallel to that of the diaphyseal axis d. The peripheral surface of the ulnar head (A: seen from the side and B: seen head on) is at its widest (h) anteriorly and slightly laterally.

The inferior surface of the ulnar head (D) is semi-lunar with its point of maximal width corresponding to the highest point (h) on its periphery. Thus are aligned along the plane of symmetry (arrow): the insertion of the medial fibres of the extensor retinaculum (square), the main insertion of the apex of the triangular articular disc (star), the centre of curvature of the distal surface (cross) and the highest point on its periphery (h).

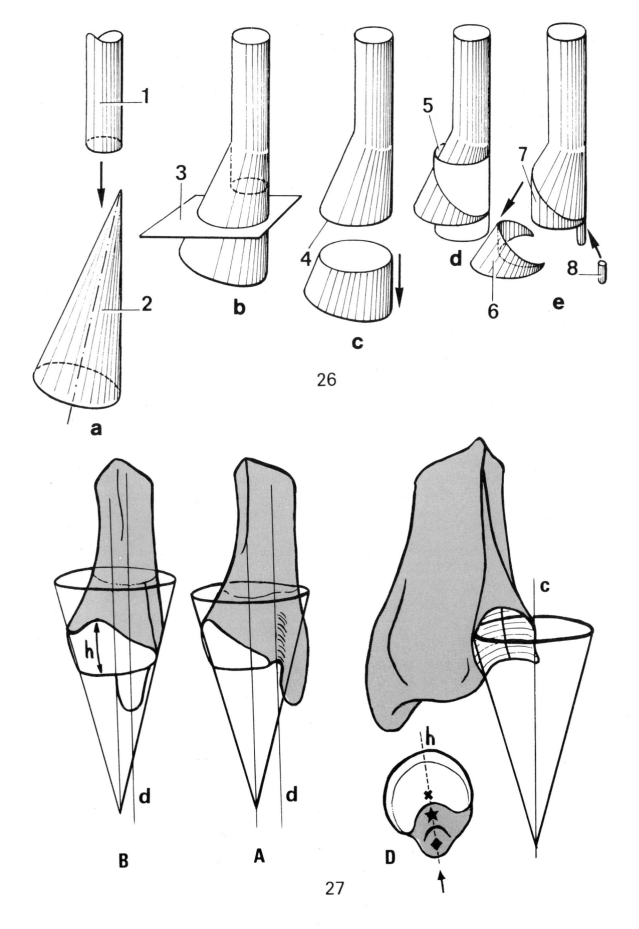

1

3

2

b

4

c

5

d

6

7

8

e

a

26

h

B

A

d

d

c

h

D

27

109

THE FUNCTIONAL ANATOMY OF THE INFERIOR RADIO-ULNAR JOINT (continued)

(the numbers have the same meaning in all the diagrams)

The **second surface**, the ulnar notch of the radius (3), lies at the distal end of the bone (Figs. 28 and 29), between the two edges of its interosseous border (2). It faces (3) medially (Fig. 29) and is concave anteroposteriorly and plane or slightly concave proximodistally. It can be inscribed on the surface of an inverted cone (27, c). It is at its widest in its mid-portion and articulates with the cylindrical portion (4) of the ulnar head.

At its distal edge is inserted the **articular disc** (5), which lies in a horizontal plane (Fig. 30: frontal section) and whose apex is inserted medially into:

- the fossa between the styloid process of the ulna and the inferior surface of the ulnar head
- the lateral aspect of the ulnar styloid process
- the deep aspect of the medial ligament of the wrist.

The articular disc thus fills the gap between the ulnar head and the os triquetrum and acts as an elastic cushion, which is compressed during adduction of the wrist. Its anterior and posterior borders are thickened so that it appears biconcave on section (Fig. 29: antero-supero-medial view). Its proximal surface, covered by articular cartilage, is in contact with the distal surface (7) of the ulnar head (Fig. 28). Its distal surface, covered by articular cartilage, is flush with the carpal surface of the radius (8), which is bounded laterally by the radial styloid process (1), and forms the medial part of the wrist (13).

Thus the articular disc fulfils three functions:

— it *binds together* the radius and the ulna

— it provides a *dual articular surface*: proximally with the ulnar head, distally with the carpal bones. Note that *the ulnar head* is not in contact with the carpal bones.

— it separates the radio-ulnar joint from the radio-carpal joint (Fig. 30), so that these joint cavities are anatomically distinct except if:

— the articular disc is markedly biconcave and is perforated in the middle;

— the insertion of its base (Fig. 28 and 29) is incomplete and a slit is present (6), an age-related change, probably degenerative in origin.

Thus with the ulnar notch of the radius it provides the ulnar head with a recess, which is partly flexible.

It corresponds to a true '**suspended meniscus**' between the superior radio-ulnar and the radio-carpal joints and is subjected to a variety of stresses (Fig. 31): traction (horizontal arrow), compression (vertical arrow) and shearing (horizontal arrows), acting individually or in combination.

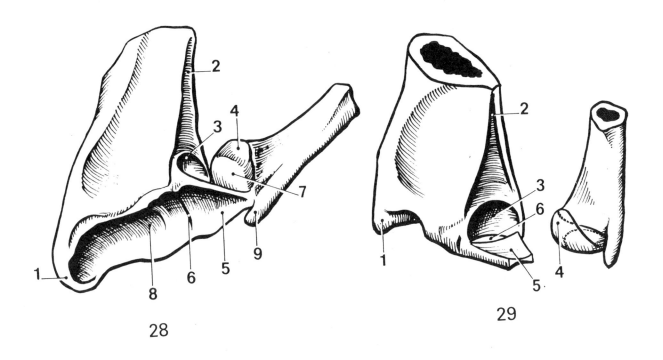

28

29

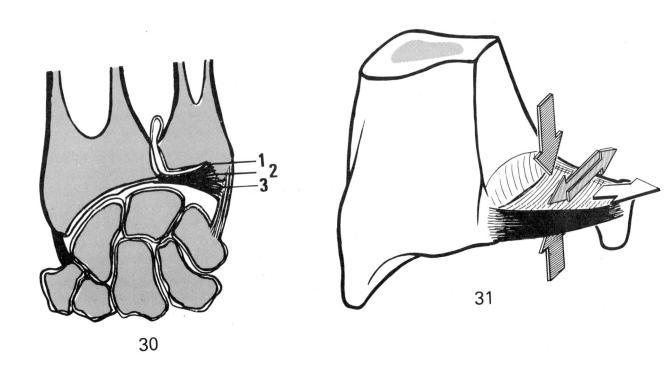

30

31

111

THE DYNAMICS OF THE SUPERIOR RADIO-ULNAR JOINT

(in Figs. 32 to 35 the upper row (a) refers to supination and the lower row (b) to pronation; the numbers have the same meaning throughout)

The **main movement** (Fig. 32) is *rotation of the head of the radius* (1) about *its axis xx'* within the fibro-osseous ring (2), formed by the annular ligament and the radial notch of the ulna. This movement is limited (Fig. 33) by the tension developed in the quadrate ligament, which therefore acts as a brake (3).

The head of the radius is not quite cylindrical but slightly oval: its great axis, lying obliquely antero-posteriorly (a, Fig. 34) (Fig. 29a), measures 28 mm and its short axis 24 mm. This explains why the annular cuff of the radial head cannot be entirely bony and rigid: *the annular ligament, which constitutes about three-quarters of the cuff, is flexible and allows some stretching*, while holding the head in perfect fit.

There are **four accessory movements** related to the radio-ulnar joint:

1. The *cup-shaped surface of the radial head* (*1*) *rotates* in relation to the capitulum humeri (Fig. 36).

2. The *bevelled ridge of the head of the radius* (*2*) (cf. p. 82) *glides* in contact with the capitulo-trochlear groove of the humerus (Fig. 36).

3. *The axis of the radial head is displaced laterally* during pronation (Fig. 35) because of the oval shape of the head. During pronation (b) the great axis of the radial head comes to lie transversely so that the long axis of the radius xx' is displaced laterally by a distance e equal to half the difference between the two axes of the radial head, i.e. 2 mm. This lateral displacement has great mechanical significance: it allows room for the *medial movement of the radial tuberosity*, into which the supinator is inserted. The white arrow (Fig. 32b) shows this movement of the radial tuberosity 'between' the radius and the ulna.

4. *The plane of the proximal surface of the radial head is tilted distally and laterally during pronation* (Fig. 37). *This is due to rotation of the radius about the ulna during pronation as follows:*

— At the beginning of pronation, i.e. while still in supination (a), the long axis of the radius is vertical and parallel to that of the ulna;

— At the end of pronation, the long axis now runs obliquely distally and medially so that the plane of the radial head, which is perpendicular to this axis, is now tilted distally and laterally at an angle y with the horizontal plane.

During pronation the long axis of the radius has 'swept' over part of the surface of a cone whose axis (finely hatched) is the same as *the common axis of the two radio-ulnar joints*.

The carrying angle of the arm (cf. also Fig. 26, p. 85), which is prominent during supination (c), becomes negligible during pronation (d) owing to the change in direction of the radial axis with the result that *the long axes of the arm and forearm become continuous*.

112

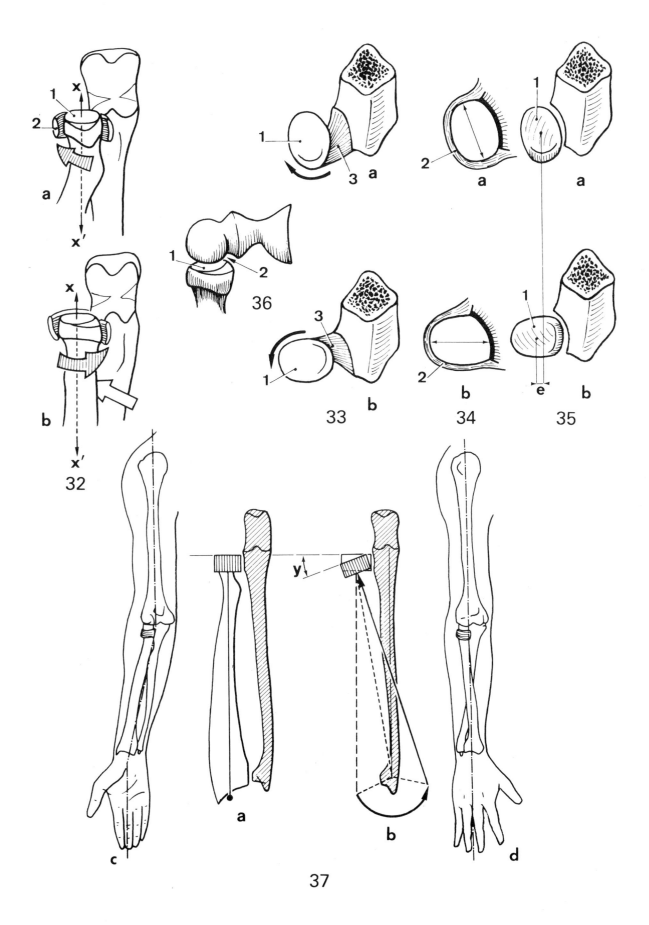

32

33

34

35

36

37

113

THE DYNAMICS OF THE INFERIOR RADIO-ULNAR JOINT

Let us first assume that **the ulna remains stationary** and only the radius moves. In this case (Fig. 38) *the axis of rotation* (marked with a black cross) *runs through the small finger and the medial edge of the ulna*. This is the case when the forearm lies in contact with the table all the time during rotation.

The **main movement** (Fig. 39) is a *rotational displacement* of the lower end of the radius about the ulna:

— supination: the radius and the ulna can be seen from below after the removal of the wrist and articular disc. Range = 90°.

— pronation: Range = 85°.

This movement of rotational displacement of the radius is well demonstrated by comparing the radius to a *crank* (Figs. 40, 41). The path covered by one arm (the other remaining stationary) is an example of rotational displacement:

— the displacement is along the arc of a circle (striped arrow, Fig. 40, crank in 'supination') around a cylinder corresponding to the head of the ulna.

— in Fig. 41 the movement is a rotation of the forearm about its own axis, as shown by the change in direction of the white arrow (Fig. 41). Note that the styloid process of the radius points laterally during supination and ulnaward during pronation.

When the radius turns around the ulna from supination to pronation the degree of articular congruence, i.e. geometric correspondence of the articular surfaces, varies because:

— on the one hand, the articular surfaces are not perfect geometrically and have variable radii of curvature, which tend to be shortest centrally;

— on the other, the radius of curvature of the ulnar notch of the radius is slightly greater than that of the ulnar head.

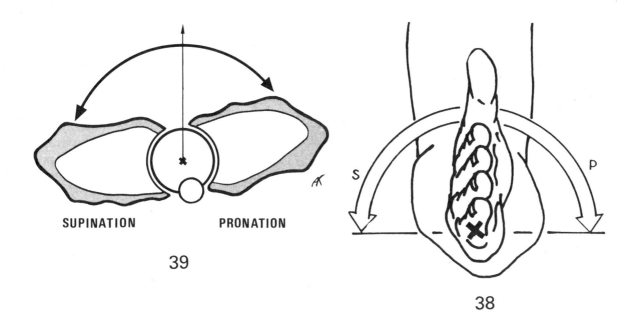

SUPINATION   PRONATION

39

38

S   P

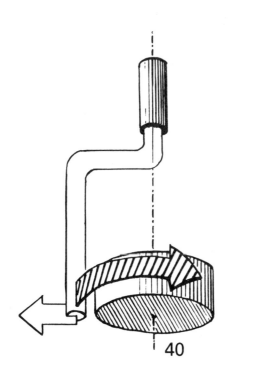

40

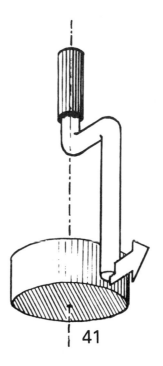

41

THE DYNAMICS OF THE INFERIOR RADIO-ULNAR JOINT (continued)

There are thus *positions of articular incongruence* (Fig. 42). In supination (B), the ulnar head is in contact with the ulnar notch of the radius over a very short distance and their radii of curvature are out of line. In full pronation (C) there is almost a true posterior subluxation of the ulnar head. The *position of maximal congruence (A) corresponds by and large to the intermediate position of rotation or the zero position*, when there is maximal contact between the surfaces and their radii of curvature are colinear.

During pronation and supination, the articular disc literally 'sweeps' the inferior surface of the ulnar head (Fig. 43) like a windscreen wiper. As a result of the eccentricity of its point of insertion into the ulna, its degree of tension varies considerably:

— it is minimal in full supination and pronation (B and C)

— it *is maximal when the correspondence of the articular surfaces is maximal*, i.e. in the position when the ligament is maximally stretched (D).

Thus there is a *position of maximal stability* for the inferior radio-ulnar joint, corresponding roughly to the intermediate position of pronation-supination. It is the 'close-packed' position of Mac Conaill with maximal correspondence of articular surfaces and maximal tension in the ligaments. Being an intermediate position it cannot be viewed as a truly locked position. The roles of the articular disc and interosseous membrane can be defined as follows:

— *in full pronation and supination*, the triangular disc is relaxed while the interosseous membrane is stretched. Note that the anterior and posterior ligaments of the inferior radio-ulnar joint, which are weak condensations of the capsule, play no role in keeping the articular surfaces together or in limiting the joint movements.

— in *the position of maximal stability*, close to the intermediate position, the articular disc is stretched and the interosseous membrane is relatively slack, *except in so far as it is stretched by the muscles attached to it*.

In sum, the articular surfaces of the inferior radio-ulnar joint are kept together by two anatomical structures, which often receive scant attention during the treatment of traumatic lesions of the forearm: the interosseous membrane, which is essential, and the triangular ligament.

Pronation is limited by the impact of the radius on the ulna. Hence the significance of the slight anterior concavity of the radial shaft, which delays the impact.

Supination is limited by the impact of the posterior end of the ulnar notch of the radius on the ulnar styloid process through the tendon of the extensor carpi ulnaris. It is not restricted by any ligaments but is limited by the tonus of the pronator muscles.

116

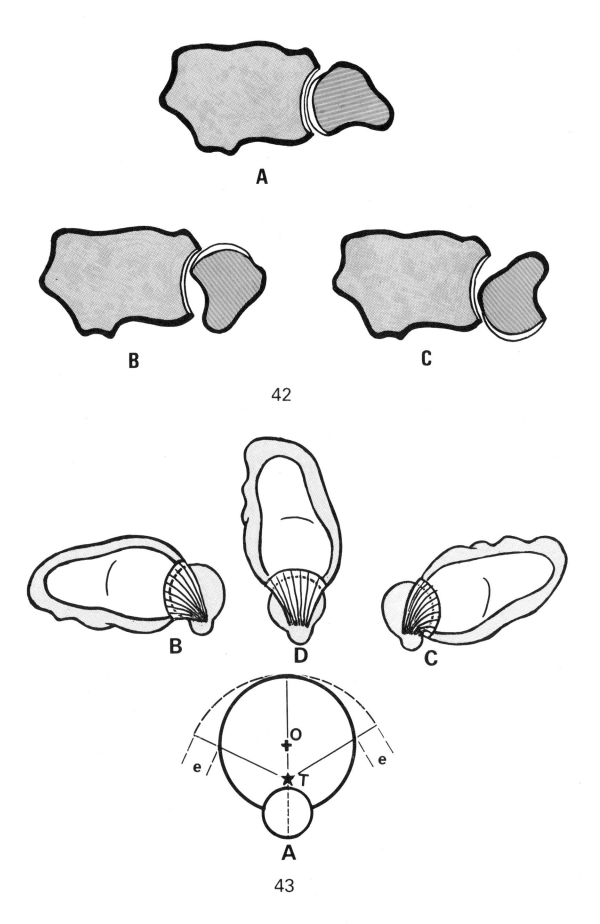

A

B   C

42

B   D   C

e   O
+
★ T
e

A

43

THE AXIS OF PRONATION-SUPINATION

So far the function of the inferior radio-ulnar joint has been discussed in isolation but it is easy to understand that there is a *functional coupling between the inferior and superior radio-ulnar joints*, which are *mechanically linked* since one joint needs the other to function.

This functional coupling depends on the coupling of the joint axes and the coupling of articular congruence.

The **two radio-ulnar joints are coaxial**: they can only function normally when their axes of movement (Fig. 44) are collinear (XX') and coincide with the *fulcrum of pronation-supination*, which passes through the heads of the ulna and radius.

When the radius moves around this axis relative to the ulna, its path traces out the surfaces of a segment of a cone, which is concave posteriorly and has its base inferiorly and its apex at the elbow.

Supposing that the ulnar head stays put, pronation-supination is due to the rotation of the distal radius around the axis of the inferior radio-ulnar joint, which is identical with that of the superior radio-ulnar joint. In this unique situation the axis of pronation-supination coincides with the fulcrum of pronation-supination.

The two radio-ulnar joints are coaxial just like the two hinges of a door (Fig. 45): their axes are collinear. The door can thus open freely (a).

When these joints are no longer coaxial following a poorly reduced fracture of one or both bones, pronation-supination is compromised from the start, because there are now *two separate fulcra* for the same moving segment, like a door with misaligned hinges. It must be sawn in half before it can be opened (b).

If pronation-supination occurs around an axis passing through the thumb, the radius rotates on either side of the styloid process (Fig. 46) of the ulna around an axis which does not correspond with the fulcrum of pronation-supination. As a result the inferior end of the ulna moves along a half circle downwards and outwards first and then upwards and outwards, while staying parallel to itself. The vertical component of this displacement can easily be explained by a concurrent movement of extension and then of flexion at the elbow. Its lateral component was previously considered to be due to a concurrent lateral movement at the elbow but it is unlikely that a movement of such range (nearly twice the width of the wrist) could occur in such a tight joint as the humero-ulnar joint. M.C. Dbjay has proposed a more mechanical and satifactory explanation. It is *concurrent lateral rotation of the humerus on its longitudinal axis* (Fig. 47) which displaces the ulnar head laterally (A), while the radius rotates on itself (B).

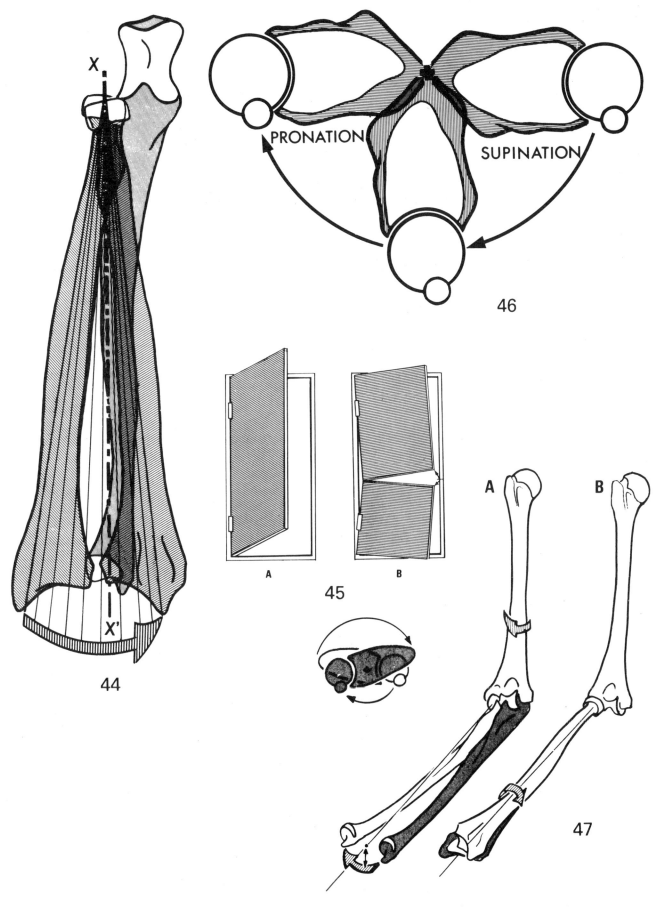

PRONATION

SUPINATION

46

A

B

45

A

B

44

47

119

THE AXIS OF PRONATION-SUPINATION (continued)

This hypothesis will only be confirmed when accurate radiographic and electromyographic studies demonstrate such a lateral rotation, ranging from 5° to 20°. If confirmed experimentally, this hypothesis could only apply to pronation-supination with the elbow at right angles, i.e. when its range is maximal (supination 90°, pronation 80°–85°). When the elbow is fully extended, the ulna is fixed by the olecranon fitting snugly in its fossa and if the elbow is fully immobilised it is clear that no pronation occurs while supination is not affected. This loss of pronation is made up for by *medial* rotation of the humerus. Thus during elbow extension there is a 'transition point' at which there is no associated rotation of the humerus.

Pronation is also reduced to 45° when the elbow is flexed. Then the humerus can barely rotate on its long axis and the lateral displacement of the ulnar head must be explained by lateral movement at the elbow joint.

In the two extreme cases of pronation-supination the axis of pronation-supination passes through the ulnar or radial end of the wrist. In the usual movement of pronation-supination, *centred on the dynamic tripod of prehension* (Fig. 48), the axis is intermediate and passes through the lower end of the radius near the ulnar notch (Fig. 49). The radius rotates on itself for nearly 180° and the ulna is displaced without rotation along an arc of the same circle, a displacement made up of a component of extension (E) and a component of lateral movement (L).

The axis of pronation-supination ZZ', which cannot be materially represented in space, is thus quite *distinct from the fulcum of pronation-supination* (Fig. 50). The latter, displaced from XX' and YY' by the ulnar head, traces out the surface of a segment of a cone, concave anteriorly.

In sum there is *a series of pronations-supinations*, the commonest occurring about an axis which passes through the radius and around which both bones 'rotate'. The *axis* of pronation-supination, *generally distinct from the fulcrum of pronation-supination*, is *variable, adaptable* and *cannot be physically defined in space*.

It does not follow that this axis does not exist; by the same token the axis of rotation of the earth would not exist either. From the fact that pronation-supination is a movement of rotation it can be deduced with certainty that its axis exists in reality though it cannot be physically defined, that it is rarely identical with the fulcrum of pronation-supination and that its position relative to the bones depends on the type and stage of pronation-supination performed.

120

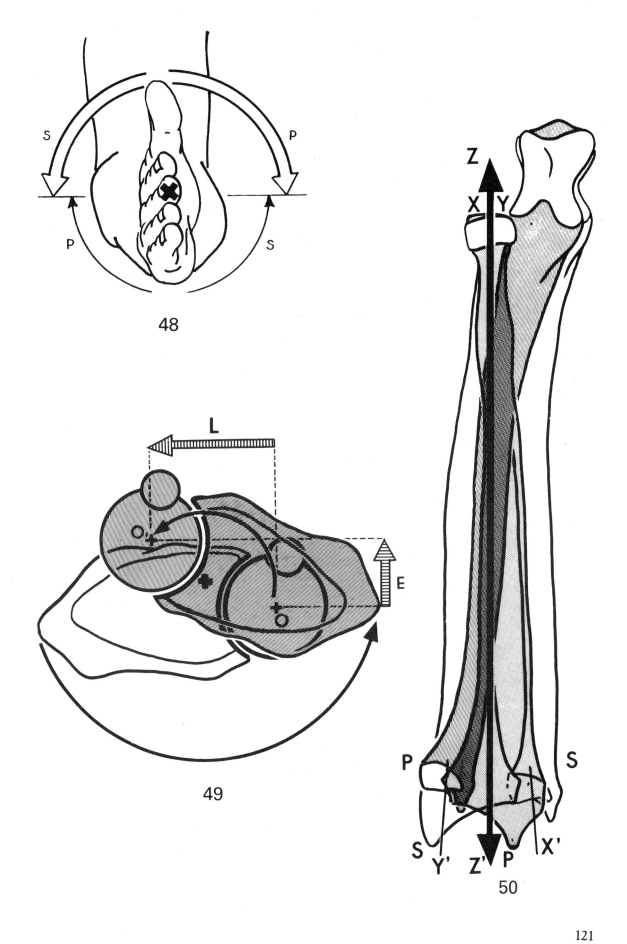

48

49

50

121

THE TWO RADIO-ULNAR JOINTS ARE CO-CONGRUENT

The functional coupling of the radio-ulnar joints also depends on *their articular cocongruence*. Thus the position of maximal stability for both joints is attained at the same degree of pronation-supination (Fig. 51).

In other words, when the maximal width of the ulnar head (h) is in contact with the ulnar notch of the radius, the same applies to the radial head (i) and the radial notch of the ulna. The planes of symmetry of the ulnar notch of the radius (s) and of the radial head (T), passing through the highest points on their peripheral surfaces, form a solid angle open medially and anteriorly. This *angle of torsion of the radius is equal to that of the ulna*, correspondingly measured through the ulnar head and the radial notch.

This angle varies from person to person (Fig. 52), as observed by looking at the lower end of the ulna along its long axis. Thus, depending on the position of the ulnar styloid process and the highest point on the peripheral surface of the ulna, three types can be defined:

(a) the styloid lies *exactly posteriorly*. The plane of symmetry S of the ulnar head then coincides with the sagittal plane F, which contains the blunt edge of the radial notch. Pronation is neither 'advanced' nor 'delayed' and the *position of maximal stability coincides with the intermediate position of pronation-supination*.

(b) the styloid lies posteriorly and *slightly medially*. The plane of symmetry of the ulnar head (S) forms with the sagittal plane (F) an angle open anteriorly and laterally, i.e. 20°. The angle is given as −20° and *pronation is said to be delayed* by 20°. The position of maximal stability does not coincide with the intermediate position but occurs at 20° supination. Note also that the range of pronation is smaller than in the previous case.

(c) The styloid lies posteriorly and *slightly laterally*. This time *pronation is 'advanced' by an angle of 15°*, given as +15°, and the position of maximal stability is in 15° pronation. The range of full pronation is greater than in the other two cases.

For each of these types there is an angle of torsion of the ulna, which is greater the more 'advanced' pronation is. But in all these cases the angle of torsion of the ulna (u) is equal to that of the radius (r), thereby ensuring cocongruence of the two radio-ulnar joints.

A large statistical study will no doubt help to establish the full spectrum of these variations.

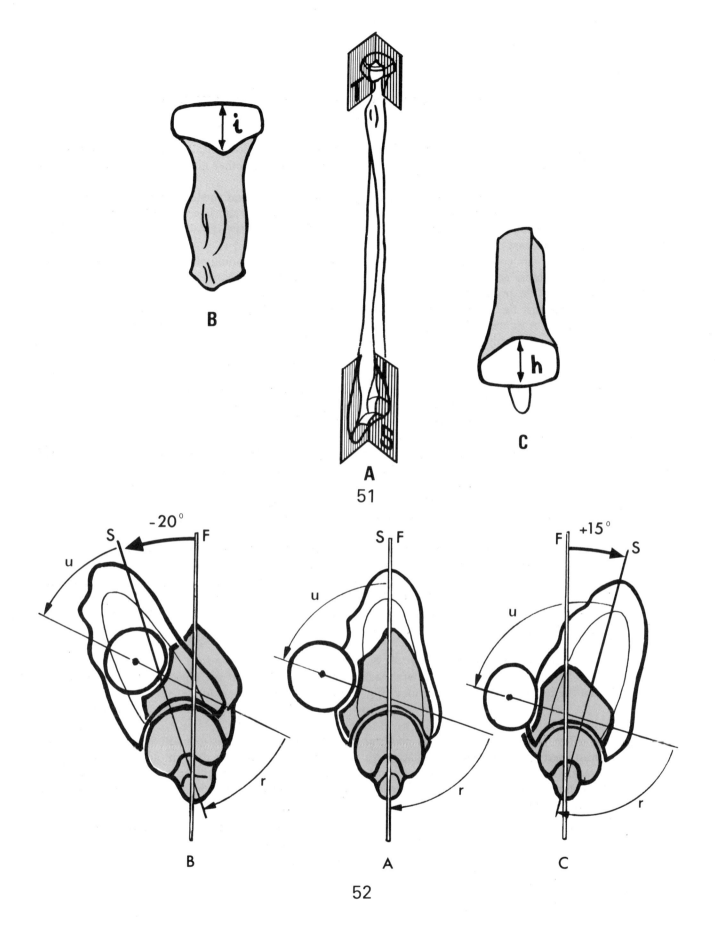

B

A
51

C

−20°

S   F
u
r
B

S F
u
r
A

F   +15°
S
u
r
C

52

123

THE MUSCLES OF PRONATION AND SUPINATION

To understand the mode of action of these muscles one must mechanically analyse the **shape of the radius** (Fig. 53). The radius comprises *three segments* which together give it roughly the shape of a *crank*.

The neck (the upper segment running obliquely distally and medially) joins the intermediate segment (the upper half of the shaft running obliquely distally and laterally) at an obtuse angle to form the *'supinator bend'* of the radius. This is at the level of the radial tuberosity (arrow 1), into which is inserted the biceps.

The intermediate segment also joins the lower segment (running obliquely distally and medially) at an obtuse angle to form the *'pronator bend'* of the radius (arrow 2). This is at the level of the insertion of the pronator teres.

Note that the 'radial crank' is *tilted at an angle* to its long axis xx' (small diagram), which also is the axis of rotation. Therefore this axis passes through both ends of the arms of the crank without passing through the arms themselves. Thus the apices of the two 'bends' lie on either side of this axis.

The axis xx' is shared by both radio-ulnar joints and this *common axis is essential* for the movements of rotation, provided the bones are not fractured either simultaneously or separately.

To move this 'crank' two mechanisms are available (Fig. 54):
1. To 'unwind' a cord coiled around one of the arms of the crank (arrow 1)
2. To pull on the apex of one of the bends (arrow 2).

These mechanisms form the basis of the mode of action of the musles of rotation.

These muscles are **four** in number and fall into two groups of two. For each of these movements there is:

— a short and flat muscle which acts by 'unwinding' (cf. arrow 1)
— a long muscle inserted into the apex of a 'bend' (cf. arrow 2).

Motor muscles of supination (Figs. 55 and 56: right side; seen from below)

1. *The supinator* (1), wound round the neck of the radius, acts by 'unwinding' (Fig. 56a).

2. The *biceps* (2), inserted into the apex of the 'supinator bend', i.e. the radial tuberosity (Fig. 56b), acts by traction and attains maximal efficiency when the elbow is flexed at 90°. This is the most powerful of the muscles of rotation; hence people screw by supinating the forearm with the elbow flexed.

Motor muscles of pronation (Figs. 57 & 58):

1. The *pronator quadratus* (1), wrapped around the distal end of the ulna, acts by 'unwinding' so that the radius moves round the ulna (Fig. 58: inferior view, right side).

2. The *pronator teres* (2) inserted into the apex of the 'pronator bend' of the radius, acts by traction; its action is weak, especially when the elbow is extended.

The *pronator muscles are less powerful than the supinators* so that to undo a jammed screw one must increase the power of pronation by simultaneously abducting the arm at the shoulder. The brachio-radialis is not a supinator but a flexor of the elbow. It can only supinate from the position of complete pronation to that of zero rotation. Paradoxically, it is a pronator from the position of complete supination to that of zero rotation.

There is only one nerve for pronation — the median nerve, and two nerves for supination — the radial nerve and the musculotaneous nerve (supplying the biceps).

124

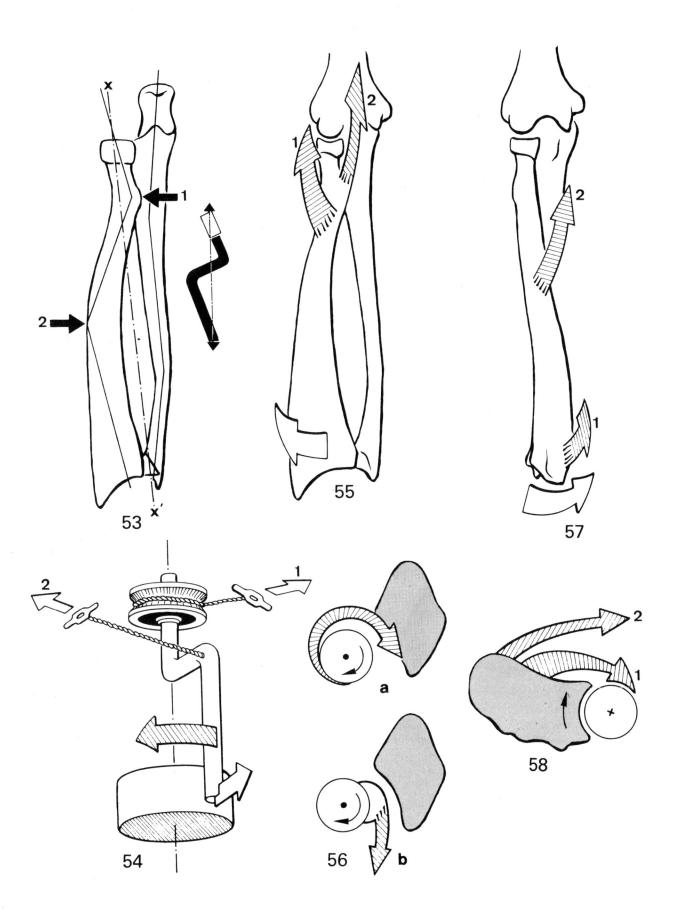

53

54

55

56

57

58

a

b

x

x′

1

2

125

Fractures of the two bones of the forearm (Figs. 59 & 60), according to Merle d'Aubigné).

The displacement of the fragments varies according to the level of the fracture and is determined by the resultant muscular pull:

1. *If the fracture occurs in the upper third of the radius* (Fig. 59), each fragment is acted upon by muscles with a corresponding effect, i.e. supinators acting on the upper fragment and pronators on the lower fragment. Therefore the relative displacement of the fragments (rotation of one with respect to the other) will be *maximal* with the upper fragment in extreme pronation and the lower in extreme supination.

2. *If the fracture occurs in the middle of the radial shaft* (Fig. 60), the displacement is less marked and is *reduced to half the maximum*, since pronation of the inferior fragment is due only to the pronator quadratus and supination of the upper fragment is checked by the pronator teres.

Therefore reduction must aim not only at the correction of the angular displacement but also the restoration of the normal 'bends' of the bones, especially of the radius:

— *The bend in the sagittal plane*, concave anteriorly. If it is flattened or reversed, pronation is curtailed in range.
— *The bends in the frontal plane*, especially 'the pronator bend'. If this is distorted, pronation is reduced owing to decreased efficiency of the pronator teres.

Dislocations of the radio-ulnar joints

1. *Dislocation of the inferior radio-ulnar joint*
This can occur alone or along with a fracture of the radial shaft. It is difficult to treat and treatment may involve either a resection of the ulnar head (Darrach's operation) or its repositioning.

The ulnar head can only be repositioned and pinned (Fig. 61) if a false joint is created by segmental resection of the ulna above the fracture (Kapandji & Sauvés operation).

2. *Dislocation of the radial head*
This is often associated (Fig. 62) with an ulnar fracture (white arrow) produced by direct violence (Monteggia's fracture). The proximal dislocation (black arrow) is produced by contraction of the biceps (striped arrow). To counteract this biceps-induced dislocation the annular ligament must be reconstructed surgically.

Fractures of the lower end of the radius.

When the lower end of the radius is broken (Fig. 63) it is tilted (A) laterally and this leads to incongruence in the lower radio-ulnar joint with excessive stretching of the articular disc. If the displacement is not reduced exactly and if repair is associated with an exuberant callus, pronation-supination can be severely impaired, as also happens if the trauma is violent enough to smash the articular disc, a lesion which cannot be detected radiographically.

In some cases (B), the insertion of the articular disc is torn off the ulnar styloid (Gérard-Marchant's fracture) with the following results:

— dislocation of the inferior radio-ulnar joint with diastasis, limited only by the interosseous membrane.
— severe sprain of the medial collateral ligament of the wrist.

When the distal end of the radius is broken (Fig. 64) it is also tilted posteriorly, severely impairing pronation-supination:

(a) normally the axes of the articular surfaces of the radius and ulna coincide.
(b) when the distal fragment of the radius is tilted posteriorly, the axis of the radial surface now forms with that of the ulnar surface a solid angle open inferiorly and posteriorly. As a result the congruence of the articular surfaces is lost.

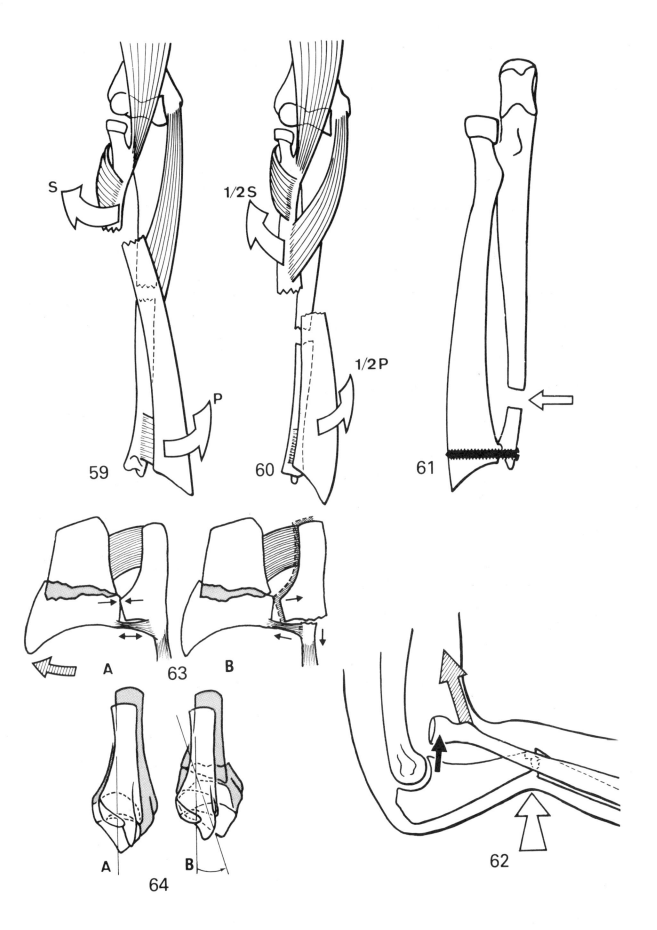

59

60

61

63   A   B

64   A   B

62

THE POSITION OF FUNCTION AND COMPENSATORY MOVEMENTS

Supination with the forearm (Fig. 65)

In fact, because the upper limb usually hangs beside the trunk, supination can only be achieved at the radio-ulnar joints i.e. true supination. This is the movement involved in unlocking a door with a key. The shoulder does not participate in supination and this explains why paralysis of the movement of supination is not easily compensated. There is some compensation, however, because complete paralysis rarely occurs, the biceps having a different nerve supply (musculocutaneous nerve) from the supinator (radial nerve).

Pronation with the help of the shoulder (Fig. 66)

On the other hand, during pronation the action of the pronator muscles can be *supplemented or amplified by abduction of the shoulder*. This movement is involved when one empties a saucepan.

The functional position of the forearm.

This lies between the position of neutral rotation (Fig. 67) (e.g. while holding a hammer), and the position of semi-pronation (Figs. 68, 69) (e.g. while holding a spoon or when writing).

The functional position corresponds to a state of *natural equilibrium* between the antagonistic muscle groups so that expenditure of muscular energy is at a minimum.

The movement of rotation is *essential for carrying food to the mouth*. In fact, when one picks up a piece of food lying on a horizontal plane (on a table or on the ground), grasping takes place with the arm *pronated* and the elbow extended. To carry it to the mouth the elbow must be bent and the hand *supinated* so as to 'present' it to the mouth

Two points are worth noting:

Supination 'spares' flexion of the elbow: if an object were brought to the mouth with the arm pronated, a greater degree of elbow flexion would be required.

The biceps is the best suited muscle for this 'feeding' movement because it is at once a *flexor of the elbow* and a *supinator of the forearm*.

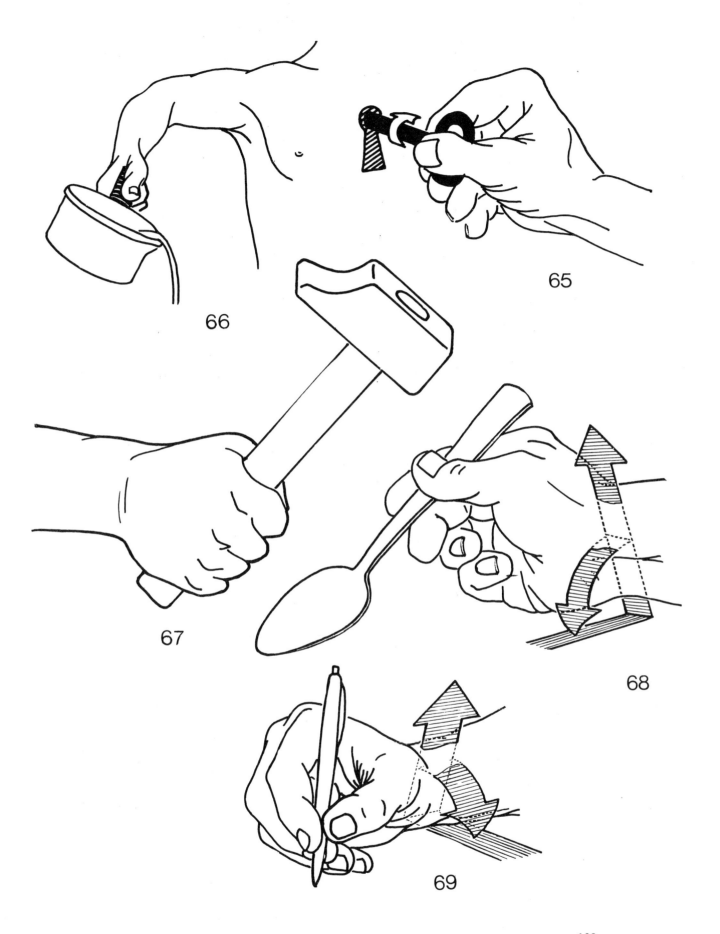

65

66

67

68

69

THE WRIST

SIGNIFICANCE

The wrist is the *distal joint of the upper limb* and allows the hand, which is the effector segment, to assume the optimal position for prehension.

The articular complex of the wrist has basically **two degrees of freedom**. When these are compounded with pronation and supination, i.e. rotation of the forearm around its long axis, *the hand can be oriented at any angle to grasp or hold an object*.

The articular complex consists of two joints:

— the radio-carpal (RC) joint (wrist joint), between the radial head and the proximal row of carpal bones.

— the mid-carpal (MC) joint between the proximal and distal rows of carpal bones.

130

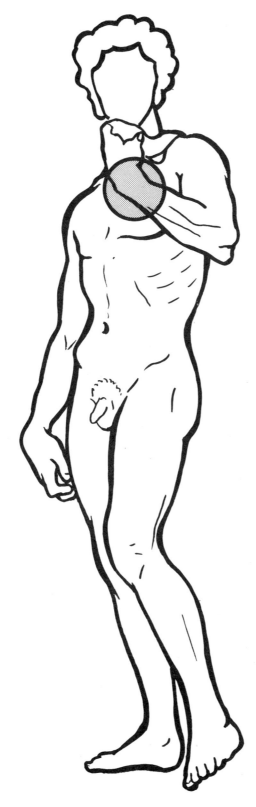

The WRIST

131

MOVEMENTS OF THE WRIST

Movements of the wrist (Fig. 1) occur around **two axes** when the hand is in the anatomical position, i.e. in full supination:

— A **transverse** axis AA' lying in the *frontal plane* (hatched vertically) and controlling movements of *flexion and extension*, which take place in the **sagittal plane** (hatched horizontally):

   — **Flexion** (arrow 1): the anterior (palmar) surface of the hand moves towards the anterior aspect of the forearm.

   — **Extension** (arrow 2): the posterior (dorsal) surface of the hand moves towards the posterior aspect of the forearm. (It is better to avoid the terms dorsiflexion and palmar flexion)

— An **antero-posterior** axis BB', lying in the *sagittal plane* (hatched horizontally) and controlling movements of *adduction* and *abduction*, which take place in the **frontal** plane (hatched vertically).

   — **Adduction** or ulnar deviation (arrow 3): the hand moves towards the axis of the body and its medial (ulnar) border forms an obtuse angle with the medial border of the forearm;

   — **Abduction** or radial deviation (arrow 4): the hand moves away from the axis of the body and its lateral (radial) border forms an obtuse angle with the lateral border of the forearm.

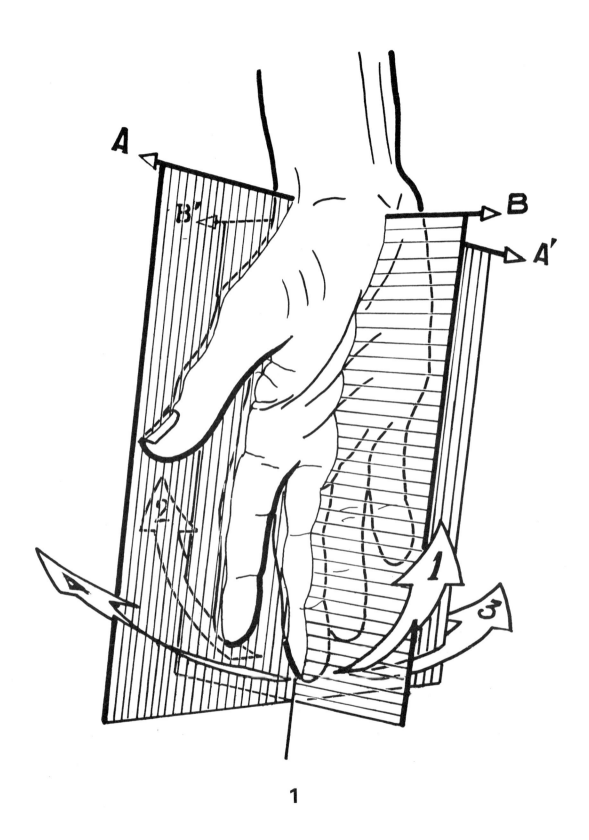

1

RANGE OF THE MOVEMENTS OF THE WRIST

Movements of abduction and adduction (Fig. 2)

The range of these movements is measured from the **reference position** (a), achieved when the axis of the hand, which lies in a plane through the middle finger and the third metacarpal, and the axis of the forearm are collinear.

The range of **abduction** (b) does not exceed 15°.

The range of **adduction** (c) is 45° when measured as the angle between the reference line and a line joining the middle of the wrist and the tip of the middle finger (broken line). However, this range varies, being 30° if reference is made to the axis of the hand and 55° if reference is made to the axis of the middle finger. These variations are due to the fact that adduction of the hand is compounded with adduction of the fingers. For practical purposes the range is taken as 45°.

Note the following points:

Adduction has a range *two to three times as great* as that of abduction.

Adduction has a greater range *in supination than in pronation* (Bunnel), when it falls short of 25°–30°.

In general, *the range of adduction and abduction is minimal when the wrist is fully flexed or extended*, because of the tension developed in the carpal ligaments. It is maximal when the hand is in the plane of reference or slightly flexed, because then the ligaments are relaxed.

Movements of flexion and extension (Fig. 3)

The range of these movements is measured from the **position of reference** (a), which is achieved when the posterior aspect of the hand is in line with the posterior surface of the forearm.

The range of **flexion** (b) is 85° and falls short of the right angle; that of **extension** (c) is also 85° and short of the right angle. As in the case of adduction and abduction the range of these movements depends on the degree of relaxation of the carpal ligaments:

Flexion and extension are maximal when the hand is in the neutral position, i.e. neither abducted nor adducted.

Flexion and extension are *minimal* when the wrist is *in pronation*.

134

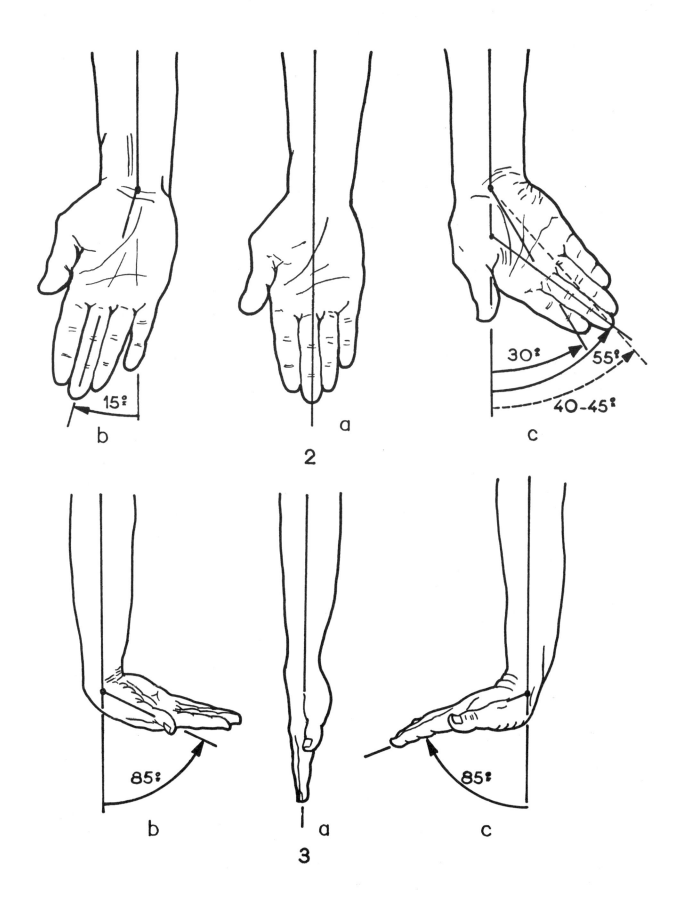

2

b 15°

a

c 30° 55° 40-45°

3

b 85°

a

c 85°

THE MOVEMENT OF CIRCUMDUCTION

This is defined as the *combination of the movements of flexion, extension, adduction and abduction*. Therefore it takes place simultaneously about the two axes of the wrist.

When circumduction is at its greatest, the axis of the hand traces in space a conical surface known as the '*cone of circumduction*' (Fig. 4). This cone has its apex O at the 'centre' of the wrist and a base shown in the diagram by the points F, R, E, C, which trace the path covered by the middle finger during maximal circumduction.

This cone is not regular and its base is not circular because the range of the various simple movements constituting circumduction is not symmetrical about the axis of the forearm 00'. Since the range of movement is maximal in the sagittal plane FOE and minimal in the frontal plane ROC the cone is flattened from side to side and *its base is ellipsoidal* with its great axis FE running postero-anteriorly (Fig. 5c).

This ellipse is also distorted medially (C) because of the greater range of ulnar deviation. Therefore the *axis of the 'cone of circumduction'* OA does not coincide with 00' but lies on its ulnar side at an angle of 15°. Besides, the position of the hand in 15° adduction is that of equilibrium for the muscles of adduction and abduction and so is one of the elements of the position of function.

In addition to the base of the cone of circumduction (c). Figure 5 shows:

— A frontal section of the cone (a) including a position of abduction (R), a position of adduction C and the axis of the cone of circumduction OA.

— A sagittal section (b) of the cone with a position in flexion F and a position in extension E.

Since the range of the movements of the wrist is less in pronation than in supination the cone of circumduction is more 'flattened' in pronation. However, *with the help of the associated rotation*, the flattening of the cone of circumduction is partially compensated and so *the axis of the hand can lie anywhere* within a cone with an angle of aperture of 160° to 170°.

In addition, as typically occurs in all biaxial joints with two degrees of freedom, (see later the trapezo-metacarpal joint), concurrent or successive movement about these axes gives rise to an *automatic rotation, the conjunct rotation of Mac Conaill*, around the long axis of the mobile segment, i.e. the hand. As a result, the palm comes to lie obliquely with regard to the plane of the anterior aspect of the forearm. This is clear-cut only during combined extension-adduction and flexion-adduction. Its functional significance is different when the thumb is involved.

136

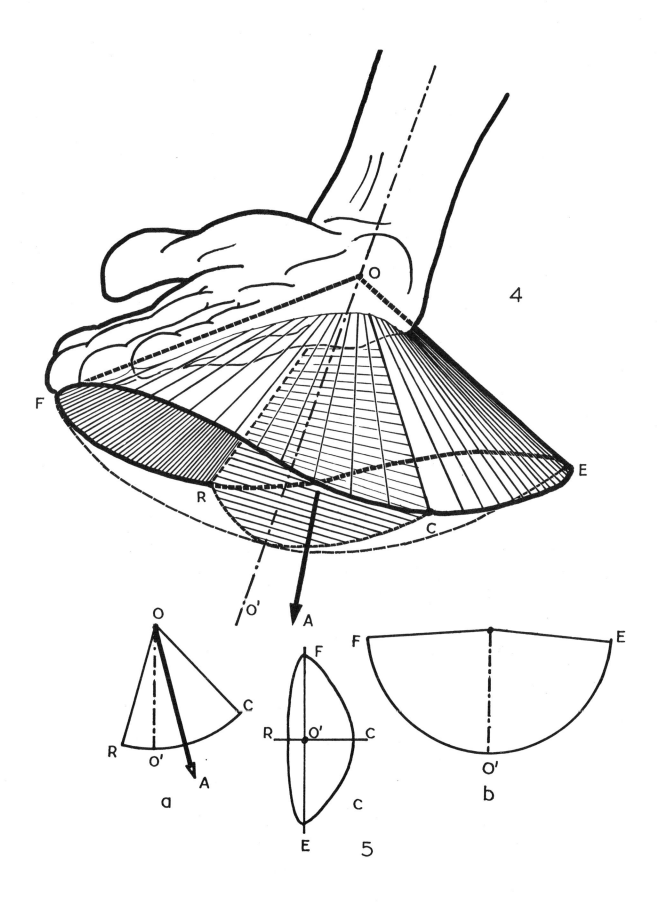

137

THE ARTICULAR COMPLEX OF THE WRIST

The articular complex of the wrist (Fig. 6) contains **two joints:**

1. **The radio-carpal joint** between the radial head and the proximal row of carpal bones.
2. The **mid-carpal joint** between the proximal and distal rows of carpal bones.

The radio-carpal joint

This is an **ellipsoidal joint** (Fig. 7) and the carpal aspect presents the following *two convexities*:

— A **transverse convexity** (arrow 1) of radius of curvature R and antero-posterior axis BB'; it is related to movements of *adduction* and *abduction*.
— An **antero-posterior convexity** (arrow 2) of radius r (smaller than R) and transverse axis AA': it is related to movements of *flexion and extension*.

On the skeleton (Fig. 8)

— The axis AA' of flexion and extension *passes between the lunate and the capitate bones.*
— The axis BB' of adduction and abduction *passes through the head of the capitate bone* near its intercarpal articular surface.

The **ligaments of the radio-carpal joint** are arranged in *two groups*:

The collateral ligaments (Fig. 8):

The *lateral* (1) is attached to the styloid process of the radius and the scaphoid bone.

The *medial* (2) is attached to the styloid process of the ulna and the pisiform and triquetrum bones.

Note that the distal attachments of these ligaments lie near the 'exit point' of the axis AA'.

The anterior and posterior ligaments (Fig. 11: diagrammatic lateral view), which will receive further attention later:

— the *anterior* ligament (or rather anterior ligamentous complex) (3) is attached to the anterior edge of the distal surface of the radius and the neck of the capitate.
— the *posterior* ligament (or the posterior ligamentous complex) (4) also forms a strap posteriorly.

Both anterior and posterior ligaments are anchored on the carpus at the 'exit' points of the axis BB' of abduction and adduction.

If, to a first approximation, the wrist is considered to be made up of a single structure, which is not true as will be shown later, the **actions of the ligaments** of the radio-carpal joint can be broken down as follows:

— During **adduction-abduction** (Figs. 8, 9 and 10: anterior views), the *medial and lateral ligaments are active*. Starting from the rest position (Fig. 8):
— during adduction (Fig. 9), the lateral ligament is stretched while the medial ligament is slackened.
— during abduction (Fig. 10), vice versa.

The anterior ligament, attached close to the centre of rotation, is little involved.

— During **flexion-extension** (Figs. 11, 12, 13: lateral views) the *anterior and posterior ligaments are most active*. From the rest position (Fig. 11):
— the posterior ligament is stretched during flexion (Fig. 12);
— the anterior ligament is stretched during extension (Fig. 13).

The medial and lateral ligaments are little involved.

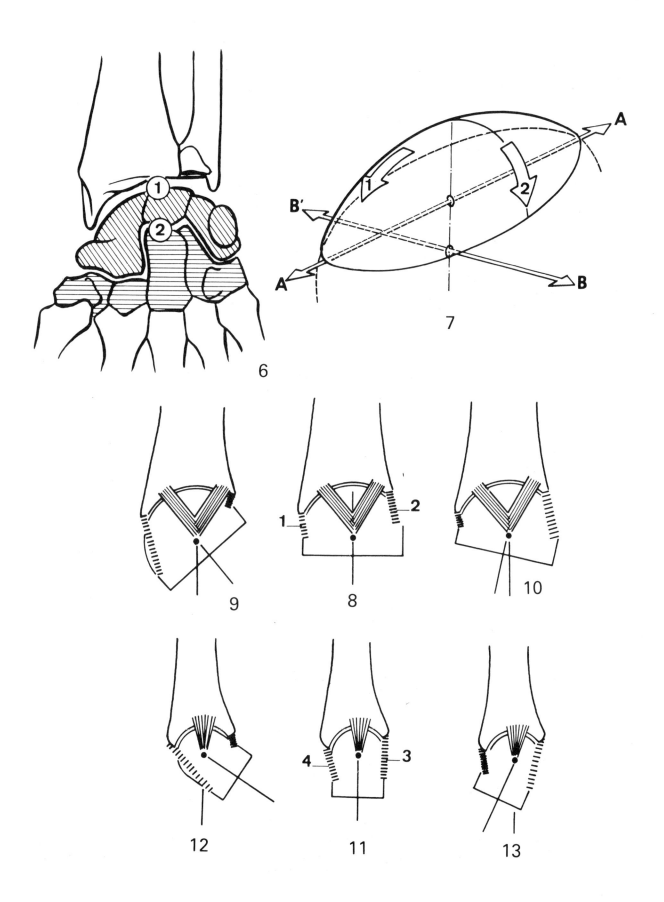

6

7

9

8

10

12

11

13

139

THE ARTICULAR SURFACES OF THE RADIO-CARPAL AND MID-CARPAL JOINTS

The **articular surfaces of the radio-carpal joint** (Fig. 14 and 15: the numbers have the same meaning in both figures) are: the proximal row of carpal bones and the distal surface of the radius and the articular disc.

The **carpal surface** (Fig. 15: anterior aspect, with the bones pulled apart) consists of the juxtaposed proximal surfaces of the *three proximal carpal bones*, arranged latero-medially as follows:

the scaphoid (1), the lunate (2) and the triquetrum (3), joined together by interosseous ligaments (scapho-lunate = s.l. and lunato-triquetral = l.t.).

Note that the pisiform bone (4) and the distal row of carpal bones, i.e. the trapezium (5), the trapezoid (6), the capitate (7) and the hamate (8), do not belong to the radio-carpal joint. These bones are linked by interosseous ligaments (trapezo-trapezoidal = t.t., trapezoido-capitate = t.c. and the capito-hamate = c.h.).

The proximal surfaces of the scaphoid, lunate and triquetrum and of their interosseous ligaments are *covered by cartilage to form a continuous surface*.

In Fig. 14 (the joint has been opened, according to Testut) can be seen the distal aspect of the joint, i.e. the articular facets of the scaphoid (1), the lunate (2) and the triquetrum (3), and its **concave proximal aspect** consisting of:

— the *distal surface of the radius* (9) laterally, concave, coated with cartilage and divided by a blunt ridge into the scaphoid impression (10) laterally and the lunate impression medially (11);
— *the distal aspect of the articular disc* (12) medially, concave, cartilage-coated. Its apex is inserted at the foot of the ulnar styloid process (13) so that the ulnar head (14) overreaches it anteriorly and posteriorly. Its base, inserted at the infero-medial ridge of the radius, is at times incomplete (15), allowing a communication between the radio-ulnar and the radio-carpal joints.

The capsule (16), shown intact posteriorly, binds together these two sets of articular surfaces. The **mid-carpal joint** (Fig. 16: opened posteriorly, according to Testut), lying between the two rows of carpal bones, consists of:

— the **proximal surface** (postero-inferior view), made up of three bones arranged latero-medially as follows:
— the *scaphoid* with two slightly convex surfaces distally, one (1) for the trapezium and the other (2) in the middle for the trapezoid, and a deeply concave medial facet (3) for the capitate;
— the distal surface of the *lunate* (4), with its semilunar cavity for the capitate.
— the distal surface of the *triquetrum* (5), concave distally and laterally, related to the proximal surface of the hamate.

The pisiform bone, in contact with the palmar surface of the triquetrum, does not belong to the mid-carpal joint.

— the **distal surface** (postero-superior view) consists of the following bones latero-medially:
— the proximal surfaces of the *trapezium* (6) and *trapezoid* (7);
— the head of the *capitate* (8) in contact with the scaphoid and the lunate;
— the proximal surface of the *hamate* (9), which is mostly in contact with the triquetrum, and its small lateral facet (10) in contact with the lunate.

If one considers each row of carpal bones as a single structure, then the *mid-carpal joint is made up of two parts*:

— a **lateral part,** consisting of two plane surfaces (trapezium and trapezoid in contact with the scaphoid), i.e. a *plane joint*.
— a **medial part,** consisting of the surfaces of the head of the capitate and the hamate, convex in all planes and fitting into the concavity offered by the three proximal carpal bones, i.e. a *condyloid joint*.

The movements at this joint are influenced by the variable *elasticity of the ligaments* which allows a certain degree of 'play'. These movements, including flexion-extension, adduction-abduction and rotation around the long axis, will be studied in detail later.

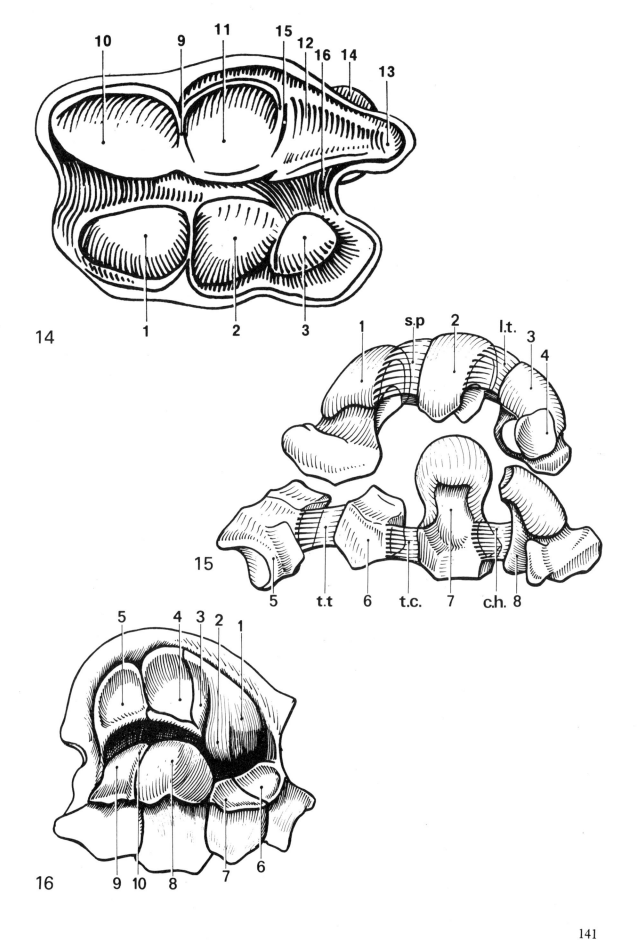

14

15

16

141

THE LIGAMENTS OF THE RADIO-CARPAL AND MID-CARPAL JOINTS

This account of these ligaments is based on the recent studies of Kuhlman (1978). As will be evident later, this modern view provides a better explanation of the role of these ligaments in maintaining the stability of the carpus and ensuring its adaptation to constraints imposed upon it by movements at the wrist.

Figure 17 (**anterior view**) shows:
— the *medial ligament* of the radio-carpal joint, attached proximally to the ulnar styloid and intricately mixed with the fibres of the apex of the articular disc (1). It then divides into a *posterior band* (2) inserted into the triquetrum and an *anterior band* inserted into the pisiform (3).
— the *lateral ligament* of the radio-carpal joint, also made up of two bands attached to the radial styloid: a *posterior band* (4), running from the styloid to below the lateral aspect of the proximal articular surface of the scaphoid; an *anterior band* (5), very thick and strong, stretching from the anterior edge of the radial styloid to the scaphoid tubercle.

— the *anterior ligament of the radio-carpal joint*, composed of two bands:
  — laterally, the *radio-lunate band* bridging the radius and the lunate (6), and running obliquely distally and medially from the anterior edge of the distal surface of the radius to the anterior horn of the lunate; hence its name of *anterior brake of the lunate*.
  — medially, the *radio-triquetral band* (7), recently recognised by Kuhlman. It is attached proximally to the anterior border of the distal surface of the radius and its fibres are interwoven with those of the anterior ligament (8) of the inferior radio-ulnar joint. Distally it is inserted into the anterior surface of the triquetrum just lateral to its zone of contact with the pisiform. This triangular, stout, highly resistant ligament runs distally and medially to form part of the 'sling of the triquetrum' (see p. 144);

— the *ligaments of the mid-carpal joint:*
  — the *radio-capitate ligament* (9), running obliquely distally and medially from the lateral portion of the anterior border of the distal surface of the radius to the anterior aspect of the neck of the capitate. It is continuous with the two bands of the anterior ligament of the radio-carpal joint and thus belongs to both joints of the wrist.
  — the *lunato-capitate ligament* (10), stretching vertically from the anterior horn of the lunate to the anterior aspect of the neck of the capitate and directly continuous distally with the medial band of the anterior ligament of the radio-carpal joint.
  — the *triquetro-capitate ligament* (11), running obliquely distally and laterally from the anterior aspect of the triquetrum to the neck of the capitate, where it helps to form a true ligamentous complex with the other preceding ligaments.
  — the *scapho-trapezial ligament* (12), short but broad and stout, linking the scaphoid tubercle and the anterior aspect of the trapezium above its oblique crest.
  — the *triquetro-hamatal ligament* (13), in effect constituting the medial ligament of the mid-carpal joint.
  — finally, the *piso-hamate ligament* (14), running from the pisiform to the hook of the hamate and the *piso-metacarpal ligament* (15), which belongs to the carpo-metacarpal joint.

Figure 17a (**posterior view**) shows:
— the *posterior band* (4) of the *lateral ligament of the radio-carpal joint.*
— the *posterior band* (2) of *the medial ligament of the radio-carpal joint*, with its fibres interwoven with those of the articular disc (1);
— the *posterior ligament of the radio-carpal joint*, consisting of two bands running obliquely distally and medially:
  — the *radio-lunate band* (16), called the posterior 'brake' of the lunate
  — the *radio-triquetral band* (17), with its mode of insertion similar to that of its anterior homologue, including the dove-tailing of its fibres with the posterior ligament of the radio-ulnar joint (18) on the posterior border of the distal surface of the radius. This band forms part of the 'sling of the triquetrum':

— the *two deep transverse ligaments of the carpus:*
  — the *proximal band* (19), running transversely from the posterior aspect of the triquetrum to that of the scaphoid. It is partially inserted into the posterior horn of the lunate, whence it sends fibres to the lateral ligament (20) and to the posterior ligament (21) of the radio-carpal joint.
  — the *distal band* (22), stretching obliquely laterally and slightly distally from the posterior aspect of the triquetrum to that of the trapezoid (23) and to that of the trapezium (24) along the posterior surface of the capitate.

— finally, the *triquetro-hamate ligament* (13), inserted posteriorly into the posterior surface of the triquetrum, which acts as a relay station for posterior ligaments of the posterior carpus, even as the neck of the capitate is the relay station for the anterior ligaments of the carpus.

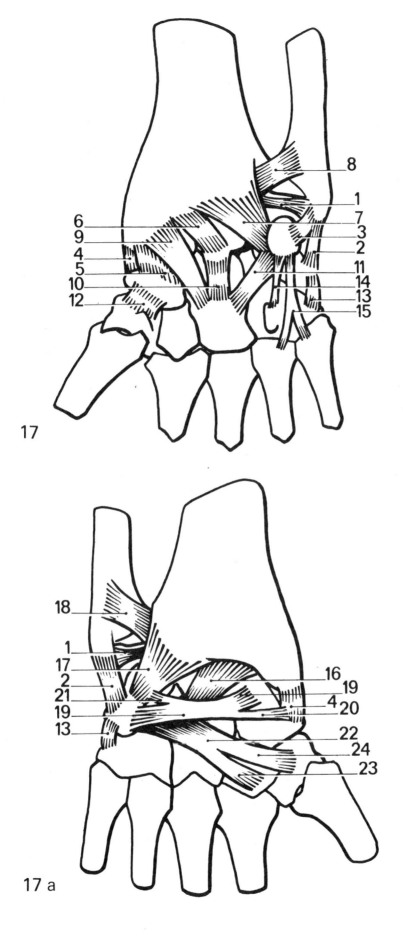

17

17 a

143

THE STABILIZING FUNCTION OF THE LIGAMENTS

Stabilization in the frontal plane

The prime function of the ligaments of the wrist is to stabilize the carpus in the frontal and sagittal planes.

In the frontal plane, the ligaments are essential, because the distal surface of the radius (Fig. 18, diagrammatic view from the front) faces distally and medially, so that as a whole it can be represented by a plane running obliquely proximo-distally and medio-laterally at an angle of 25° to 30° with the horizontal plane. Under the pull of the longitudinal muscles, the carpus in the neutral position tends to slip proximally and medially in the direction of the white arrow.

On the other hand, when the wrist is *adducted* to approximately 30° (Fig. 19), the pull of the muscles now acts perpendicular to the plane of slippage described above. As a result the carpal bones are pushed back into the joint cavity and the carpus is stabilized. This position of slight adduction is the natural position of the wrist, the position of function, coinciding with the position of maximal stability.

Conversely (Fig. 20), when the wrist is *abducted*, however slightly, the pull of the long muscles accentuates the instability and tends to displace the carpal bones proximally and medially.

The medial and lateral ligaments of the radio-carpal joint, running lengthwise like the muscles themselves, cannot counteract this dislocating effect. As shown by Kuhlmann, the full brunt is borne by the *two radio-triquetral bands of the anterior and posterior ligaments of the radio-carpal joint* (Fig. 21). As they run obliquely proximally and laterally, they keep the carpal bones in position and prevent their medial displacement.

In Fig. 22 (postero-medial view) the distal end of the radius is viewed from behind after removal of the distal end of the ulna. One can see the distal surface of the radius (1) and the triquetrum (2), flanked by the pisiform (3) (the other carpal bones are not shown) The triquetrum and the radius are linked by two radio-triquetral ligaments, anterior (4) and posterior (5), which constitute the **"triquetral sling"**, responsible for pulling the triquetrum proximally and medially. They also vitally influence (see later) the internal movements of the carpus during abduction.

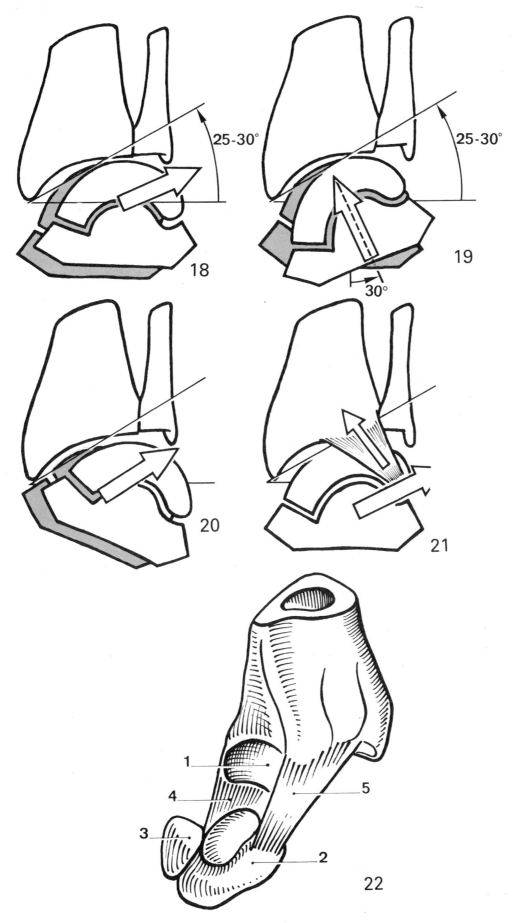

25-30°

25-30°

18

19

30°

20

21

1

4

5

3

2

22

145

THE STABILISING FUNCTION OF THE LIGAMENTS (continued)

Stabilisation in the sagittal plane

In the **sagittal plane** roughly similar events take place.

Because the distal surface of the radius points distally and anteriorly (Fig. 23: lateral view), the carpal bones tend to slide proximally and anteriorly in the direction of the white arrow, i.e. in a plane parallel to that of the distal surface of the radius and at an angle of 20–25° with the horizontal.

When the wrist is *flexed* 30° to 40° (Fig. 24), the muscular pull tends to displace the carpal bones in a plane perpendicular to that of the distal surface of the radius, thus repositioning and stabilising these bones.

Thus the ligaments play a relatively unimportant part (Fig. 25). The 'posterior' brake of the lunate' (the radio-lunate band, p. 142) and the proximal band of the transverse ligament of the carpus are stretched, thus bringing the lunate and the distal surface of the radius closer together. The anterior ligaments are relaxed and inactive.

In the *neutral position* (Fig. 26) the tension in the posterior and anterior ligaments is balanced and as a result the lunate is closely applied to the distal surface of the radius.

On the contrary, during *extension* (Fig. 27), the tendency for the carpal bones to be displaced proximally and anteriorly is reinforced.

Under these circumstances, the ligaments become essential (Fig. 28), not so much the posterior ones, which are slackened, as the anterior, which develop a tension proportional to the degree of extension. Their deep surfaces displace the lunate and the head of the capitate proximally and posteriorly, thereby repositioning and stabilising the carpus. This position corresponds to that of maximal tension in the ligaments and coaptation of the articular surfaces, the 'close-packed position' of Mac Conaill.

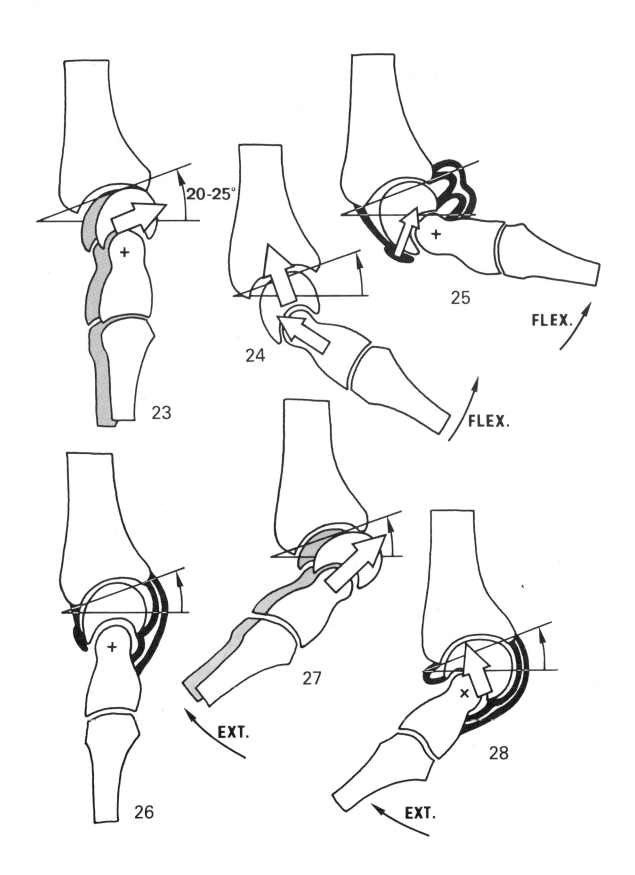

20-25°

23

24 FLEX.

25 FLEX.

26 EXT.

27

28 EXT.

147

THE DYNAMICS OF THE CARPUS

The lunate pillar

It is convenient, to a first approximation, to consider the carpus as made of a single unchanging structure but recent studies in functional anatomy have shown that this monolithic view is incorrect. It is best to have in mind a **geometrically variable carpus,** which alters its shape under the influence of the relative movements of the bones and the constraints imposed by the ligaments.

These elementary movements have been studied by Kuhlmann, as they occur in the median pillar of the lunate and capitate and in the lateral pillar of the scaphoid, trapezium and trapezoid.

The **dynamics of the median pillar** depends on *the asymmetrical shape of the lunate*, which is *bulkier and thicker anteriorly than posteriorly.* Thus the head of the capitate is capped by a *Phrygian cap* (Fig. 29), a *Cossack's hat* (Fig. 30) or a *turban* (Fig. 31). Rarely is it capped by a symmetrical *two-pointed hat* (Fig. 32) and in this case the head of the capitate is asymmetrical with a greater obliquity anteriorly. In about 50 per cent of cases it is the 'Phrygian cap' that lies between the capitate and the distal surface of the radius in the fashion of a wedge. Thus the *effective distance* between the capitate and the distal articular surface of the wrist varies according to the degree of flexion and extension of the wrist.

In the **neutral position** (Fig. 33), that distance corresponds to the mean thickness of the lunate.

In **extension** (Fig. 34), that distance is less as it corresponds to the smallest thickness of the lunate.

In **flexion** (Fig. 35), that distance is increased because it corresponds to the full thickness of the bulkier portion of the lunate.

However, the *obliquity of the distal articular surface* of the wrist also influences this effective distance. Thus it is in the *neutral position* that the distance between the centre of the head of the capitate and the distal articular surface of the wrist is maximal, when measured along the long axis of the radius. In *extension* (Fig. 34), the proximal 'ascent' of the head of the capitate is partly cancelled by the distal 'descent' of the posterior edge of the distal articular surface of the wrist. In *flexion* (Fig. 35), the distal 'descent' of the head of the capitate is partly cancelled by the proximal 'ascent' of the anterior border of the distal articular surface of the wrist. Thus the centre of the head of the capitate is in effect displaced proximally by a distance h from its location in the neutral position.

On the other hand, during flexion (Fig. 35), this centre shows an *anterior displacement* a equal to twice the posterior displacement p occurring in extension. As a result, the tensions and moments of forces developed by the flexor and extensor muscles of the wrist are inversely affected.

Classically, flexion is greater at the radio-carpal (50°) than at the mid-carpal joint (35°) and conversely extension is greater at the mid-carpal (50°) than at the radio-carpal joint (35°). This is certainly true for extreme ranges of movement but in movements of small range the degree of flexion and extension is almost equal in both joints.

Because of its asymmetry the lunate plays an important role in determining the architecture of the carpus at rest. In the neutral position (Fig. 36) the lunate is held securely by anterior and posterior radio-lunate ligaments (see p. 142). If then the lunate is titled forwards (Fig. 37) or backwards (Fig. 38), the centre of the head of the capitate is displaced proximally (e) and posteriorly (c) or anteriorly (b) respectively. Hence *primary instability of the lunate*, caused by rupture or stretching of the anterior (Fig. 37) or posterior (Fig. 38) radio-lunate ligament, will secondarily spread to the capitate and thence to the entire carpus.

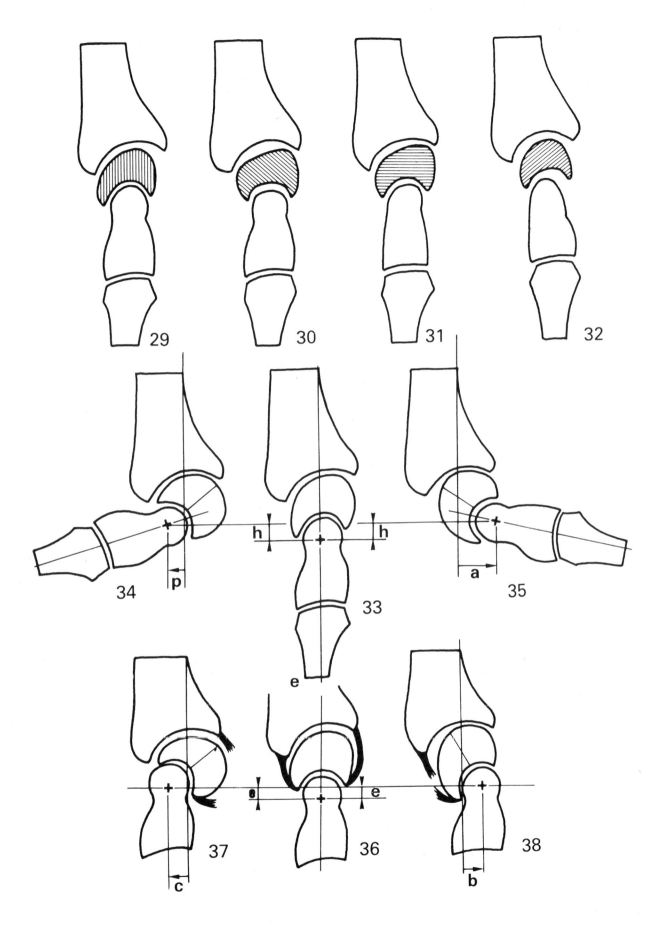

29 30 31 32

34 p h h a 35

33

e

37 c 36 e e 38 b

149

THE DYNAMICS OF THE CARPUS (continued)

The scaphoid pillar

The shape and spatial orientation of the scaphoid dominates the **dynamics of the lateral pillar of the carpus.**

The scaphoid (Fig. 39: lateral view) is *kidney-shaped* with its upper rounded end corresponding to its convex proximal surface in contact with the distal surface of the radius and its distal end forming the tubercle in contact with the trapezoid (not shown) and the trapezium. It lies clearly anterior to the trapezoid and the capitate and thus *is responsible for the position of the thumb and the first metacarpal anterior to the plane of the palm*. Thus the scaphoid is *jammed obliquely between the radius and the trapezium* with its degree of obliqueness depending on its shape. Thus the scaphoid can be *kidney-shaped* and *'lying down'* (Fig. 39), *bent* and *'sitting'* (Fig. 40) or *nearly straight* and *'erect'* (Fig. 41). The 'lying down' scaphoid is the most frequent and will be shown in the diagrams.

Because of its elongated shape, the scaphoid has a *long diameter* and *a short diameter* (Fig. 42), which are variably related to the distal surface of the radius and the proximal surface of the trapezium. This underlies the variations in the *effective distance* between the radius and the trapezium.

It is in the *neutral position* (Fig. 43) that this distance is maximal. Then the scaphoid and the radius are in contact at a and a' and the scaphoid and the trapezium at b and g, the mid-point of the proximal surface of the trapezium.

In *extension* (Fig. 44), the distance is reduced as the scaphoid rears itself up between radius and trapezium. Contact between radius and scaphoid occurs at c' and c and that between trapezium and scaphoid at d and g.

In *flexion* (Fig. 45), the distance is also reduced as the scaphoid 'lies down' flat and the trapezium slides anteriorly. Contact points are now e and e' and f and g.

It is worth noting that:

1. the *contact points* move along the distal surface of the radius and the scaphoid (Fig. 46):

   — on the *radius* the contact point is extension c' lies anterior to contact point a' in the neutral position, both lying anterior to the contact point e' in flexion.
   — on the *proximal surface of the scaphoid* the contact point e in flexion lies anterior, the contact point c in extension posterior and the contact point a in the neutral position lies in between;
   — on the *distal surface of the scaphoid* the same disposition of contact points is noted (f anterior, d posterior and b in between).

2. The *effective diameters of the scaphoid* ab, cd and ef corresponding to the neutral position, extension and flexion are almost parallel and practically equal.

   — cd and ef are parallel
   — ab and ef are equal, cd being slightly shorter.

3. The *displacement of the trapezium relative to the radius* (Fig. 47):

   During flexion (F) and extension (E) from the neutral position (N) the trapezium moves along the arc of a circle concentric with that of the distal surface of the radius and also rotates on itself through an angle almost equal to the angle of displacement. Hence its proximal surface always points towards the centre of the circle C.

So far we have discussed concurrent movements of the scaphoid and trapezium. Later isolated movements of the scaphoid will be discussed.

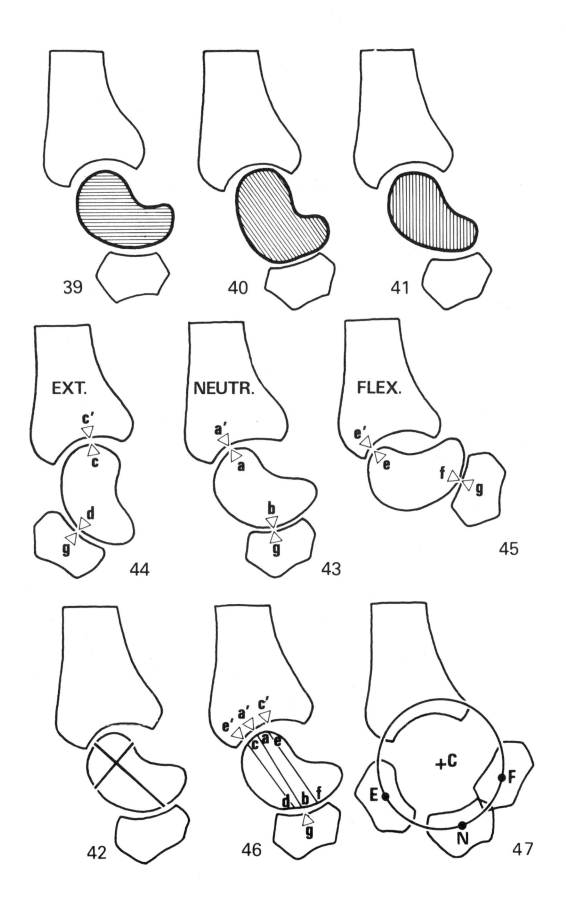

39

40

41

EXT.

c'
c
d
g
44

NEUTR.

a'
a
b
g
43

FLEX.

e'
e
f
g
45

42

e' a' c'
c a e
d b f
g
46

+C
E
F
N
47

151

THE SCAPHOID-LUNATE COUPLE

During flexion and extension of the wrist (Fig. 48), the movement can be divided into **four sectors** (Kuhlmann):

— the *sector of maximal utility* (I) extending to 20°. The elementary movements are small and difficult to appreciate, the ligaments remain slack and the pressure on the articular surfaces is minimal. It is in this sector that take place the commonest movements and that normal mobility must be restored after operation or trauma.

— the *sector of free mobility* (II) extending up to 40°. The ligaments begin to tense up and intraarticular pressures begin to rise. Up to this point the ranges of the movements occurring at the radio-carpal and the mid-carpal joints are roughly the same.

— the *sector of increasing physiological constraints* (III), extending up to 80°. The tensions in the ligaments and the intraarticular pressures rise to a maximum, eventually achieving the *locked* or the close-packed position (Mac Conaill).

— the *sector of pathological displacement* (IV) above 80°. From this point onwards movement can only occur if ligaments are ruptured or forcefully overextended. This occurrence, often clinically undetected, may then lead to instability of the carpus and secondary fracture or dislocation, as will be discussed later.

These notions of constraint and locking of joints are essential for the understanding of the *asynchrony of the locking mechanism in extension* of the lunate and scaphoid pillars.

In effect, *the locking in extension of the scaphoid pillar* (Fig. 49), due to maximal stretching of the radio-scaphoid (1) and scapho-trapezoidal (2) ligaments and jamming of the scaphoid between trapezium and radius, *occurs earlier than that of the lunate pillar*, which is due to stretching of the anterior radio-lunate (3) and lunato-capitate (4) ligaments and the impact of the posterior aspect of the neck of the capitate on the posterior edge of the distal surface of the radius. Thus extension goes on in the lunate pillar while it has already been checked in the scaphoid pillar.

Starting from the position of flexion (Fig. 51: the lunate and scaphoid are seen from the side), at first (Fig. 52) the scaphoid and lunate move together during extension and then (Fig. 53) the scaphoid comes to a halt, while the lunate moves on for another 30° thanks to the elasticity of the interosseous scapho-lunate ligament. Thus the range of movement of the lunate (1) is 30° greater than that of the scaphoid.

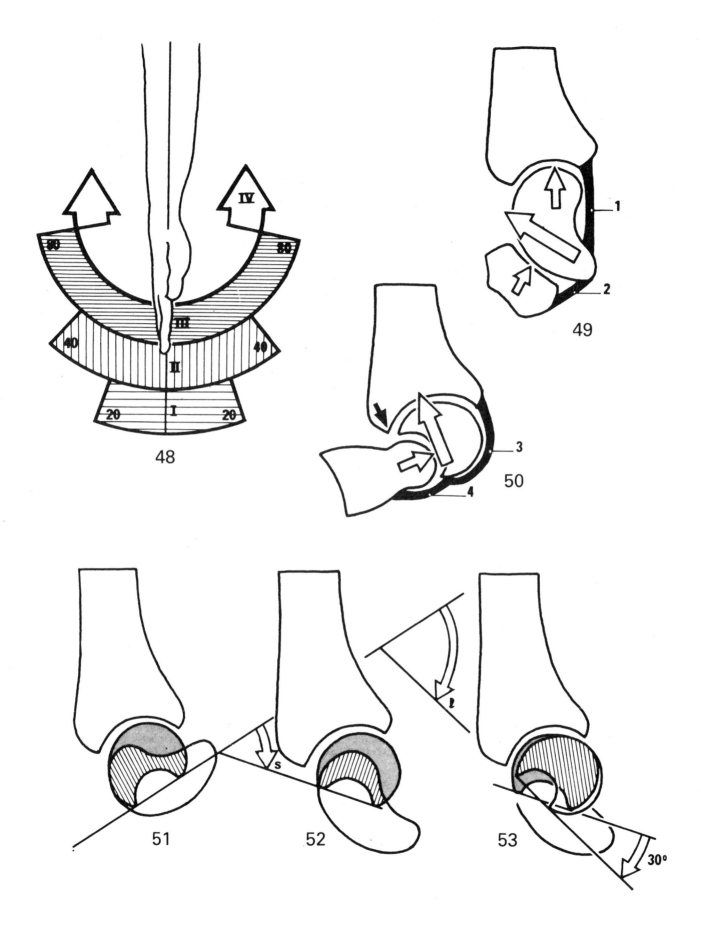

48

49

50

51   52   53

30°

THE GEOMETRICALLY VARIABLE CARPUS

(Abduction and adduction)

The carpus must be viewed as a bag of marbles rather than a single structure, especially during abduction and adduction, when its shape is altered by bony interactions and tensions developed in the ligaments. This is well brought out by careful study of anteroposterior radiographs of the wrist taken in abduction and adduction. The following diagrams are based on these findings.

During abduction (Fig. 54) the carpus as a whole at first rotates around a centre located in the head of the capitate, while the proximal row of carpal bones (arrow 1) moves proximally and medially so that the lunate comes to lie partly distal to the ulnar head and the triquetrum pulls away from the lunate distally. But this displacement of the triquetrum is soon checked by the medial ligament of the radio-carpal joint (I) and above all by the 'triquetral sling' F. Thus halted, the triquetrum now acts as a check for the lunate. If abduction goes on, only the distal row of carpal bones can move:

— the trapezium and trapezoid (arrow 2) move proximally closer to the radius. Compressed between trapezium (2) and radius, the scaphoid sinks by 'lying down', causing flexion (f) in the radio-carpal joint (Fig. 56) and extension in the mid-carpal joint (e);

— the capitate 'descends' distally (arrow 4), increasing the available space for the lunate, which, held in check by the anterior radio-lunate ligament, tilts posteriorly (Fig. 57) as a result of flexion at the radio-carpal joint. At the same time, the capitate moves posteriorly as a result of extension (e) at the mid-carpal joint. As the scaphoid sinks the capitate and the hamate can slide upwards against the proximal bones (arrow 1). The triquetrum, held in check by its three ligaments, 'climbs' over the hamate towards the head of the capitate. When the carpal bones stop moving relative to one another, the *locked or close-packed position in abduction* is attained.

During adduction (Fig. 53) the carpus starts to turn as a whole but this time the proximal row moves distally and laterally while the lunate slips completely under the radius and the trapezium and the trapezoid (arrow 1) move distally, thereby increasing the space available for the scaphoid. The latter, pulled distally by the scapho-trapezial ligament, rears itself up (Fig. 58) anteriorly (e) causing extension at the radio-carpal joint and fills the gap under the radius. Concurrently the trapezium slips anteriorly (f) under the scaphoid, causing flexion at the mid-carpal joint. As the 'descent' distally of the scaphoid (arrow 2) is checked by the lateral ligament of the radio-carpal joint (E), abduction proceeds only in the distal bones, which move relative to the proximal bones as follows (black arrows): the head of the capitate slips under the concave surface of the scaphoid, the lunate slips under the head of the capitate to hit the hamate and the triquetrum 'descends' distally along the slanting surface of the hamate. At the same time, the triquetrum rises anteriorly (arrow 3) as it hits the ulnar head (arrow 4) via the articular disc, thus transmitting stresses from the hand to the forearm. The capitate moves proximally (arrow 5) reducing the available space for the lunate, which, as a result of slackening of the anterior radio-lunate ligament, can tilt anteriorly (Fig. 59) with extension (e) at the radio-carpal joint. Meanwhile the capitate also moves anteriorly with flexion at the mid-carpal joint (f).

When the carpal bones come to a halt, *the locked or close-packed position in adduction* is attained.

In sum (inset), if the scaphoid-lunate couple is compared in abduction (grey) and in adduction (white), it is clear that both bones undergo inverse changes. During abduction the active surface of the scaphoid decreases while that of the lunate increases and vice versa in adduction. These changes result from movements of flexion and extension in the two joints of the carpus:

— in abduction (Figs. 56 & 57), flexion in the radio-carpal is cancelled by extension in the mid-carpal joint.

— in adduction (Figs. 58 & 59), conversely, extension in the radio-carpal joint is compensated for by flexion in the mid-carpal joint.

Thus logically the corollary follows:

— wrist flexion is associated with abduction at the radio-carpal and adduction at the mid-carpal joint.

— wrist extension implies adduction at the radio-carpal and abduction at the mid-carpal joint.

Thus is confirmed the mechanism proposed by Henke.

154

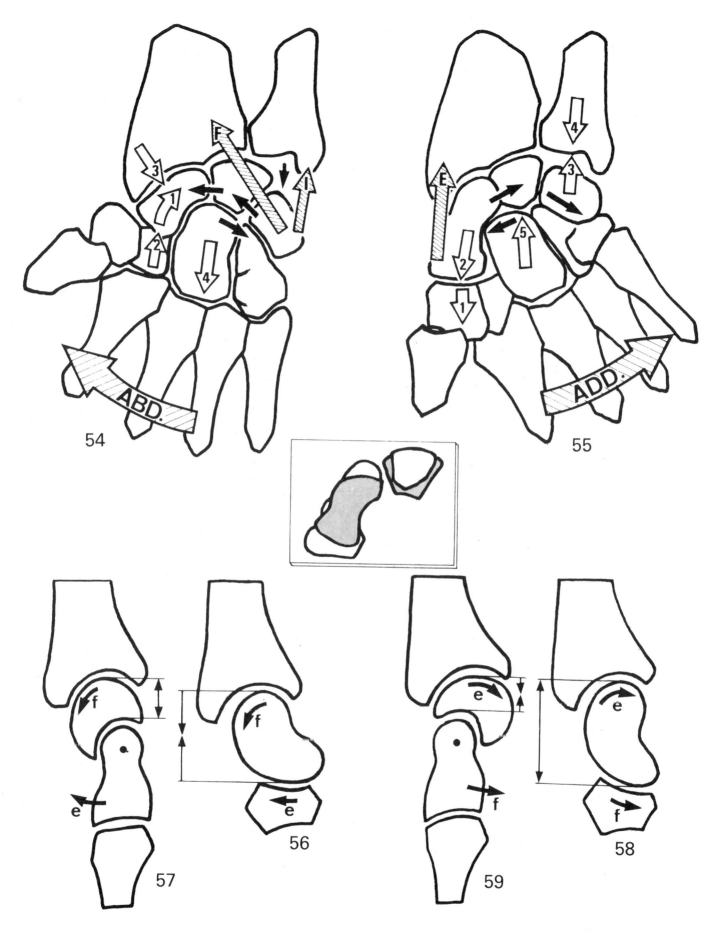

54

ABD.

55

ADD.

56

57

58

59

ABNORMAL MOVEMENTS

Anatomical damage is most often caused by abduction and extension often in combination.

Abduction past the locked position causes two types of damage:

— *fracture of the distal end of the radius* (Fig. 60). As the scaphoid is pressed against the lateral buttress of the distal end of the radius, the latter breaks, especially in the aged patient with osteoporosis. The bony fragment is displaced laterally and posteriorly as a result of extension of the wrist (Fig. 61). This type of fracture only occurs because the scaphoid resists crushing, as it is well protected in its 'lying down' position beneath the distal surface of the radius, and also because the anterior ligaments do not snap. The ulnar styloid, pulled by the articular disc and the medial ligament of the radio-carpal joint, often breaks at its base.

— *fracture of the scaphoid* (Fig. 62), which this time is 'surprised' in extension and allows its full length to hit the lateral buttress of the distal end of the radius. The radial styloid strikes the lateral surface of the scaphoid, which fractures as a result of shearing forces.

Extension, when exaggerated, most often causes a Colles' fracture (Fig. 61). More rarely it causes damage to ligaments (Fig. 63) with primary rupture of the lunato-capitate ligament and secondarily:

— *retrolunate dislocation of the carpus* (Fig. 64): the capitate rears itself in extension and its head is jammed posterior to the posterior horn of the lunate, which has not moved.

— *anterior dislocation of the lunate* (Fig. 65). The posterior radiolunate ligament, stretched by hyperextension and pressure from the head of the capitate, snaps with anterior displacement of the lunate, which, still attached by its anterior horn, rotates on itself for 90° to 120° around a transverse axis, so that its distal surface faces proximally. The head of the capitate moves proximally towards the radius and displaces the lunate anteriorly into the carpal tunnel with compression of the median nerve.

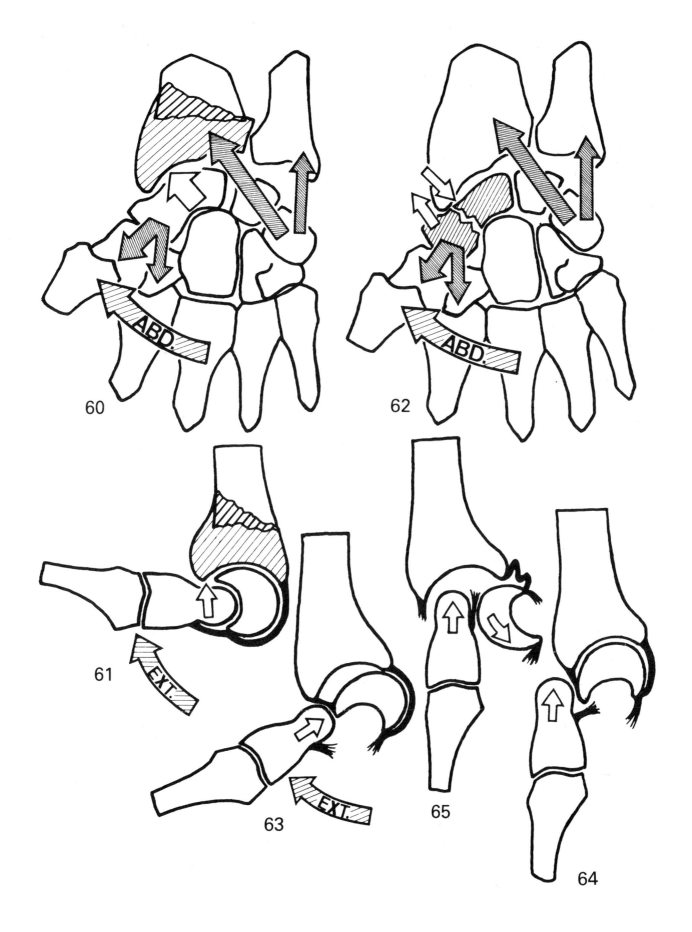

60

62

61

63

65

64

THE MOTOR MUSCLES OF THE WRIST

In Fig. 66 (**anterior aspect of the wrist**) can be seen:

— the **flexor carpi radialis** (1), which runs through a special groove deep to the flexor retinaculum and is inserted chiefly into *the base of the second metacarpal* and also into the trapezium and the base of the third metacarpal.

— the *palmaris longus* (2), less powerful, is inserted vertically into the *flexor retinaculum* and also into the apex of the palmar aponeurosis.

— the **flexor carpi ulnaris** (3), which passes anterior to the styloid process of the ulna and is inserted mainly into the *proximal surface of the pisiform* and also into the flexor retinaculum, the hook of the hamate and the bases of the fourth and fifth metacarpals.

To simplify the diagram the tendons of the digital flexors, flanking the median nerve in the carpal tunnel, are not shown:

— the four tendons of the flexor digitorum profundus

— the four tendons of the flexor digitorum sublimis

— the flexor pollicis longus.

They are shown in Fig. 71.

In Figure 67 (**posterior view of the wrist**) can be seen:

— **the extensor carpi ulnaris** (4), which passes anterior to the ulnar styloid process and is inserted into the posterior aspect of *the base of the fifth metacarpal*

— the **extensor carpi radialis brevis** (5) which is inserted into the *base of the third metacarpal*

— *the* **extensor carpi radialis longus** (6), which runs posterior to the 'anatomical snuffbox' and is inserted into *the base of the second metacarpal.*

For simplicity's sake, the following tendons (shown in Fig. 71) are not included:

— the four tendons of the extensor digitorum communis

— the tendon of the extensor indicis

— the tendon of the extensor digiti minimi.

In Fig. 68 (**medial view of the wrist**) can be seen:

— the **flexor carpi ulnaris** (3): its point of insertion is pulled anteriorly by the pisiform and this increases its efficiency

— **the extensor carpi ulnaris** (4).

These two tendons *lie on either side of the ulnar styloid process.*

In Fig. 69 (**lateral view of the wrist**) can be seen the tendons of:

— the **extensor carpi radialis brevis** (5) and the **extensor carpi radialis longus** (6)

— the **abductor pollicis longus** (7), inserted into the lateral aspect of *the base of the first metacarpal*

— the **extensor pollicis brevis** (8), inserted into the dorsal aspect of *the base of the proximal phalanx of the thumb*

— the **extensor pollicis longus** (9), inserted into *the second phalanx of the thumb.*

The radialis muscles and the thumb muscles encase the radial styloid process. The *anatomical snuffbox* is bounded posteriorly by the tendon of the extensor pollicis longus and anteriorly by those of the abductor pollicis longus and the extensor pollicis brevis.

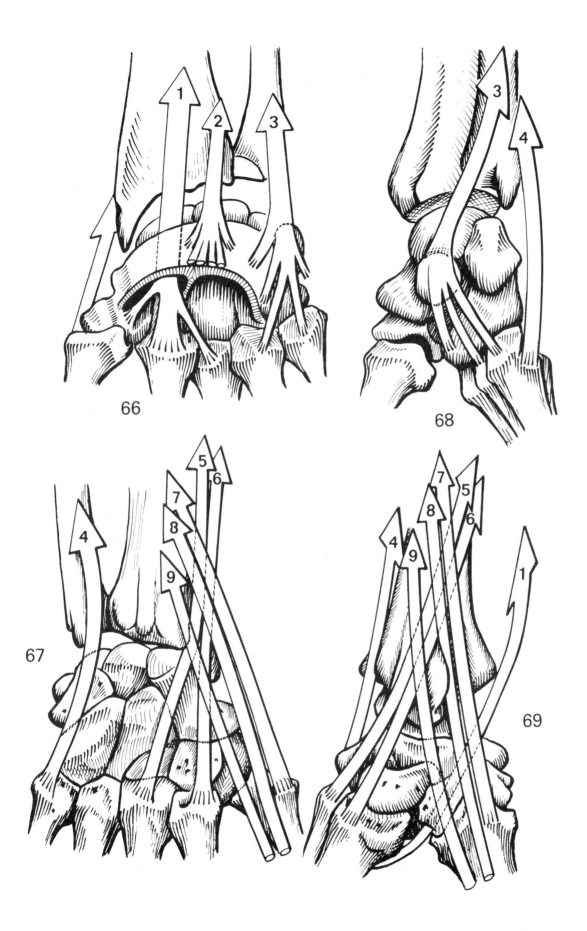

66

68

67

69

THE ACTIONS OF THE MUSCLES OF THE WRIST

Posterior to the wrist the extensor tendons, lined by their synovial sheaths, run deep to the extensor retinaculum, (Fig. 70: the same figures apply to Fig. 71), arranged medio-laterally in compartments as follows:
- that of the extensor carpi ulnaris
- that of the extensor digiti minimi
- that of the extensor digitorum and extensor indicis
- that of the extensor pollicis longus
- that of the extensors carpi radialis longus and brevis
- that of the abductor pollicis longus and extensor pollicis brevis.

The extensor retinaculum and these osteofibrous compartments act as pulleys for the extensor tendons *when the wrist is extended.*

Classically the effector muscles of the wrist fall into four groups, and Figure 71 shows diagrammatically how these muscles are related to the *two axes of the wrist joint*, AA', axis of flexion and extension and BB', axis of adduction and abduction.

(The diagram shows the distal aspect of a coronal section through the wrist: B' is anterior, B posterior, A' is lateral, A medial. The grey tendons act on the wrist, the *white ones on the fingers*).

Group I: *Flexor carpi ulnaris* (1):
- flexes the wrist (being situated anterior to axis AA') and the fifth carpometacarpal joint owing to its tendinous expansion
- adducts the hand (lying medial to axis BB') but less powerfully than extensor carpi ulnaris.
Example of flexion and adduction: left hand playing the violin.

Group II: *Extensor carpi ulnaris* (6):
- extends the wrist (lying posterior to axis AA')
- adducts the hand (being medial to axis BB').

Group III: *Flexor carpi radialis* (2) and *palmaris longus* (3):
- flex the wrist (being anterior to axis AA')
- abduct the hand (being lateral to axis BB').

Group IV: *Extensor carpi radialis longus* (4) and *extensor carpi radialis brevis* (5):
- extend the wrist (being posterior to axis AA')
- abduct the hand (being lateral to axis BB).

According to this theory, none of the muscles of the wrist has a single action. Thus, to *perform a single movement two groups of muscles must be activated so that any unwanted associated movements are suppressed* (another example of **muscle antagonism-synergism**):

Flexion (a) requires group I (flexor carpi ulnaris) and group III (flexor carpi radialis and palmaris longus).

Extension (b) requires group II (extensor carpi ulnaris) and group IV (extensores carpi radialis longus and brevis).

Adduction (c) requires group I (flexor carpi ulnaris) and group II (extensor carpi ulnaris).

Abduction (d) requires group III (flexor carpi radialis and palmaris longus) and group IV (extensores carpi radialis longus and brevis).

In practice, however, the movements of these individual muscles are more subtle and the experiments of Duchenne de Boulogne (1867) with electrical stimulation have revealed the following facts:
- Only the extensor carpi radialis longus (4) extends and abducts; *extensor carpi radialis brevis is exclusively extensor*, hence its physiological importance.
- Like the palmaris longus, the flexor carpi radialis is exclusively flexor, flexing the second carpometacarpal joint while pronating the hand. *When driven electrically it does not produce abduction* and it contracts during abduction at the wrist only to counterbalance the extensor component of carpi radialis longus, which is the main abductor muscle.

160

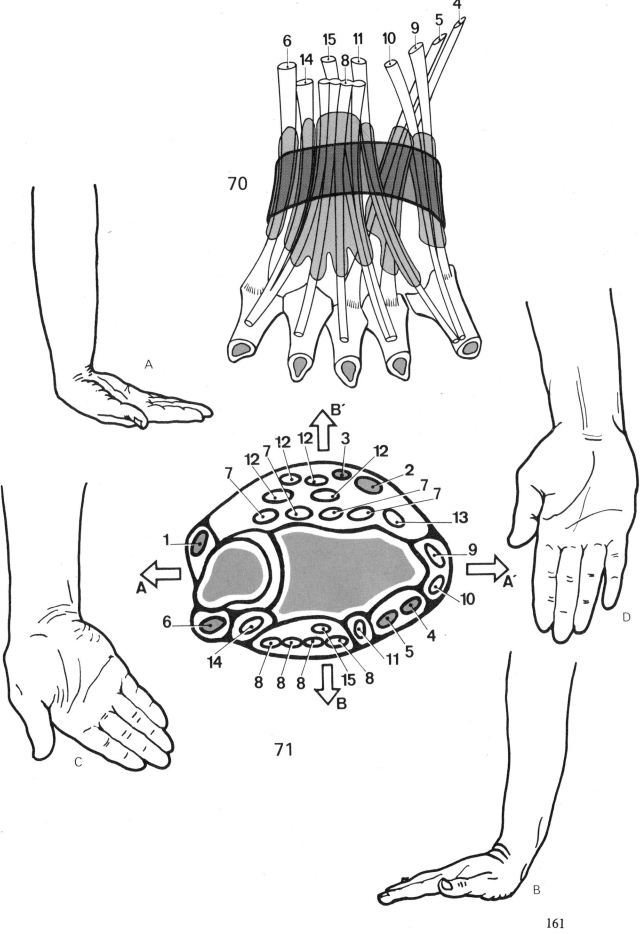

70

B´

12 7 12 12 3 12
7
7 7
1 13
9
10
6 4
14 11 5
8 8 8 15 8

A

A´

B

71

161

THE ACTIONS OF THE MUSCLES OF THE WRIST (continued)

The muscles acting on the fingers (Figs. 70 and 71) can act on the wrist only under certain conditions, such as:

— The digital flexors only flex the wrist if flexion of the fingers is stopped before the excursion of their tendons is completed during contraction. For example, *if a large object (e.g a bottle) is held in the hand*, wrist flexion is helped by the flexors of the fingers. Likewise the digital extensors (8) take part in extension of the wrist *if the fist is clenched*.

— The abductor pollicis longus (9) and extensor pollicis brevis (10) abduct the wrist unless counterbalanced by the action of the extensor carpi ulnaris (6). If the latter contracts simultaneously, only the thumb is abducted by the abductor pollicis longus. *The synergistic action of the extensor carpi ulnaris is therefore essential for abduction of the thumb* and this muscle can be called a 'stabiliser' of the wrist.

— The extensor pollicis longus (11), which produces thumb extension and retroposition, can also cause abduction and extension at the wrist when the flexor carpi ulnaris is inactive.

— Likewise the extensor carpi radialis longus (4) is essential for maintaining the hand in a neutral position and if it is paralysed there follows a permanent ulnar deviation.

The synergistic and stabilising action of the muscles of the wrist (Fig. 72):

— **The extensor muscles of the wrist act synergistically with the flexors of the fingers** (a): for example, during extension of the wrist the fingers are automatically flexed and, to extend the fingers in this position, a voluntary movement is required.

Furthermore, it is when the wrist is extended that the digital flexors can act at their best advantage because the flexor tendons are then shorter than when the wrist is either in the neutral position or in flexion. *The efficiency of the flexors of the fingers measured dynamically, when the wrist is flexed, is only a quarter of what it is when the wrist is extended.*

— **The flexor muscles of the wrist act synergistically with the extensors of the fingers** (b): when the wrist is flexed, extension of the proximal phalanx follows automatically and a voluntary movement is require to flex the fingers and this flexion is very weak. The tension developed in the digital flexors limits flexion of the wrist and the range of wrist flexion is increased by 10° by extending the fingers.

This delicate balance of muscles action can easily be upset. A deformity resulting from an unreduced Colles' fracture changes the orientation of the distal aspect of the radius and of the articular disc and, by stretching the extensors of the wrist, interferes with the efficiency of the digital flexors.

The functional position of the wrist (Fig. 36) corresponds to the position of maximal efficiency of the muscles of the fingers especially of the flexors. This position is achieved by:

— slight extension of the wrist is 40°–45°

— slight ulnar deviation (adduction) to 15°.

It is in this position of the wrist that the hand is best adapted for its function of prehension.

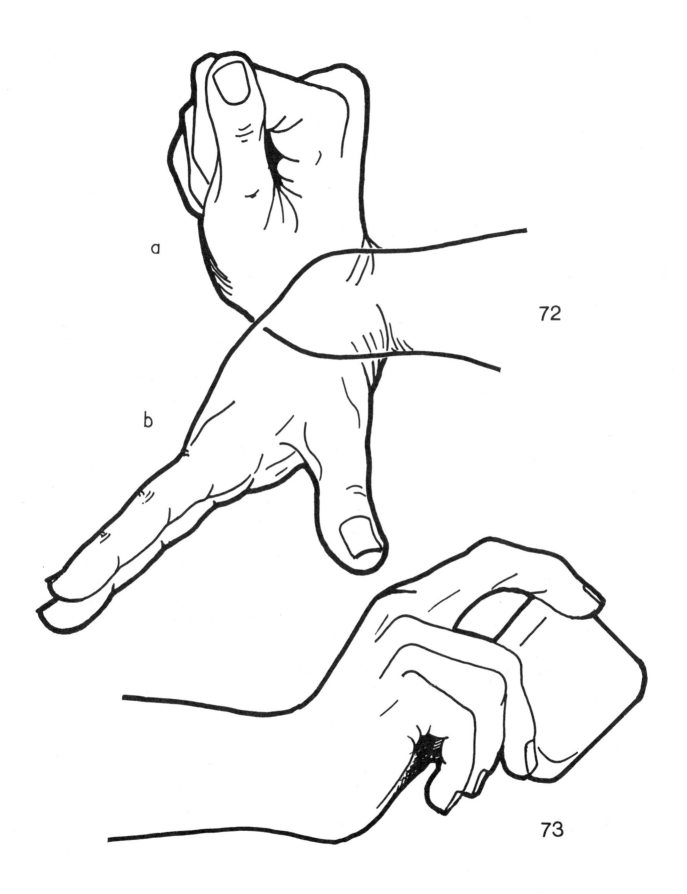

a

b

72

73

THE HAND

ITS ROLE

The hand of man is a remarkable instrument, capable of performing countless actions, owing to its essential function: prehension.

Prehension is seen in all forms of the 'hand' from the pincers of the lobster to the paw of the ape, but it attains perfection only in man. This is due to a special movement of the thumb (called opposition) which brings it into contact with each finger. Opposition is seen in the great apes, but its range is more limited than in man.

At the same time the lack of specialization in the human hand underlies its adaptability and creativity.

From the functional viewpoint the hand is the *effector organ* of the upper limb, which supports it mechanically and allows it to adopt the optimal position for any given action. However, the hand is not only a motor organ but also a very sensitive and accurate sensory receptor, which feeds back information essential for its own performance. Finally, it provides the cerebral cortex with *information regarding thickness and distance* and thus is responsible for the development of *visual appreciation* by allowing cross checking of information. Without the hand our idea of the world would be flat and lacking in contrasts.

It is essential for that particular sense, stereognosis, which is the appreciation of relief, shape, thickness, *space*. It also trains the brain in the appreciation of texture, weight and temperature. By itself the hand is able to recognise an object, unaided by the eye.

The hand therefore forms with the brain an inseparable *interacting functional pair* and this close interaction is responsible for man's ability to alter nature at will and to dominate other species.

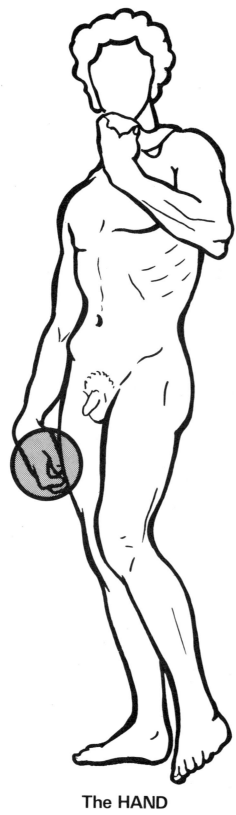

The HAND

THE TOPOGRAPHY OF THE HAND

The topography of the hand is best studied on its two surfaces, i.e. anterior (palmar) and posterior (dorsal).

The **anterior surface** (Fig. 1) consists of:

1. the *palm of the hand*, made up of three parts:
    — centrally, *the palm proper* (1) or the hollow of the hand, containing the flexor tendons, the blood vessels and the nerves and bounded by two transverse creases: the *distal palmar crease* (2), overlying the three medial metacarpophalangeal joints and the *middle palmar crease* (3), laterally overlying the metacarpophalangeal joint of the index.
    — laterally, a fleshy convex mould, lying next to the base of the thumb, *the thenar eminence* (4), bounded medially by the *proximal palmar crease* (5) (also known as the crease of thumb opposition) and holding the thenar muscles, i.e. the intrinsic muscles of the thumb. At its proximal apex can be felt the hard bony projection of *the scaphoid tubercle* (6).
    — medially, the *hypothenar eminence* (7), less prominent than the thenar eminence, contains the hypothenar muscles, i.e. the intrinsic muscles of the little finger. Proximally can be felt the hard bony projection of the *pisiform* (8), into which is inserted the tendon of the flexor carpi ulnaris.

Proximal to the palm is the **wrist** overlying the carpal bones and the radio-carpal joint, which lies deep to *the crease of the wrist* (9) and to the insertion of the *palmaris longus* (10), which lies medial to the *radial pulse* (11). The *flexor retinaculum of the wrist*, running transversely, plasters this area and the proximal part of the palm.

The *anterior surface* of the **fingers** is bounded proximally by the *digito-palmar crease* (12), lying 10 to 15 mm *proximal* to the metacarpo-phalangeal joint. The four fingers are separated from one another by the *second, third and fourth interdigital clefts* (13), which are deeper dorsally. The *proximal interphalangeal crease* (14) is double, lies slightly proximal to the distal interphalangeal joint and separates the *first phalanx* (15) from *the second* (16). The distal interphalangeal crease (17) is single, lies slightly distal to the distal interphalangeal joint and proximally bounds the pulp (18), i.e. the palmar surface of the terminal phalanx. The **thumb,** attached to the base of the lateral border of the hand, is separated therefrom by the wide and deep *interdigital cleft* (19). Its site of attachment to the thenar eminence is surface-marked by *the two pollici-palmar creases* (20), which 'encase' its metacarpophalangeal joint. Its *proximal phalanx* (21) is separated from *the pulp* (22), i.e. the palmar surface of the second phalanx, by *the inter-phalangeal crease* (23), lying just distal to the interphalangeal joint.

2. **The dorsal or posterior surface of the hand** (Fig. 2) also consists of two regions, i.e. the dorsal surface of the hand proper and the dorsal aspect of the fingers.
    — The *dorsum of the hand* is covered by thin and mobile skin, traversed by the venous plexus draining the hand and the fingers, raised by the extensor tendons (24), bounded distally by the hard and rounded *heads of the metacarpals* (25) and by *the interdigital clefts* (26), which are fairly deep dorsally.

Medially the *ulnar aspect of the hand* (27) is carpeted by the adductor digiti minimi.

The lateral (Fig. 3) border of the had bears the *first interdigital cleft* (19) and the slightly concave anatomical snuffbox (28), which lies at the junction of the wrist and the thumb, is bounded by the *apposed tendons of the abductor longus and extensor brevis of the thumb* (29) and by that of *the extensor pollicis longus* (30) and contains in its depths the *radial styloid process*, the *trapezo-metacarpal joint* (31) and the radial artery, arranged proximo-distally. The tendons converge on to the dorsal surface of the *first metacarpal* (32) at the level of the *metacarpophalangeal joint of the thumb* (33).

On the medial aspect of the dorsum of the wrist can be seen, only in *pronation*, the hard and rounded projection of the ulnar head (34).

— **The posterior surface of the fingers** shows *the proximal interphalangeal creases* (35), which directly overlie the interphalangeal joints. The distal phalanx carries the nail bounded by the periungual margins (37). The space between the nail and the distal interphalangeal creases covers the base of the nail (38).

Functionally the hand can be divided into three components (Fig. 4):
    — the thumb (I), which by itself fulfils most of the functions of the hand because of its *movement of opposition.*
    — **the index and the middle finger** (II), which help the thumb of achieve *the precision grips*, i.e. *the bi- or tri-digital pollici-digital pincers.*
    — **the ring finger and the little finger** (III) which, along with the rest of the hand, are essential for solidly grasping tool-handles on the ulnar side of the hand and thus are vital in strengthening the *grip.*

166

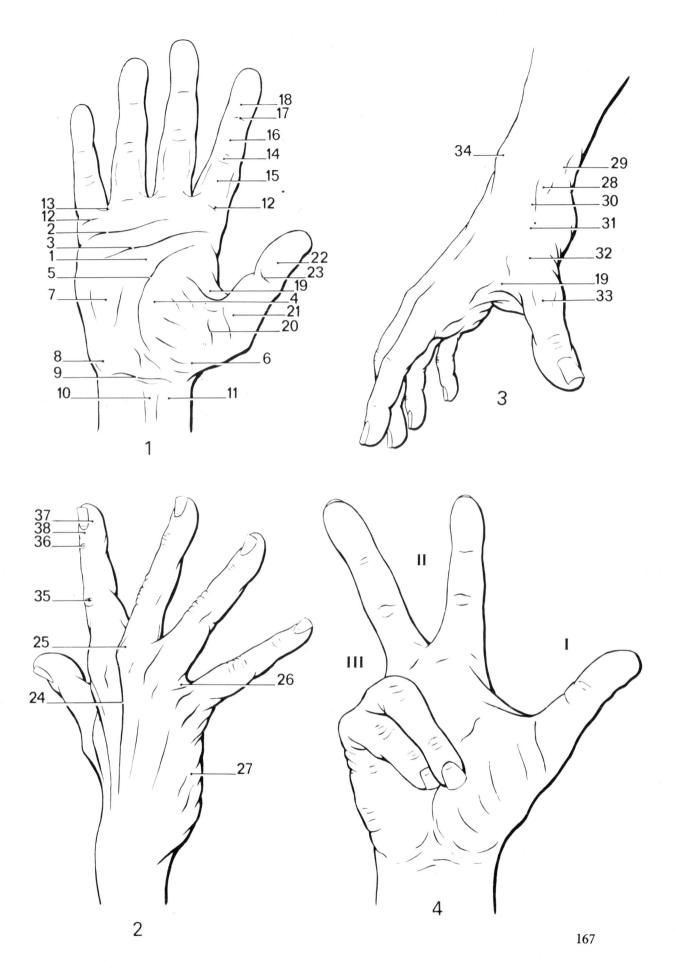

1

2

3

4

167

THE ARCHITECTURE OF THE HAND

For grasping objects **the hand must change its shape.**

On a flat surface, for example a glass pane (Fig. 5), *the hand spreads out and becomes flattened,* making contact (Fig. 6) at the thenar eminence (1), the hypothenar eminence (2), the metacarpal heads (3) and the palmar surfaces of the phalanges (4). Only the infero-lateral aspect of the palm does not touch the glass.

When a large object is being grasped, *the hand becomes hollow* with the formation of three arches running in three different directions:

— *Transversely* (Fig. 7): the **carpal arch** XOY corresponds to the concavity of the wrist. It is continuous distally with the **metacarpal arch** formed by the metacarpal heads. The long axis of the carpal gutter traverses the lunate, the capitate and the third metacarpal bones.

— *Longitudinally* (Figs. 7 & 8): the **carpometacarpo-phalangeal arches** fan out from the wrist (cf. Fig. 10) and are formed for each finger by the corresponding metacarpal bone and phalanges. The arches are concave on the palmar surface and *the keystone of each arch lies at the level of the metacarpo-phalangeal joint,* so that any muscular imbalance at this point interferes with the concavity of the arch. The two most important **longitudinal arches** are the following:

— The *arch of the middle finger* OD_3 (Fig. 7) which is continuous with the axis of the carpal gutter.

— The *arch of the index finger* OD_2 (Fig. 8), which most often comes into opposition with the thumb.

— *Obliquely* (Figs. 7, 8 and 9): the **arches formed by the thumb during opposition with the other fingers.** The *most important* of these arches is the one linking the thumb and index finger D_1-D_2 (Fig. 8) and the *most extreme* is that linking the thumb and the little finger, D_1-D_5 (Figs. 7, 8 and 9).

In general, when the hand becomes hollow, it comes to form a *gutter, concave anteriorly,* whose sides bear the following landmarks: the thumb (D_1), which alone forms the lateral side, and the index finger (D_2) and the little finger (D_5) which represent the two extreme points of the medial side.

Across the two sides of the gutter lie the **four oblique arches formed by the movements of opposition.**

This *palmar gutter,* which is set obliquely at all levels (shown by the large arrow in Figs. 8 and 9) runs perpendicular to the various arches formed during thumb opposition. It stretches from the base of the hypothenar eminence X (Fig. 7) — where the pisiform bone can be palpated — to the second metacarpal head Z (Fig. 7) and corresponds roughly to the palmar crease, known as 'the line of life'. This is also the direction taken by a cylindrical object (e.g. the handle of a tool) when fully grasped by the hand.

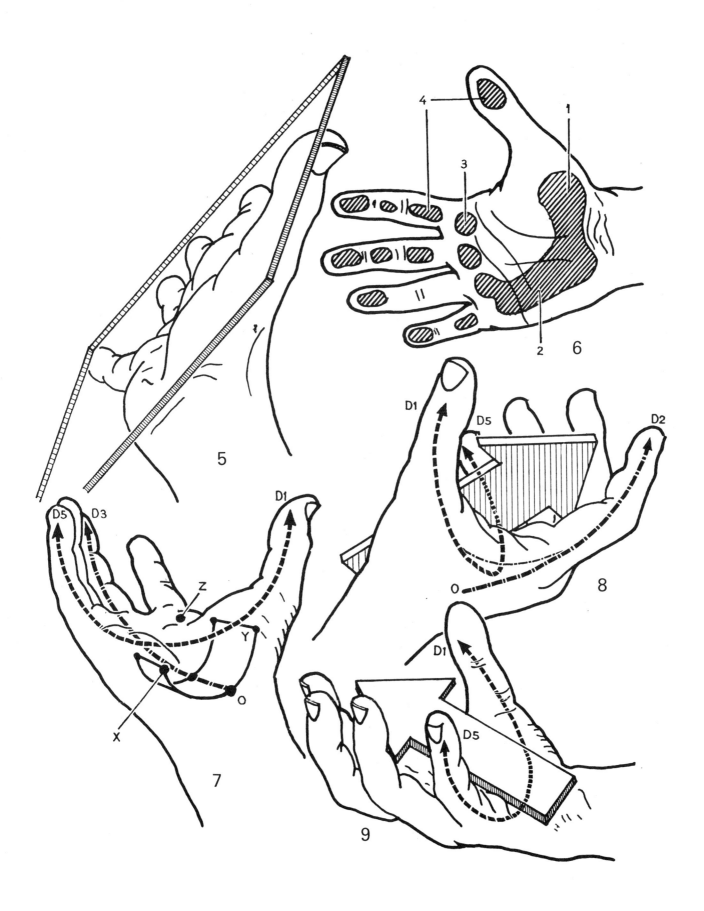

5

6

4

3

1

2

II

7

D5   D3

D1

Z

Y

X

O

8

D1

D5

D2

O

9

D1

D5

169

THE ARCHITECTURE OF THE HAND (continued)

When the *fingers are voluntarily spread out* (Fig. 10) the axes of the five fingers converge towards the base of the thenar eminence, deep to which lies the easily palpated tubercle of the scaphoid. In the hand the movements of the fingers in the frontal plane are referred not to the plane of symmetry of the body as a whole (i.e. adduction and abduction) but *to the axis of the hand* which runs through **the third metacarpal bone and the middle finger**. Therefore the movements of the fingers should strictly be called approximation for *adduction* (Fig. 12) and separation for *abduction* (Fig. 10). During these movements the middle finger does not move appreciably, though it is possible to abduct and adduct this finger voluntarily (i.e. with respect to the axis of the body).

When the fingers are *voluntarily brought together* (Fig. 12), their axes are not parallel but *converge towards a point lying far distal to the hand*. This is due to the fact that the fingers are not cylindrical but taper distally.

When the fingers are allowed to take a *natural position* (Fig. 11), i.e. a position from which they can be both approximated (adducted) and separated (abducted) — they lie a short distance away from one another but their axes do not meet at one point. In the example given the last three fingers are parallel and the first three fingers diverge from one another while the middle finger represents the axis of the hand and also the 'zone of transition'.

When the *fist is clenched* with the distal interphalangeal joints still extended (Fig. 13), the axes of the two distal phalanges of the four fingers and the axis of the thumb (discounting its terminal phalanx) converge to a point corresponding to the 'radial pulse'. Note that in this situation the axis of the index is parallel to the long axis of the hand while *the axes of the other fingers become progressively more oblique the farther they are from the index*. The cause and significance of this will be discussed later (p. 188).

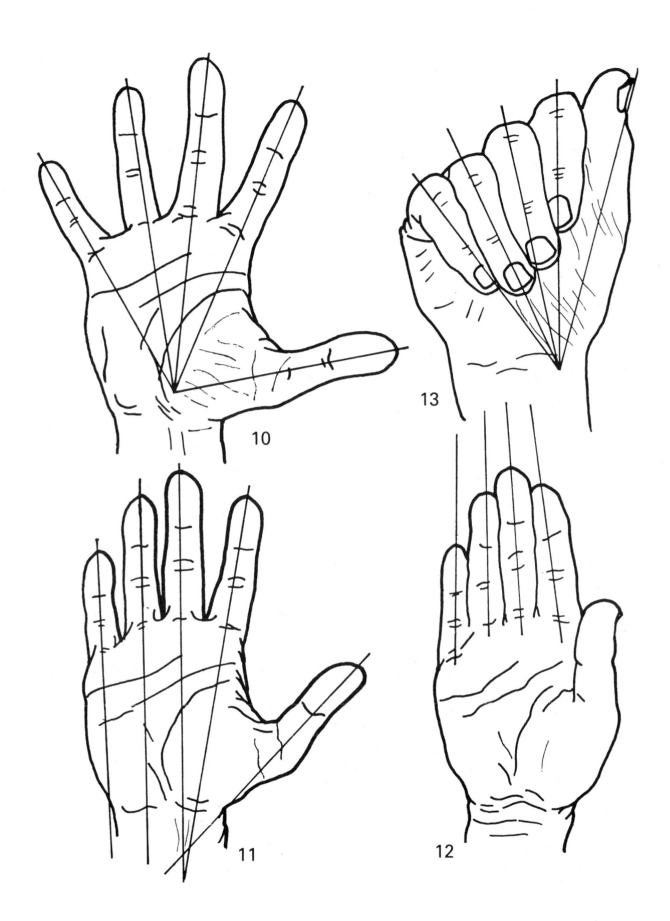

10

13

11

12

171

THE CARPAL BONES

The carpal bones form *a gutter which is concave on the anterior (palmar) side* and is transformed into a tunnel by the flexor retinaculum inserted on either side of the gutter.

This gutter is easily seen when one examines the skeleton of the hand with the wrist in hyperextension (Fig. 14) and it corresponds to the axis of the carpal tunnel. Its two sides consist of:

laterally: the tubercle of the scaphoid (1), and the crest of the trapezium (2);

medially: the pisiform (3), and the hook of the hamate (4).

This is confirmed by the following *two horizontal sections*:

The first section (Fig. 15) passes through the *proximal row of carpal bones* (level A, Fig. 17) and shows latero-medially: the scaphoid, the head of the capitate bounded by the two horns of the lunate, the triquetrum and the pisiform:

The second section (Fig. 16), passing *through the distal row* (level B, Fig. 17), shows latero-medially: the trapezium, the trapezoid, the capitate and the hamate.

The flexor retinaculum is shown in broken lines in both sections.

When the palmar concavity deepens, the *carpal tunnel also deepens* owing to the slight movements at the various intercarpal joints. The concavity of the scaphoid slips over the convexity of the capitate distally and anteriorly in a 'corkscrew' fashion. The triquetrum and the hamate are symmetrically displaced anteriorly while the trapezoid (especially) and the trapezium glide over the articular facets of the distal surface of the scaphoid. The trapezium moves anteromedially over the cylindrical articular facet, which extends up to the distal aspect of the scaphoid tubercle. These movements are initiated by the thenar (arrow X) and the hypothenar (arrow Y) muscles, which arise from the flexor retinaculum and, by tensing up the ligament (Fig. 16), *approximate the two sides of the tunnel* (displacements dotted in).

Lengthwise the carpal bones (Fig. 17) can be considered to consist of three columns (Fig. 18):

The *lateral column* (a) (vertically striped) is the most important and corresponds to the column of the thumb (Destot). It is made up of the scaphoid, the trapezium and the first metacarpal. From the scaphoid springs the column of the index consisting of the trapezoid and the second metacarpal.

The *intermediate column* (b) (obliquely striped) consists of the lunate, the capitate and the third metacarpal and corresponds to the axis of the hand.

The *medial column* (c) (horizontally striped), ending on the last two fingers, consists of the triquetrum and the hamate, which articulates with the fourth and fifth metacarpals. The pisiform lies superficial to the triquetrum and does not transmit any stresses.

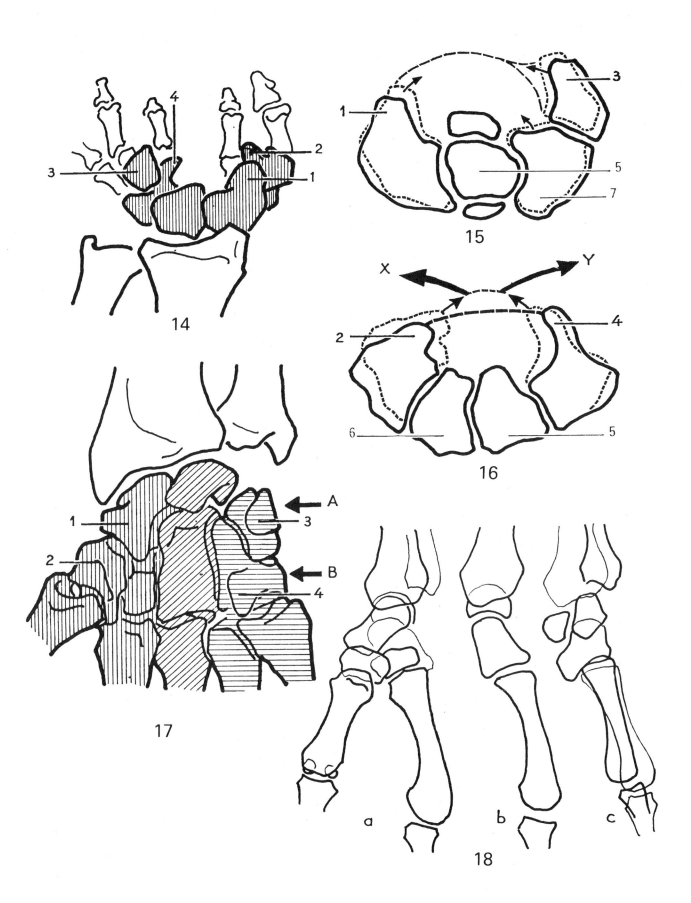

14

15

16

17

18

THE HOLLOWING OF THE PALM

This is due essentially to movements of the last four metacarpal bones (the first metacarpal bone is ignored for the time being) with respect to the wrist. These movements, occurring at the *carpometacarpal joints*, consist of **weak** movements of flexion and extension, as typical of plane joints. But the range of these movements increases from the second to the fifth metacarpal:

— When the hand is flat the heads of the last four metacarpal bones lie on a straight line AB (Fig. 20: hand seen 'end on');

— When the palm 'hollows', the heads of the last three metacarpal bones move anteriorly (Fig. 19) and the more so as the last finger is approached. Then the metacarpal heads lie on a curved line A'B (Fig. 20), which is *the transverse metacarpal arch.*

The following points are worth noting:

(a) the second metacarpal head B does not move appreciably and the *flexion and extension movements at the trapezoid-second metacarpal joint are negligible;*

(b) the fifth metacarpal head A, which is the most mobile, moves not only anteriorly but also *slightly laterally* to position A'.

This brings us to the analysis of **the fifth carpometacarpal joint** (between the hamate and the fifth metacarpal).

It is a saddle joint (Fig. 22) with slightly cylindrical surfaces. The axis is oblique in two planes and this explains why the metacarpal head moves laterally:

1. Figure 21 (distal surface of the distal row of the carpus) shows that the axis XX' of the medial facet of the hamate is *oblique lateromedially and posteroanteriorly.* Therefore any movement about this axis must carry the fifth metacarpal head anteriorly and laterally (white arrow).

2. *The axis XX' of this joint is not quite perpendicular to the longitudinal axis OA of the metacarpal* but forms an acute angle XOA with it (Fig. 22). This is also responsible for the lateral movement of the fifth metacarpal head for the following reason, illustrated in geometrical terms as follows:

If a segment OA (Fig. 23) rotates about an axis YY' which is at right angles to it, the point A describes a circle with centre O and lying in a plane P perpendicular to axis YY'. After rotation the point A reaches the position A'.

If the same segment OA turns about an axis XX', which is not at right angles to it, the point A will now describe not a circle but a cone with apex A and lying tangential to the plane P. After the same degree of rotation as above the point A is now in position A' which, with respect to the plane P, lies on the same side as the acute angle formed by the axis XX' and the segment OA.

If one now refers back to the diagram of the joint (Fig. 22), it becomes clear why the fifth metacarpal head leaves the sagittal plane P and moves slightly laterally.

This anterior and lateral movement of the fifth metacarpal, associated with a slight degree of supination due to automatic longitudinal rotation, is similar to a *movement of opposition* towards the thumb and thus takes part in the *symmetrical opposition of fifth finger and thumb.*

174

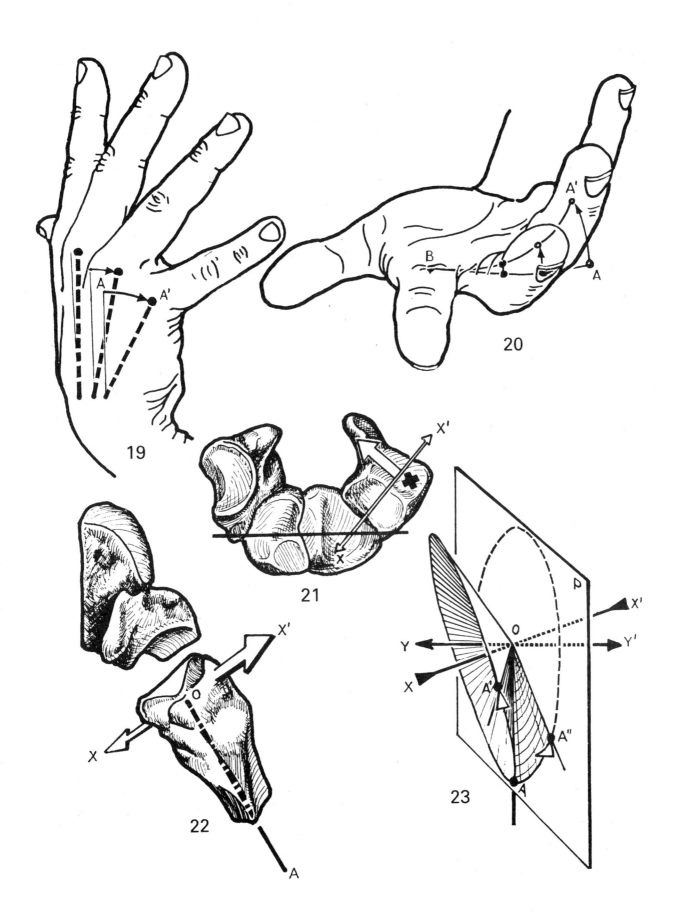

19

20

21

22

23

175

THE METACARPO-PHALANGEAL JOINTS

These joints are of the **condyloid type** (Fig. 24) with movements about two axes at right angles and **two degrees of freedom:**

— *Flexion* and *extension* in the sagittal plane about the transverse axis YY'.

— *Adduction* and *abduction* in a frontal plane about the antero-posterior axis XX'.

The **metacarpal head** is a *biconvex* articular surface which is broader anteriorly than posteriorly.

The **base of the proximal phalanx** contains a *biconcave* articular surface (B) which is much smaller in surface area than the head of the metacarpal. This surface is increased anteriorly by the *fibro-cartilaginous plate or ligament* (2), which is attached to the anterior surface of the base of the phalanx. Its attachment to the articular cartilage of the phalanx is formed by a small fibrous band, called 'the incisura' (3), which functions like a *hinge*.

In fact (Fig. 25), during extension (a) the medial cartilaginous half of the fibro-cartilaginous plate articulates with the metacarpal head. During flexion (b) the plate *moves past the metacarpal head* and turns upon its hinge-like 'incisura' *to glide along the palmar surface of the metacarpal*. It is clear that if the fibro-cartilaginous plate were replaced by a bony plate firmly attached to the base of the phalanx, flexion would be checked earlier by contact of the bones. Therefore the fibro-cartilaginous plate fulfils two apparently mutually exclusive requirements:

1. maximal contact between the two bony surfaces, and

2. absence of any movement-limiting impact between the bones.

There is also, however, another essential condition for freedom of movement, i.e. a certain degree of 'give' of the capsule and synovium. This is provided by the posterior (4) and anterior (5) recesses of the capsule, and the *deep recess is essential for the gliding movement of the fibro-cartilaginous plate during flexion*. On the posterior surface of the base of the phalanx is inserted the deep attachment (6) of the extensor tendon.

On each side of the joint are present *two types of ligaments:*

— A **ligament joining the metacarpal to the fibro-cartilaginous plate** and controlling the movements of the latter (see later).

— The **collateral ligaments** seen sectioned (1) in Figure 20. These keep the articular surfaces together and restrain their movements.

Their insertion into the metacarpal head (Fig. 26, according to Dubousset) is clearly posterior to the centre of curvature of the articular surface, which, because of the variable radius of curvature of the metacarpal head, is really a *series of centres of curvature* arranged spirally. Thus the distance between the proximal attachment of the collateral ligament and its distal attachment to the first phalanx B (in extension) and B' (in flexion) ranges from 27 to 34 mm. Hence the collateral ligament is *slackened in extension and tightened in flexion*.

Footnote: For the sake of brevity the following abbreviations will be used both in the text and in the diagrams: P_1 = proximal phalanx, P_2 = middle phalanx, P_3 = distal phalanx; MP = metacarpo-phalangeal joint, PIP = proximal interphalangeal joint, DIP = distal interphalangeal joint; FDS = flexor digitorum sublimis, FDP = flexor digitorun profundus, EDC = extensor digitorum communis.

M_1, M_2, ... = Metacarpals.

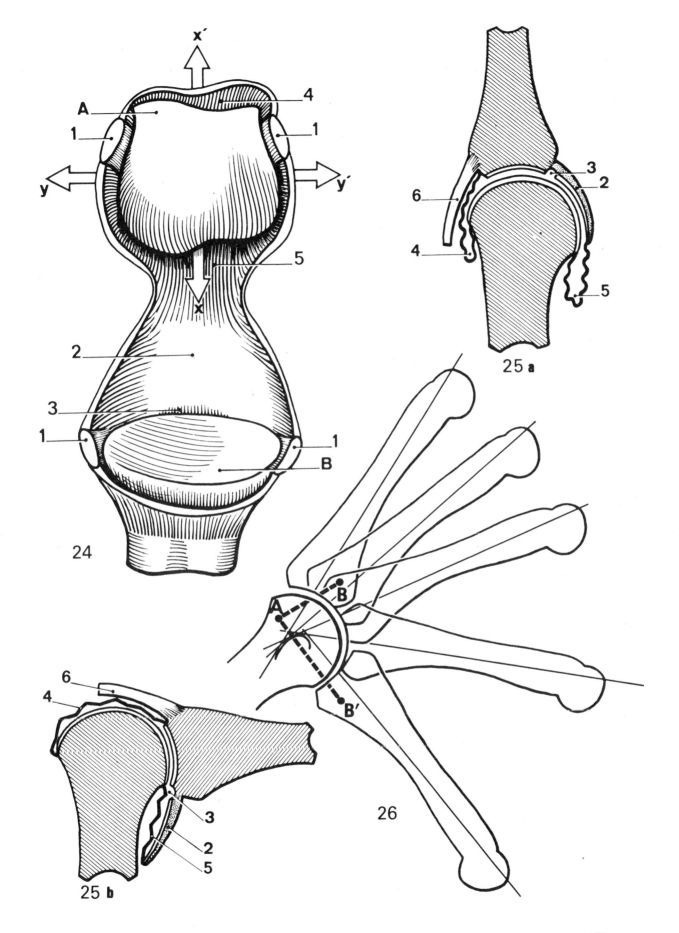

24

25 a

25 b

26

THE METACARPO-PHALANGEAL JOINTS (continued)

It is easy to understand (Fig. 27: frontal section) that during extension (a) the slackening of the collateral ligaments allows side to side movements at the joints (b); thus one ligament is stretched while the other is slackened.

Thus stabilization of the MP joint is secured by the collateral ligaments during flexion and by the interosseous muscles during extension.

Another important consequence of this state of affairs is that the MP joints *must never be immobilised in extension* for fear of producing almost irreversible stiffness. The slack collateral ligaments can retract in extension but cannot do so in flexion.

The shape of the metacarpal heads (Figs. 28, 29, 30, 31: heads of metacarpals II, III, IV, V, right side) and the length and direction of the ligaments influence at once the obliquity of flexion of the fingers (see later) and their ulnar deviations in rheumatoid arthritis (according to Tubiana).

The head of M_2 (Fig. 28) is clearly asymmetrical, being significantly swollen posteromedially and flattened laterally. The medial ligament is thicker and longer than the lateral, which is inserted more posteriorly.

The head of M_3 (Fig. 29) is similarly asymmetrical but its asymmetry is even more marked. Its ligaments are identical.

The head of M_4 (Fig. 30) is more symmetrical with posterior swellings equal on both sides. Its ligaments are similar in their thickness and obliquity, with the lateral being slightly longer.

The head of M_5 (Fig. 31) shows a pattern of asymmetry opposite to that of M_2 and M_3. The collateral ligaments are identical to those of M_4.

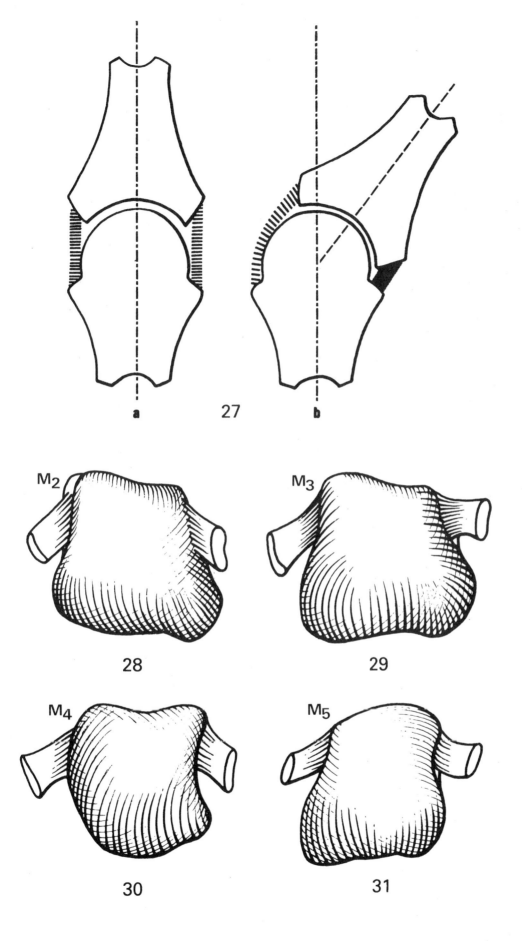

27

28

29

30

31

179

THE LIGAMENTS OF THE METACARPO-PHALANGEAL JOINTS

The collateral ligaments of the MP joints belong to a more complex **ligamentous system**, which holds and 'directs' the tendons of the extensors and flexors.

In Fig. 32 (the joint viewed from behind, above and outside):

— the **EDC** (1), which dorsal to the capsule sends a *deep expansion* (a) to be inserted into the base of P_1. It then divides into the *medial slip* (b) and the *two lateral slips* (a) which receive the insertions of the interossei (not shown). Just before the deep expansion leaves the tendon, small *sagittal bands* become detached from the main tendon and cross the lateral aspects of the joint before gaining insertion into the *deep transverse ligament of the palm* (4). Thus, during flexion at the joint, the extensor tendon is kept in the axis of movement as it crosses the convex dorsal surface of the metacarpal head.

— the **FDP** (2) and **FDS** (3) enter the *metacarpal pulley* (5), which starts at the level of the *fibro-cartilaginous plate* (6) and extends to the palmar surface of P_1, where the FDS tendon splits into *two slips* (3') before being perforated by the FDP tendon (2). The ligamentous complex is made up of:

(a) the **articular capsule** reinforced by

(b) the **collateral ligament**, attached to the lateral tubercle (8) of the metacarpal head posterior to the line of the centres of curvature (see p. 176) and composed of three components:

— a *metacarpophalangeal bundle* (9) running obliquely distally and anteriorly towards the base of P_1.

— a *bundle linking the metacarpal and the fibrocartilaginous plate* (10), running anteriorly to insert into the edges of the fibrocartilaginous plate, which is thus pressed against the metacarpal head and stabilised;

— a *thin bundle linking the phalanx and the fibrocartilaginous plate* (11), which helps keep the plate in position during extension.

(c) the **deep transverse ligament of the palm** (4), attached to the adjacent borders of the fibrocartilaginous plates of the MP joints, so that its fibres span the entire width of the hand at the level of these joints. It contributes to the formation of the fibrous tunnels for the interossei (not shown) and lies posterior to the tendon of the lumbrical (not shown).

The **metacarpal pulley** (5), attached to the lateral borders of the fibrocartilaginous plate, is thus literally *suspended from the metacarpal head*. It plays an important role *during flexion at the MP joint:*

— *when intact* (Fig. 33), the pulley, with its fibres rolled up distally, redirects the tendon-detaching component of force (white arrow) towards the metacarpal head (small black arrow). Hence the flexor tendons stay close to the joint and the phalangeal head is stabilised.

— *in disease states* (Fig. 34), when the ligaments are overstretched and finally ruptured as in rheumatoid arthritis, this 'detaching' component of force is directed not towards the metacarpal head but towards the base of P_1, with anterior and proximal subluxation of the metacarpal head, which becomes more prominent.

— *treatment of this condition* (Fig. 35) can to some degree be achieved by resection of the proximal part of the metacarpal pulley but this leads to loss of efficiency of the flexor muscles.

180

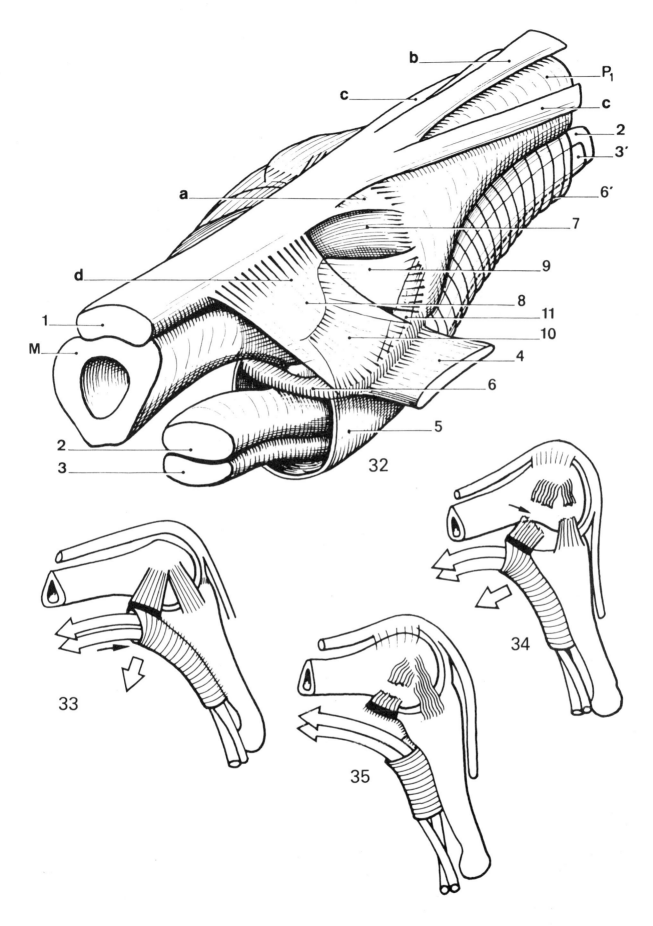

32

33

34

35

181

THE LIGAMENTS OF THE METACARPO-PHALANGEAL JOINTS (continued)

The tendons of the EDC (Fig. 36), which are closely set on the dorsum of the wrist, tend to be pulled towards the ulna (white arrows) because of the angle between the metacarpal and P_1. This angle is greater for the little finger (14°) and the ring finger (13°) than for the index (8°) and the middle finger (4°). Only the sagittal bands of the extensor tendon, lying on the radial side, will oppose this tendency of the extensor tendon to be displaced ulnaward on the convex dorsal surface of the metacarpal head.

In rheumatoid arthritis (Fig. 37: seen at the level of the metacarpal heads), the collateral ligaments (10) degenerate releasing the fibrocartilaginous plate (6), which gives attachment to the metacarpal pulley (5) holding the tendons of the FDP (2) and FDS (3). The sagittal bands on the radial side are also loosened or ruptured, resulting in the ulnar displacement of the extensors into the intermetacarpal gutters. The intermetacarpal gutter normally contains only the tendons of the interossei (12) and that of the lumbrical, which lie anterior and posterior respectively to the intermetacarpal ligament (4).

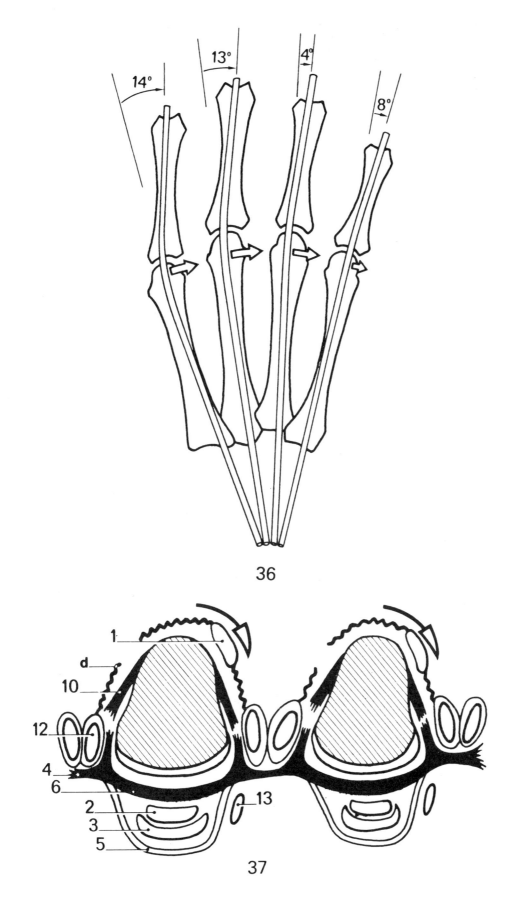

36

37

183

THE RANGE OF MOVEMENTS OF THE METACARPO-PHALANGEAL JOINTS

Flexion has a range of about 90° (Fig. 38). It falls just short of 90° for the index but *increases progressively with the other fingers*. Also, isolated flexion of the finger (here of the middle finger) is checked (Fig. 39) by the tension developed in the palmar interdigital ligament.

Active extension is variable and can reach up to 30° or 40° (Fig. 40). **Passive extension** can reach up to 90° in people with very lax ligaments (Fig. 41)

Of all the fingers (except the thumb) the index finger has the *greatest range of side-to-side movement* (30) and, as it can easily be moved alone, the terms *abduction* (A) and *adduction* (B) strictly apply here. It is to this great mobility that the index owes its name: **index = indicator.**

By a succession of the simple moveements (Fig. 43) of abduction, (A), adduction (B), extension (C) and flexion (D) the index performs the **movements of circumduction** which take place within the **cone of circumduction.** This is defined by its base (ACBD) and its apex (metacarpo-phalangeal joint). This cone is flattened transversely because of the greater range of the movements of flexion and extension. Its axis (white arrow) corresponds to *the position of equilibrium or function* of the MP joint of the index.

Condyloid joints do not normally show axial rotation and this applies to the MP joints of the four fingers as regards *active rotation*. However, owing to the laxity of the ligaments, a measure of **passive axial rotation** is possible with a range of about 60° (Roud).

Note that with the *index finger* the range of medial rotation — or pronation — is much greater (45°) than that of lateral rotation — or supination — which is trivial.

Even if a true active axial rotation is not seen at the MP joints, there is an **automatic rotation** in the direction of supination, resulting from the asymmetry of the metacarpal head and the unequal length and tension of the collateral ligaments. This movement, which is similar to that seen in the IP joint of the thumb, is more marked in the more medial fingers and is maximal for the little finger, where it contributes to the movement of that finger towards the opposing thumb.

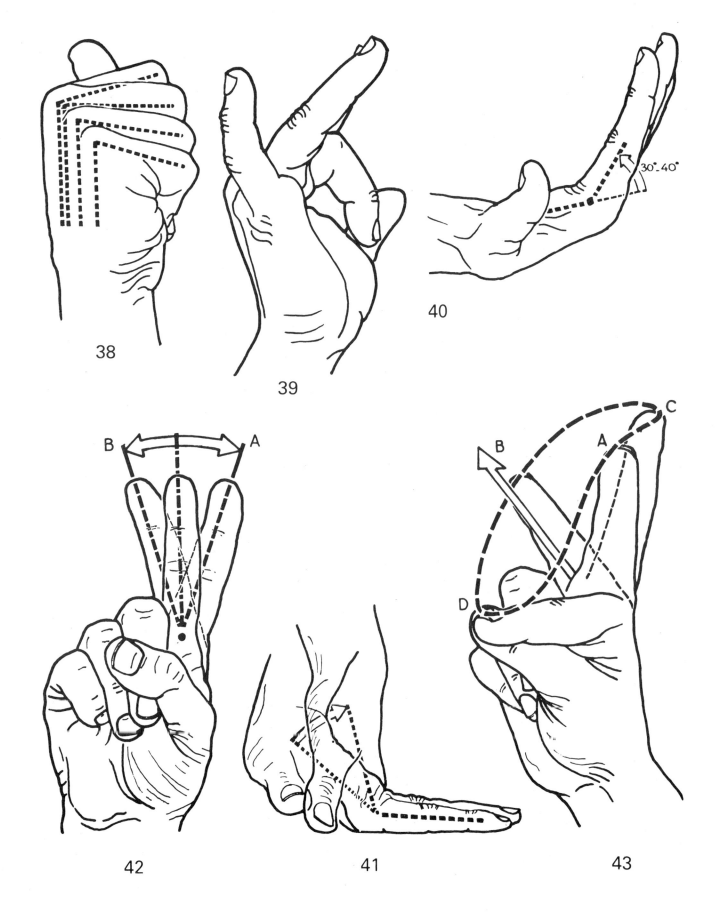

38

39

40

30°-40°

42

41

43

185

THE INTERPHALANGEAL JOINTS

These are **hinge** joints with movement about one axis only and **one degree of freedom**.

The **head of the phalanx** (Fig. 44 and A, Fig. 45) is *pulley-shaped* with *only one transverse axis* about which flexion and extension take place in the sagittal plane.

The **base of the immediately distal phalanx** (B) bears two *shallow facets* separated by a median ridge. The facets articulate with the pulley-shaped head of the proximal phalanx and the shallow crest comes to rest within the central groove.

As in the MP joints and for the same mechanical reasons the articular surface is widened by a *fibro-cartilaginous plate* (2). (The numbers have the same meaning as in Fig. 24.)

During flexion (Fig. 46) the plate glides along the palmar surface of P_1.

Figure 47 (lateral view) shows the *collateral ligaments* (1), the expansions of the extensor tendons (6) and the *anterior capsular* ligaments (7), joining P_1 to the fibrocartilaginous plate.

Note that *the collateral ligaments tense up during flexion* to a greater degree than those of the MP joints.

The *pulley-shaped phalanx* (A, Fig. 45) is broader anteriorly than posteriorly so that the tension in the ligaments is enhanced and a larger articulating surface is offered to the head of the distal phalanx. *No lateral movements are possible when the joint is flexed.*

Note that they are also stretched in full extension, which is also a *position of absolute lateral stability*. On the contrary they become slack in intermediate positions of flexion, which must never be used during immobilisation for fear of causing retraction of the ligaments and subsequent restriction of movement.

Stiffening in flexion can also be due *to retraction of the check rein ligaments* recently described by Anglo–Saxon authors. They consist (Fig. 48: PIP joint, viewed from the palm and from above) of bundles of longitudinal fibres (8) coursing over the palmar surface of the fibrocartilaginous plate (2) on either side of the tendons of the FDP (11) and FDS (12), bridging the 'ligamentous pulleys' of P_1 (10) and P_2 (not shown) and forming the lateral edge of the diagonal fibres (9) of the pulley of the PIP joint. These check rein ligaments prevent hyperextension of the PIP joint and, when they retract during immobilisation in flexion, they are primarily responsible for restriction of movement. They must then be resected surgically.

In sum, the IP joints, especially the proximal, must be immobilised in a position close to full extension.

The *range of flexion* in the PIP joints (Fig. 49) is **greater than 90°** so that in flexion P_1 and P_2 form an acute angle (in Fig. 49 the phalanges are seen obliquely from the side so that the angles appear obtuse). As in the case of the MP joints, flexion increases in range from *the second to the fifth finger* to reach a maximum of 135° with the latter.

The *range of flexion* at the DIP joints (Fig. 50) is *slightly less than 90°* so that the angle between P_2 and P_3 remains obtuse. As with the proximal joints, this range increases from the second to the fifth finger to attain **a maximum of 90°** with the latter.

The *range of active extension* (Fig. 51) at the IP joints is: **nil** at the PIP joints (P); **nil** or trivial (5) at the distal IP joints (D).

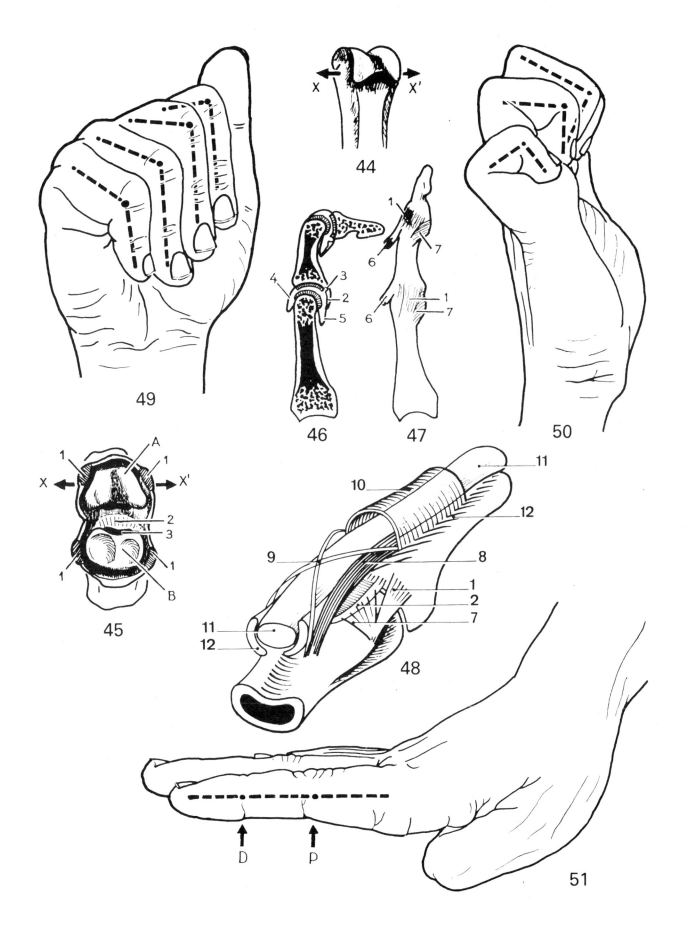

44

49

46   47   50

45

A
X ← → X'
1   1
1   1
2
3
B

9
11
12

10   11
12
8
1
2
7

48

D   P

51

187

THE INTERPHALANGEAL JOINTS (continued)

Passive extension (Fig. 52) is nil at the PIP joint (P), but appreciable (30°) at the DIP joint (D).

Since the IP joints have only one degree of freedom, there is no active, but only *slight passive side-to-side movement* (Fig. 53), especially at the DIP joint.

The *plane of movement of flexion* of the last four fingers is worth discussing (Fig. 54).

The index is flexed in *a strictly sagittal plane* (P) towards the base of the thenar eminence (long white arrow).

As shown previously (Fig. 13), the axes of the fingers during flexion all converge to a point corresponding to the 'radial pulse'. This can only occur if the other fingers are flexed not in a sagittal plane like the index, but *in an increasingly oblique plane.*

The little finger shows maximal obliquity of its plane of flexion (shown as small white arrow).

The significance of this 'oblique' flexion lies in the fact that it allows the more medial fingers to oppose the thumb like the index.

How this 'oblique' flexion occurs is demonstrated in diagram 55.

A narrow piece of cardboard (a) represents the whole finger with the metacarpal (M) and the three phalanges (P_1, P_2, P_3).

If the fold in the cardboard, representing the axis of flexion of an interphalangeal joint, is perpendicular (xx″) to its long axis, the phalanx will bend in the sagittal plane and cover exactly the proximal phalanx. If, on the other hand, the fold is *slightly oblique* medially (xx′), flexion will not occur in the sagittal plane and the flexed phalanx will *move past* the proximal phalanx *laterally.*

Therefore, only a slight obliquity of the axis of flexion is required because it is multiplied by a factor of 3 (xx′, yy′, zz′), so that when the little finger is fully flexed (c) the obliquity of the movement brings it into contact with the thumb.

The same demonstration applies, though to a lesser extent, to the ring finger and the middle finger.

In reality, the axes of flexion of the MP and IP joints are not fixed and unchanging. They are perpendicular to the joints in full extension and become progressively more oblique during flexion.

This change in the orientation of the axis of flexion is due to the asymmetry of the articular surfaces of the metacarpals (see above) and of the phalanges and also because the collateral ligaments are stretched differentially, as will be shown later with respect to the MP and IP joints of the thumb.

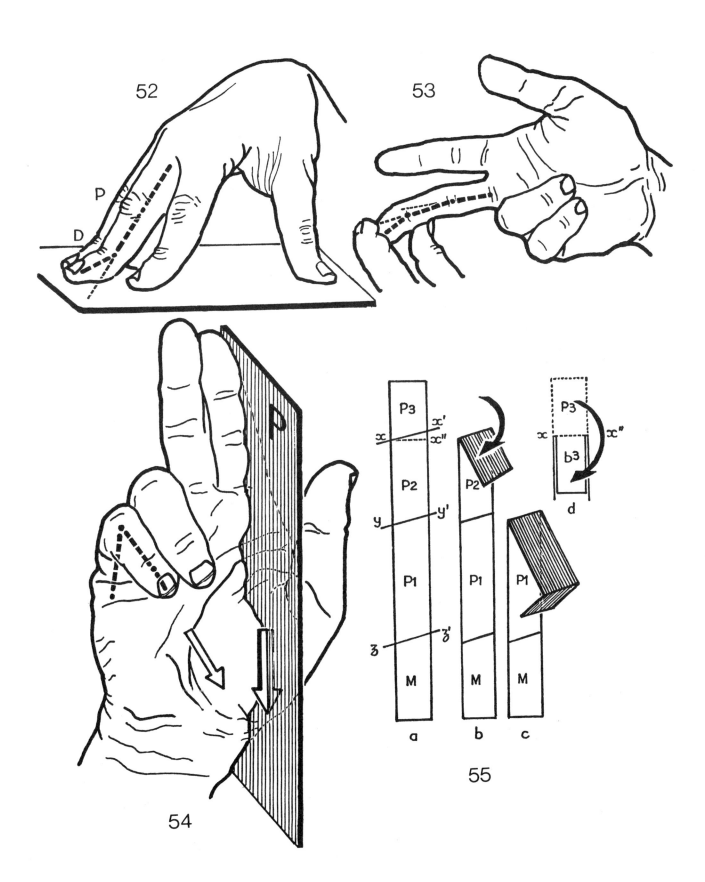

52

53

P

D

54

P

55

P3   x'
x   x''
P2

y   y'

P1

3   3'

M

a

P2

P1

M

b

P1

M

c

P3
x   x''

b3
d

189

THE TUNNELS AND SYNOVIAL SHEATHS OF THE FLEXOR TENDONS

During their course through the concavities of the hand these tendons have to be tethered to the bones by **fibrous tunnels** or else they would under tension assume a straight path rather than follow the arches formed by the bones. This would mean a relative lengthening of the tendons with respect to the skeleton and so a decrease in efficiency.

The two sides of the carpal gutter are bridged (Fig. 56) by the **flexor retinaculum** and this forms the first fibro-osseous tunnel of the hand, the **carpal tunnel** (Fig. 57, according to Rouvière). This tunnel allows through all the flexor tendons (white arrow) as they pass from the forearm into the hand.

The **section of the carpal tunnel** (Fig. 58) shows in two planes the superficial (2) and deep flexors (3) as well as the flexor pollicis longus (4). The tendon of the flexor carpi radialis (5) traverses a special compartment of its own before reaching its insertion into the second metacarpal base (Fig. 57). The median nerve (6) also traverses the carpal tunnel (where it can be compressed), unlike the ulnar nerve (7) which, with its companion artery, passes through a special canal (the canal of Guyon) in front of the retinaculum.

At the level of the fingers the flexor tendons are tethered by three **fibrous sheaths or pulleys** (Figs. 56 & 59): the first (8) lies just proximal to the metacarpal head, the second (9) on the palmar surface of P_1, the third (10) on the same surface of P_2. These form fibro-osseous tunnels along with the slightly concave palmar surfaces of the phalanges (inset, Fig. 56). Between these three sheaths the tendons are held down by annular oblique and cruciate fibres (11), which crisscross the MP and PIP joints.

The **synovial sheaths** (like brake linings) *allow smooth gliding of the tendons within their tunnels.*

The **synovial sheaths of the middle fingers** have the simplest structure (Fig. 60: simplified diagram). The tendon (only one shown for clarity) is surrounded by a **synovial sleeve** (part of which has been cut here), which consists of two layers: a *visceral layer* (a) investing the tendon and a *parietal layer* in contact with the deep surface of the fibro-osseous tunnel. Between these two layers is a potential but closed cavity (c), as the two layers are continuous with each other and have become invaginated by the tendon; section A shows this simple arrangement. During movement of the tendon within its tunnel the visceral layer, lubricated by a small quantity of synovial fluid, glides over the parietal layer. If inflammatory adhesions develop between these two layers the tendon cannot glide in its canal and becomes functionally useless, like the cable of a rusty brake.

In places (section B) this double synovial layer fails to invest the tendon completely because of the arteries of supply to the tendons and a 'mesotendon' (m) is thus formed, i.e. a sort of longitudinal sling holding the tendon within its synovial sheath (c). This description is a very simplified version, especially as regards the synovial sheaths, and for further details an anatomy textbook should be consulted.

In the palm of the hand the tendons lie embedded in **three synovial sheaths** which are, lateromedially:
— the **radiocarpal sheath** (13), investing the flexor pollicis longus and continuous with the digital sheath of the thumb.
— the **intermediate sheath** (12), investing the tendon of flexor indicis.
— the **common flexor sheath** (14), which has three prolongations anteriorly, posteriorly and between the superficial and deep tendons (Fig. 58) and eventually becomes the sheath of the flexor digiti minimi.

Anatomically, it is worth noting that:

1. The synovial sheaths of the flexor tendons start in the forearm proximal to the flexor retinaculum (Fig. 56).

2. The sheaths of the three middle fingers extend to the middle of the palm and their superficial edges correspond to the distal palmar crease (d.p.c.) for the third and fourth fingers and to the middle palmar crease (m.p.c.) for the second finger (Fig. 56).

3. The skin creases (black arrows) on the flexor aspect of the fingers (Fig. 59) — except for the proximal crease — lie immediately proximal to the corresponding joints and at this level the skin is directly in contact with the synovial sheath, which can therefore be readily infected.

Note too that the dorsal skin creases (white arrows) are also located proximal to their joints.

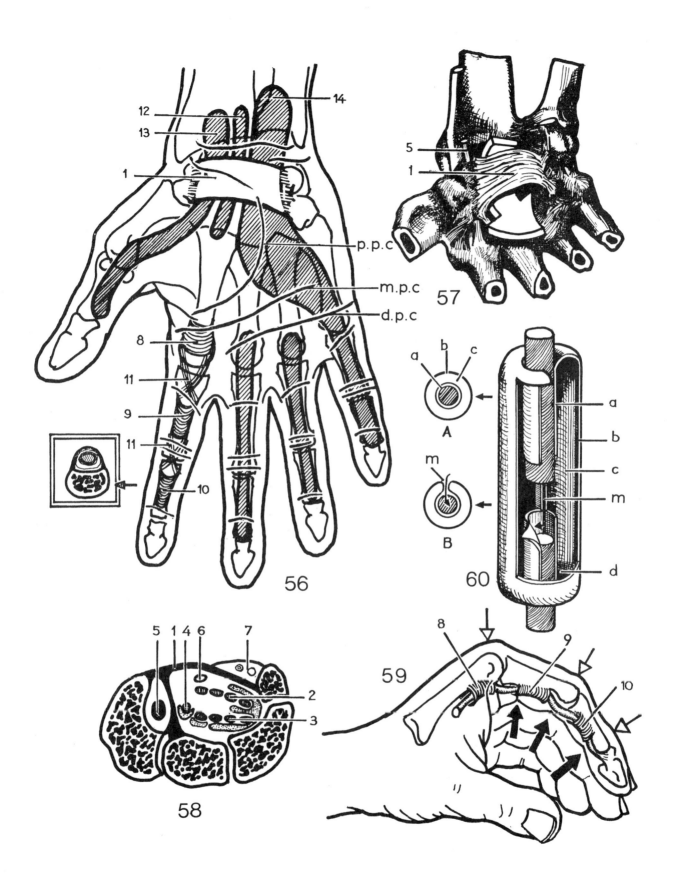

56

57

58

60

59

A

B

THE TENDONS OF THE LONG FLEXORS OF THE FINGERS

The fleshy bellies of the digital flexors lie in the anterior compartment of the forearm and so can be considered as **extrinsic musles** as regards the hand. Their course across the wrist and the palm of the hand has been studied already and their insertions and actions will now be discussed.

The most superficial muscle, the flexor digitorum sublimis (FDS) (not striped in Fig. 61a), must have its insertion proximal (i.e. on the second phalanx) to that of the deep muscle, the flexor digitorum profundus (FDP) (striped in Fig. 61a). *Therefore inevitably these two tendons must cross each other in space and they must do so symmetrically* to avoid any unwanted lateral component of force. The only way in which this can be accomplished is for **one tendon to pass through the other** and it is the *profundus* that 'perforates' the *sublimis*. This is shown as follows in the classical anatomical diagram (Fig. 61):

The sublimis tendon (b) divides into two slips at the level of the MP joint and these two slips wrap themselves round the profundus tendon (c) and re-unite at the PIP joint proximal to their insertion into the sides of the shaft of the second phalanx. This is further illustrated in the projected view (Fig. 62) which also shows the mesotendons (cf. Fig. 60).

The blood vessels for the tendons run through these *mesotendons* and are distributed as follows (Lundborg et al) (Fig. 62):

The *blood supply to FDS consists of:*

— proximally (zone A), small, longitudinal, intratendinous vessels (1) and vessels coursing down at the proximal end of the synovial sheath (2).

— distally (zone B), vessels running through the short mesotendon (3) at the level of the tendinous insertions into P_2

In the middle there is an *avascular zone* located at the point of division of the tendon.

The *blood supply to FDP consists of:*

— proximally (zone A), blood vessels (5 and 6) similar to those of the FDS

— in the intermediate zone (zone B), vessels running through the long and short mesotendons (7)

— distally (zone C), vessels running through the short mesotendons attached to the P_3 (8).

Thus for the FDP there are *3 avascular zones:*

— a short zone (9) betwee A and B

— a short zone (10) between B and C

— a peripheral zone (11), 1 mm wide and equal to a quarter of the tendon diameter, and related to the PIP joint.

The hand surgeon must be familiar with the blood supply of these tendons if he wants to preserve them in optimal condition. Moreover sutures placed in these avascular zones run a higher risk of giving way.

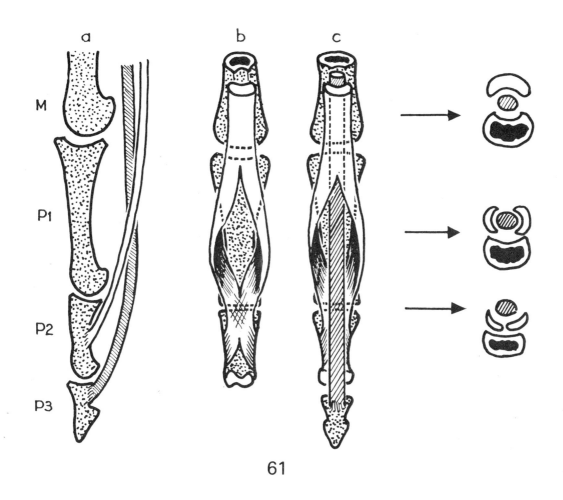

61

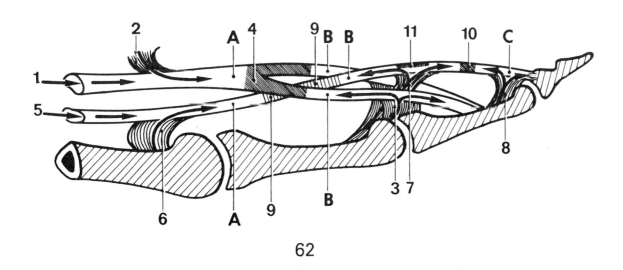

62

THE TENDONS OF THE LONG FLEXORS OF THE FINGERS (continued)

A simpler arrangement is theoretically possible (with the profundus tendons inserted into P_2 and the sublimis into P_3), and the *need for the complicated crossing of the tendons is not immediately apparent*. Without being guilty of teleological reasoning, one must point out that (Fig. 63) by staying superficial right down to its insertion, the sublimis tendon forms a *greater angle of contact with the bone* than it would be running close to the bony skeleton of the hand. This enhances its efficiency and explains why the sublimis tendon is perforated by the profundus.

The action of these two muscles can be deduced from their points of insertion:

1. **Flexor digitorum sublimis** (FDS) (Fig. 63) is inserted into P_2 and so *flexes the PIP* joint. It has no effect on the DIP joint and is a weak flexor of the MP joint, and only when the PIP joint is fully flexed.

Its *efficiency is maximal when the MP joint is extended by contraction of the extensor digitorum* (synergistic action).

Its angle of contact with P_2 increases as the proximal PIP joint is flexed and so does its efficiency.

2. **Flexor digitorum profundus** (FDP) (Fig. 64) inserted at the base of P_3, is primarily *a flexor of the DIP joint* but flexion of this joint is soon followed by flexion of the PIP joint which has no special extensor to antagonise this action. Therefore to assess the strength of the flexor profundus, *the PIP joint must be kept extended passively*.

When the MP and PIP joints are flexed passively to 90° the profundus cannot flex the distal IP joint because it has become too slack for any useful contraction: *it works at its best advantage when the MP joint is kept extended by extension of the extensor digitorum* (synergistic action).

Despite these limitations, the FDP is a functionally important muscle, as will be illustrated later. The *radial extensors* (RE), i.e. extensor radialis longus and brevis and extensor carpi ulnaris, and the *extensor digitorum communis* (EDC) are *synergistic with the flexors* (Fig. 65).

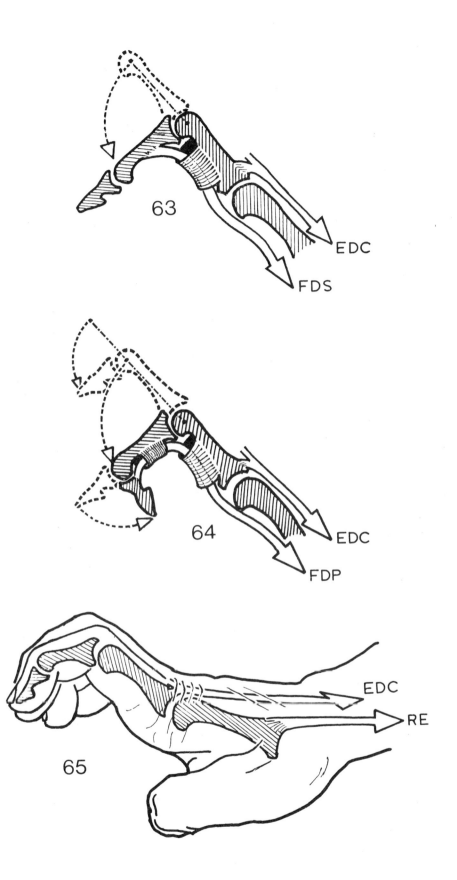

63

EDC

FDS

64

EDC

FDP

65

EDC

RE

195

THE TENDONS OF THE EXTENSOR MUSCLES OF THE FINGERS

These extensors are also **extrinsic muscles** of the hand and they also run along fibro-osseous tunnels but, since their course on the whole is convex, these tunnels are less numerous than in the case of the flexors. They are only seen at the wrist where the tendons become concave outwards during extension. The fibro-osseous tunnel is constituted by the distal ends of the radius and ulna and the **extensor retinaculum** (Fig. 66) and is **subdivided into six tunnels** by fibrous bands running from the retinaculum to the bone. These tunnels contain the following tendons, mediolaterally (from left to right in diagram):

1. The extensor carpi ulnaris

2. The extensor digiti minimi, which joins more distally the tendon of the extensor digitorum communis for the little finger

3. The four tendons of the extensor digitorum communis accompanied deeply by the extensor indicis, which joins distally the tendon of the extensor digitorum for the index

4. Extensor pollicis longus

5. Extensor radialis brevis and extensor radialis longus

6. Extensor pollicis brevis and abductor pollicis longus.

In these fibro-osseous tunnels the tendons are invested by synovial sheaths which extend beyond the retinaculum both proximally and distally (Fig. 67).

Functionally the **extensor digitorum communis is essentially an extensor of the MP joint.**

It is a powerful extensor and active *in all positions of the wrist* (Fig. 69). It extends the MP joint via the extensor expansion (Fig. 68). This expansion is 10 to 12 mm long and arises from the deep surface of the tendon, crosses the capsule of the MP joint without blending with its main fibres and is inserted at the base of P_1 along with the distal fibres of the capsule. This is shown in Figure 68a, (seen from the back), where the tendon has been partially resected to show the deep expansion (1).

On the other hand, its **action on the PIP joint** — by means of the median band (2) — and **on the DIP joint** — by means of the two lateral bands (3) — **depends on the degree of tension in the tendon** and so on **the position of the wrist** (Fig. 69). It **also depends on the degree of flexion at the MP joint**. This action is appreciable when the wrist is flexed (A), partial and weak when the wrist is straight (B) and negligible when the wrist is extended (C).

In fact, the action of the extensor digitorum communis on P_2 and P_3 depends on the degree of tension in the digital flexors:

— if these are taut because the wrist or the MP joint is extended, the extensor digitorum by itself cannot extend these IP joints.

— if, on the other hand, these flexors are relaxed by flexion of the wrist or the MP joint or are sectioned, the extensor digitorium can easily extend these IP joints.

The tendons of the **extensor indicis and extensor digiti minimi** behave in the same way as those of the extensor digitorum with which they blend. *They allow the index and little finger to be extended singly* (e.g. when 'making horns' with index and little finger).

The accessory movements of the extensor tendons of the index are (Duchenne de Boulogne) *adduction* and *abduction* (Fig. 70); the extensor indicis adducts while the extensor digitorum abducts, only when the interossei are out of action, i.e. with the PIP and DIP flexed and the MP joint extended.

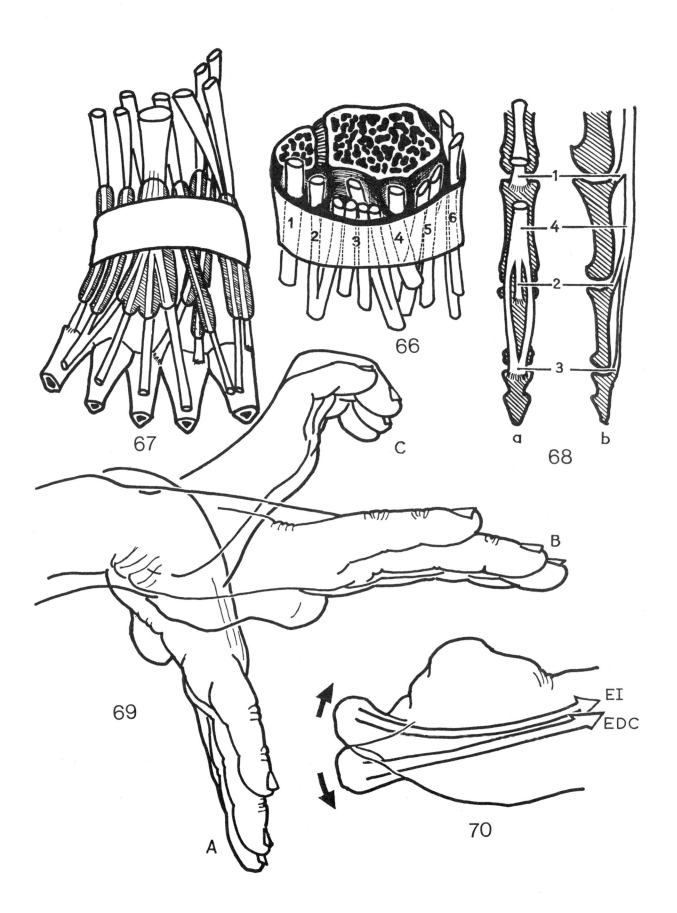

66

67

68

a   b

C

B

69

A

70

EI
EDC

THE INTEROSSEOUS AND LUMBRICAL MUSCLES

The **attachments of the interossei** (summarised diagramatically in Figs. 71–73) will not be described in detail, since we are only interested in the way these insertions influence the actions of the muscles. Functionally the interossei have **two actions**: adduction and abduction and flexion and extension.

Their **ability to adduct or abduct the fingers** depends on the attachment of part of their tendon insertion to the *lateral tuberosity of the base of P_1* (1). This action of these muscles is such a distinctive one that occasionally it is subserved by a separate belly of muscle (as seen with the first posterior interosseus, according to Winslow).

The direction of the muscle determines whether *the finger is abducted or adducted*: if the muscle *runs towards the axis of the hand*, i.e. the middle finger — e.g. **posterior interossei** (vertically striped, Figs. 71–73) — *abduction* is produced (white arrows, Fig. 71).

After giving off its tendon of insertion (1) to the lateral tuberosity of the base of P_1 the tendon of the interosseus gives off a *fibrous band* which runs on the posterior surface of P_1 to blend with similar fibres from the contralateral muscle. This is the **extensor expansion** (2). When this expansion is viewed from its deep surface (Fig. 75, with the phalanges removed) it is seen to consist of two parts: a thick part (2) and a thin part (2'). The latter, made up of *oblique fibres*, blends with the lateral bands of the extensor digitorum tendon (7). The former (2) glides on the posterior surface of P_1 and of the MP joint with an intervening *synovial bursa* (9), distal to which arises the deep median band of the extensor digitorium communis (4).

A **third expansion** of the interosseous tendon consists of a *thin fibrous band* (3), which divides into two groups of fibres before blending with the fibres of the extensor digitorum tendon: (a) the *triangular band* (10) formed by a few oblique fibres running towards the median band of the extensor digitorum; (b) the rest of the fibres which blend with the lateral band of the extensor digitorum communis tendon just before the DIP joint to form a small lateral band inserted into P_3 along with similar fibres from the contralateral muscle (12).

N.B. — (Fig. 76) — the lateral band (12) does not run posterior to the PIP joint but posterolaterally and is tethered *to the side of the capsule* by a few transverse fibres [the so-called *capsular expansion* (11)].

It is clear that if the second and third interossei contract simultaneously their action on the middle finger is balanced out. Abduction of the little finger is produced by the abductor digiti minimi (5) (Fig. 59), which is similar to a posterior interosseus. Abduction of the thumb produced by the abductor pollicis brevis (6) is of small range and is compensated by the action of the abductor pollicis longus, which acts on the first carpometacarpal joint.

When the muscles *run away from the axis of the hand* — **anterior interossei** (horizontally striped, Figs. 72–73) — they *adduct* the fingers (white arrows, Fig. 72).

The tendons of the interossei, lying within fibrous sheaths continuous with the transverse intermetacarpal ligament, cannot be subluxated anteriorly during flexion of the MP joints, as they are kept in place by the anteriorly located transverse ligament. The first posterior interosseus lacks this support and, when its fibrous sheath is damaged in rheumatoid arthritis, its tendon slips anteriorly and it is changed from an abductor to a flexor muscle.

N.B. — The posterior interossei are larger and more powerful than the anterior interossei, which are thus less efficient in approximating the fingers.

To understand fully the **actions of these muscles in flexion and extension** of the fingers the *extensor expansion* must first be described in detail (Figs. 74–76).

The four **lumbrical muscles** (Fig. 77), numbered lateromedially arise from the radial aspects of the tendons of the FDP. Their tendons (13) start to run distally and then curve medially. They are at first separated from the tendons of the interossei by the deep transverse palmar ligament so that they lie in the palmar compartment of the hand. They finally (Figs. 75 & 76) blend with the third interosseous expansion distal to the extensor expansion.

198

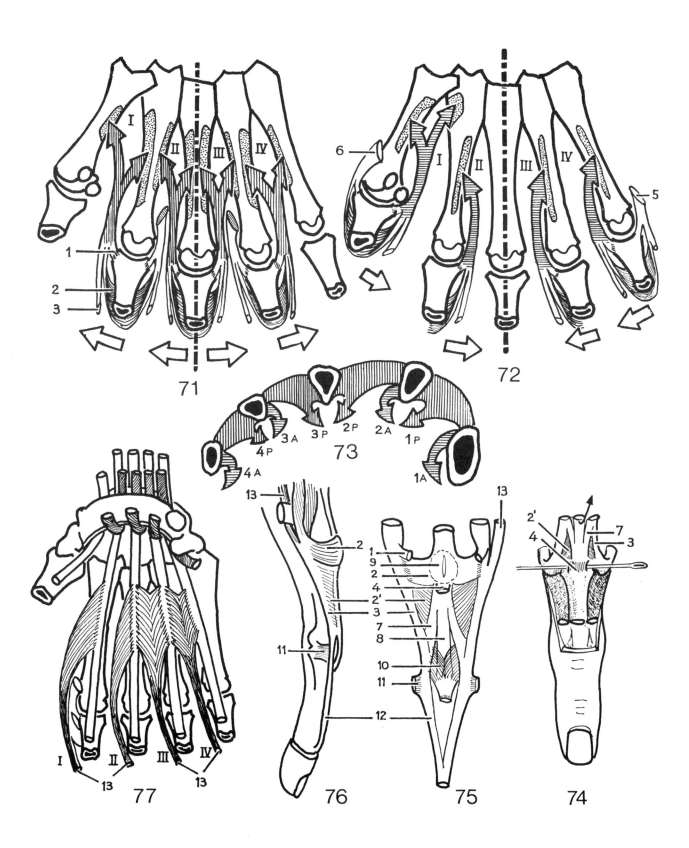

EXTENSION OF THE FINGERS

This is produced by the combined action of the extensor digitorum communis (EDC), the interossei (IO) and the lumbricals (L) and, to some extent, of the FDS. These muscles act as *synergists and antagonists*, depending on the position of the MP joint and of the wrist. The **digital retinacular ligament** plays a purely passive role in extension and coordinates the movements of the two distal phalanges.

Extensor digitorum communis (EDC)

As shown previously (p. 196), EDC is a *true extensor of the MP joint* and acts on the IP joints only when the flexors are relaxed (i.e. by wrist flexion, flexion of MP joint or surgical section of the flexor tendons). On an anatomical model traction on EDC causes complete extension of the MP joint and partial extension of the IP joints (Fig. 69, C).

The amount of tension developed in the various insertions of the EDC depends closely on the degree of flexion of the phalanges:
— Flexion of the DIP joint alone (Fig. 78) produces a 3 mm elongation of the median band and of the deep expansion of EDC so that the tendon has no longer any effect on the PIP and MP joints.
— Flexion of the PIP joint (Fig. 79) has the following two effects:

1. It produces a 3 mm elongation of the collateral expansions (a) as they 'skid' (b) forward under the pull of the capsular expansion (II, Fig. 76). During extension of the PIP joint these ligaments return to their dorsal position owing to the elasticity of the triangular band (10, Fig. 75).

2. It produces a 7 to 8 mm elongation of the deep expansion of the EDC (c), which then has no effect on the MP joint. EDC can, however, indirectly extend the MP joint by acting on the PIP joint if the latter is stabilised in flexion by the FDS, which therefore acts synergistically with the EDC during extension of the MP joint (Fig. 80). The components e'' and f'' cancel out while e' and f' add up. These last two can be further resolved into an axial component A and a normal component B (for extension); the latter therefore includes part of the force exerted by FDS (R. Tubiana and P. Valentin).

The Interossei (IO)

These *flex the MP joint and extend the IP joints* but their action on the phalanges depends on the degree of flexion of the MP joint and the state of contraction of EDC:

1. If the MP joint is extended (Fig. 81) by contraction of EDC, the extensor expansion (a) is carried proximally past the MP joint towards the posterior aspect of the metacarpal (Bunnel) and so the lateral expansion can tense up (b) and extend both IP joints.

2. If the MP joint is flexed (Fig. 82) by relaxation of EDC (a) and contraction of the lumbrical (not shown in diagram) the following consequences ensue:
— the extensor expansion is carried distally over the posterior surface of P_1 (b) for a distance of 7 mm (Bunnel);
— the interossei (c), acting on the extensor expansions, flex the MP joint powerfully;
— as a result of the latter, the lateral expansions, held down by the extensor expansions, relax (d) and can no longer extend the IP joints, the more so as the MP joint is further flexed;
— it is at this stage that the EDC becomes an efficient extensor of the IP joints.

Therefore there is a **synergistic equilibrium** (Bunnel) between EDC and the interossei as regards extension of the IP joints (Fig. 89):
— MP joint flexed at 90°: extensor action of interossei on the IP joints is nil and the action of EDC maximal.
— MP joint extended: Extensor action of EDC on the IP joints is nil and the effect of the interossei, which retighten the lateral bands (Fig. 81, b), is maximal.
— MP joint in intermediate position: additive action of EDC and interossei.

The Lumbrical Muscles (L)

These flex the MP joint and extend the IP joints but, unlike the interossei, they do so **whatever the degree of flexion of the MP joint**. They are therefore extremely important muscles for digital movements. They owe their efficiency to two anatomical factors:
— *lying on the anterior side of the interossei* they make contact with P_1 at an angle of 35° (Fig. 83), so that they can flex the MP joint even when it is hyperextended. They are therefore the **'flexor starters' of the MP joint** with the interossei acting secondarily on the extensor expansions.
— they are inserted (Fig. 84) into the lateral extensor expansions *distal to the extensor expansions* and so are not tethered by these. Hence their ability to retighten the extensor expansions of P_2 and P_3, whatever the degree of flexion of the MP joint.

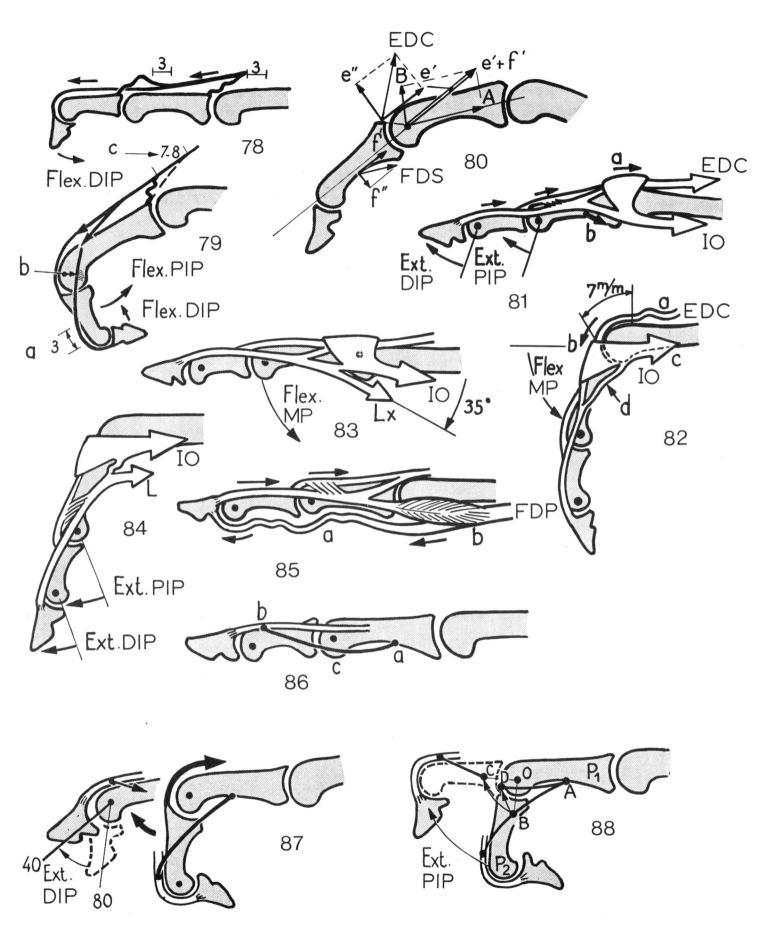

MP = metacarpophalangeal joint. PIP = proximal interphalangeal joint.
DIP = distal interphalangeal joint

Eyler and Marquee, and Landsmeer have shown that in some people the interossei contain two separate insertions, one for the extensor expansion, the other for the lateral expansion. The lumbrical muscles, according to Recklinghausen, promote extension of the IP joints (Fig. 85) by *relaxing the distal portion of the tendons of FDP* (a), from which they arise (b). Because of their **diagonal course**, contraction of the lumbrical muscles displaces '*functionally*' the insertion of FDP from the anterior to the dorsal aspect of P_3 and thus transforms FDP into an extensor muscle like an interosseus. This system is similar to a *transistor* which shunts current in one direction or the other depending on its state of excitation. This 'transistor effect' makes use of a weak muscle — the lumbrical — to divert the power of a strong muscle (FDP) into the extensor grid.

From their numerous **proprioceptive receptors** the lumbrical muscles gather essential information for **the coordination of the extensors and flexors, between which two groups they run transversely.**

The retinacular ligament of the digits (RL)

This ligament (Landsmeer 1949) consists of a band of fibres (Fig. 86) arising from the anterior surface of P_1 (a), and blending with the lateral extensor expansion over P_2 and P_3 (b). But, unlike the lateral expansions, its fibres run *anterior to the axis* of the PIP joint. Therefore (Fig. 87) **extension of this joint tenses up the fibres of the RL and causes passive extension of the DIP joint** with a range equal to half the maximum; in other words, the DIP joint moves from a position of flexion of 80° to one of 40°. This tightening of the RL by extension of the PIP joint is easily demonstrated (Fig. 88). If RL is cut at B, extension of the PIP joint is not automatically followed by extension of the DIP joint and the two cut ends of RL are separated by a distance CD (where D represents the final position assumed by B after rotation about centre A and C is that assumed by B after rotation about centre O).

Conversely, with RL intact, passive flexion of the DIP joint causes automatic flexion of the PIP joint.

Pathological retraction of RL fixes the hand in a 'buttonhole' deformity, following rupture of the extensor expansion, and causes hyperextension of the DIP joint in advanced cases of Dupuytren's contracture.

Summary of the actions of the flexor and extensor muscles of the fingers

Extension of the MP and IP joints (Fig. 89A): Synergism of EDC + Interossei + Lumbricals. RL passively and automatically active.

Extension of the MP joint: EDC
+ flexion of the PIP joints: FDS (Agonist of EDC) } relaxation of
    + flexion of the DIP joint: FDP   } interossei
+ flexion of the PIP joint: FDS (as above),
    + extension of the DIP joint: Lumbricals and interossei
                        (this movement is very difficult).

Flexion of the MP-joint: lumbricals ('flexor starters')
  + interossei (antagonism of EDC/interossei with relaxation of EDC)
  + extension of the PIP and DIP joints (Fig. 89C): lumbricals (extensors in all positions of the MP joint) + synergistic action of EDC + interossei (Fig. 89B)
  + flexion of the PIP joint: FDS,
    + extension of the DIP joint: Lumbricals (difficult movement because flexion of the DIP joint relaxes the lateral expansions),
  + flexion of the PIP joint: FDS,
    + flexion of the DIP joint (its action becomes easier because of the 'skidding' of the lateral expansions during flexion of the PIP joint).

N.B. — The everyday movements of the fingers are compounded of these elementary movements:
— during writing (Duchenne de Boulogne): when the pencil is moved forward (Fig. 90) the interosseus flexes the MP joint and extends the PIP and DIP joints; when the pencil is brought back (Fig. 91) EDC extends the MP joint and the FDS flexes the PIP joint.
— when the hand assumes the **shape of a hook** (Fig. 92) FDS and FDP both contract and the interossei relax. This movement is essential for the mountain climber as he clutches at a vertical face of rock.
— when the hand assumes the **shape of a hammer** (Fig. 93) the EDC extends the MP joint while FDS and FDP flex the PIP and DIP joints. This is the initial position of the pianist's fingers. The hand strikes the keys as a result of contraction of the interossei and lumbricals which flex the MP joint when the EDC relaxes.

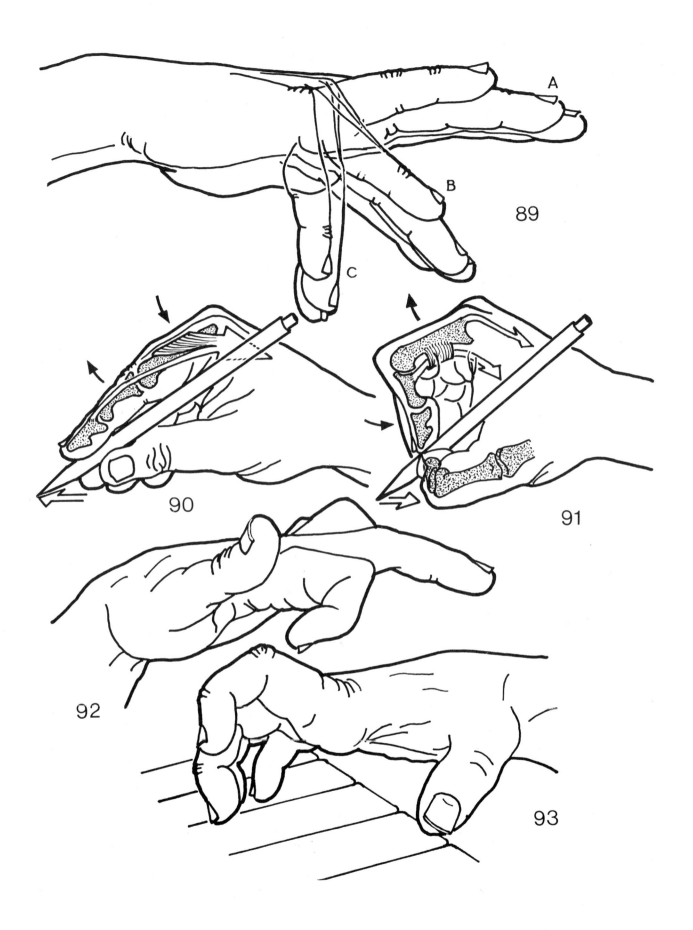

89

90

91

92

93

203

ABNORMAL POSITIONS OF THE HAND AND FINGERS

These can result from either underactivity or overactivity of the muscles described. The following conditions cause *abnormal positions* of the fingers (Fig. 94):

(a) **Tearing of the extensor expansion** at the level of the triangular band, which runs between the two lateral bands and whose elasticity is necessary to restore their dorsal position during extension of the PIP joint. This causes the posterior surface of the PIP joint to herniate through the torn expansion and the lateral bands to become displaced to the sides of the joint, which *stays in midflexion*. This can also be produced by section of the extensor digitorum communis at the PIP joint ('buttonhole deformity').

(b) **Rupture of the extensor tendon just proximal to its insertion into P₃** causes *flexion of the DIP joint* which can be reduced passively but not actively. The flexion results from the tone of the FDP now unbalanced by the EDC. This is the 'mallet finger'.

(c) **Rupture of the extensor tendon just proximal to the MP joint** leads to *flexion of the MP joint*, which results from the now predominating action of the extensor expansion.

(d) **Rupture or paralysis of FDS** leads to hyperextension of the PIP joint because of the greater activity of the interossei. This *'inverted' position* of the PIP joint is accompanied by a slight flexion at the DIP joint due to a relative shortening of the FDP following hyperextension at the PIP joint.

(e) **Paralysis or section of the FDP tendon** prevents any active flexion of the DIP joint.

(f) **Paralysis of the interossei** is followed by hyperextension at the MP joint due to the action of EDC, and by increased flexion at the PIP and DIP joints by the FDS and FDP.

Therefore paralysis of the intrinsic muscles breaks the longitudinal arch of the hand at the level of its keystone. This 'claw hand' position (Fig. 96) is seen mainly with **paralysis of the ulnar nerve** which supplies the interossei. It is also associated with atrophy of the hypothenar eminence and interosseous spaces.

The loss of the extensors of the wrist and digits, most commonly caused by **radial nerve paralysis**, produces *'wrist drop'* (Fig. 95), i.e. increased flexion of the wrist, flexion of MP joint and extension of the DIP joint due to the interossei.

In **Dupuytren's contracture** (Fig. 97), caused by shortening of the pretendinous fibres of the central palmar aponeurosis, *the fingers are irreducibly flexed* i.e. flexion of the MP and PIP joints and extension of the DIP joint. The last two fingers are usually most severely involved, the middle finger later in the disease and the thumb only exceptionally.

In **Volkmann's contracture** (Fig. 98), caused by *ischaemic contracture of the flexor muscles*, the fingers assume a hook-like position, which is obvious especially during extension (a) of the wrist and becomes less so as the wrist is flexed (b).

The hand can also adopt a hook-like position (Fig. 99) in **suppurative synovitis of the common flexor sheath**. This is most marked in the medial digits, being maximal in the small finger. Any attempt at extending the fingers is exquisitely painful.

Finally the hand may be fixed in a position of **massive ulnar drift** (Fig. 100), when all the fingers are markedly deviated medially so that the metacarpal heads are abnormally prominent. This deformity allows one to make a (retrospective) diagnosis of rheumatoid arthritis.

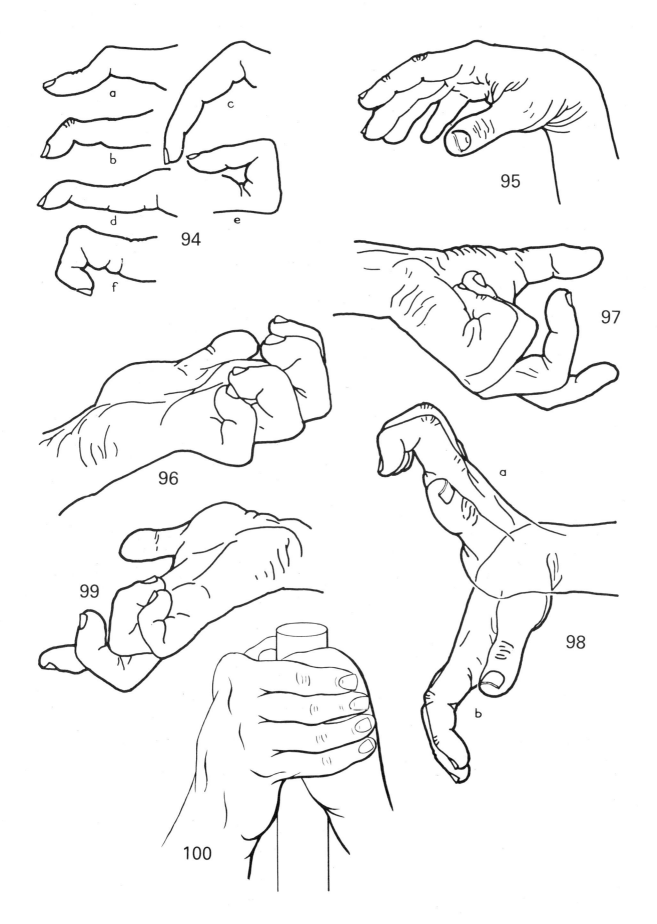

94

95

96

97

98

99

100

205

THE MUSCLES OF THE HYPOTHENAR EMINENCE

The hypothenar eminence contains *3 muscles* (Fig. 101):

1. **Flexor digiti minimi** (1) inserted into the ulnar aspect of the base of P_1, runs obliquely distally and medially from its fleshy origin from the palmar surface of the **flexor** retinaculum **and** the hook of the hamate.

2. **Adductor digiti minimi** (2), which moves the finger towards the trunk, is inserted like an interosseus. Its flat tendon divides into two slips: one is inserted (along with the **flexor digiti** minimi) into the ulnar aspect of the base of P_1 and the other into the ulnar border of the **dorsal** digital expansion of EDC. It arises from the palmar aspect of the flexor retinaculum and the **palmar** surface of the pisiform bone.

3. **Opponens digiti minimi** (3) is inserted into the whole length of the ulnar margin of the fifth metacarpal. It runs over the anterior border of the metacarpal (Fig. 102) (white arrow) distally and medially from its origin from the distal border of the flexor retinaculum and the hook of the hamate.

The **physiological actions** of these muscles are as follows:

The *opponens* (Fig. 102) *flexes the fifth carpometacarpal joint* about the axis XX′. During flexion the metacarpal is pulled *anteriorly* (arrow 1) and *laterally* (arrow 2) and this oblique direction of movement is the same as that of the long axis of the muscle. But, at the same time, it rotates the metacarpal around its long axis (marked by a cross) in the direction of the arrow 3 so that the *anterior aspect of the metacarpal now faces laterally towards the thumb*. Hence its name of opponens is justified.

Flexor digiti minimi (1) and *abductor digiti minimi* (2) have roughly similar actions (Fig. 103).

Flexor digiti minimi (1) flexes the MP joint and *abducts the fifth finger* from the axis of the hand.

Abductor digiti minimi (2) also *abducts* the finger from the axis of the hand and so can be considered as similar to a *posterior interosseus*. Like the interossei it flexes the MP joint by acting on the digital interosseous expansion and *extends the two IP joints* by acting on the lateral extensor expansions.

206

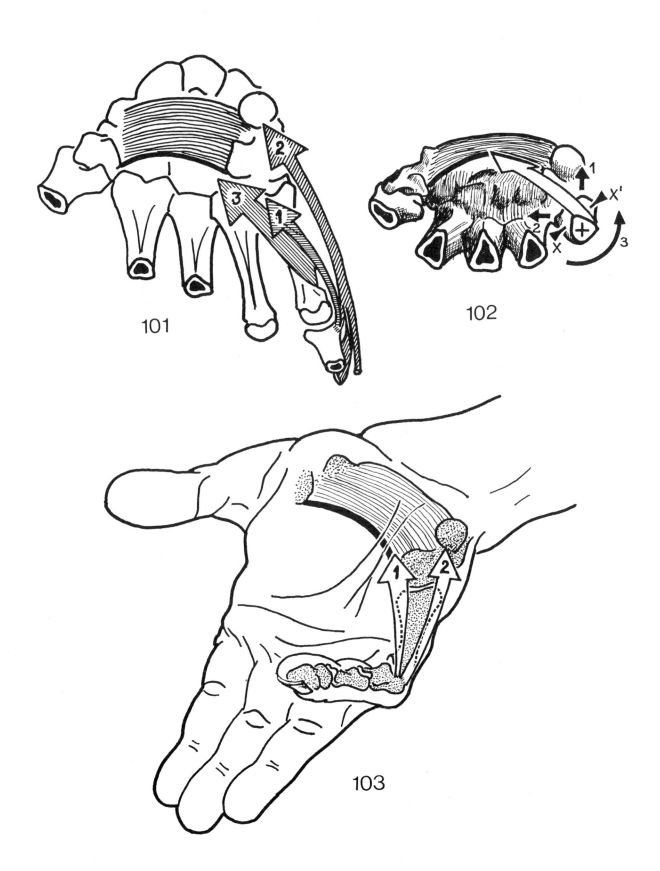

101

102

103

THE THUMB

The thumb plays a unique role in the function of the hand, being essential for the formation of the *pollici-digital pincers* and for the development of a *powerful grip* along with the other fingers. It can also take part in *dynamic grips* (grips associated with actions). Thus, without the thumb, the hand loses most of its capabilities.

This preeminent role of the thumb is partly due to its *location anterior to the palm and the other fingers* (Fig. 104), which allows the thumb to move towards the fingers individually or together (the *movement of opposition*) and away from them (the *movement of counteropposition*). It is also due to its remarkable *functional suppleness* secondary to the peculiar organization of its *osteo-articular column* and its *motor muscles*.

The **osteo-articular column of the thumb** (Fig. 105) consists of five bony structures lying along the lateral border of the hand:

— the scaphoid (S)

— the trapezium (TZ), which embryologically is homologous to a metacarpal

— the first metacarpal (M_1)

— the first phalanx (P_1)

— the second phalanx (P_2)

Anatomically the thumb has only two phalanges but, importantly so, its column is attached to the hand at a point *far more proximal* than that of the other fingers. Thus its column is far *shorter* and its tip only reaches the middle of P_1 of the index. This is in fact its *optimal length* because:

— if it is shorter (as after partial amputation), it cannot carry out opposition, being too short and unable to flex adequately so as to meet the other fingers.

— if it is longer (as the congenitally malformed thumb with three phalanges), fine opposition of termino-terminal type is hampered by the inadequate degree of flexion at the DIP joint of the finger involved.

This illustrates *Occam's principle of universal economy*, which states that optimal function is ensured by a minimum of structural components and organization. Thus for the thumb *optimal function requires five components*.

There are *four joints in the column of the thumb*:

— the scapho-trapezian joint (ST), which, as we have already seen (p. 150), allows the trapezium to move anteriorly for a short distance along the distal surface of the scaphoid bearing the tubercle. Here a movement of flexion of small range is initiated.

— the *trapezo-metacarpal* joint (TM), with *two* degrees of freedom.

— the *metacarpophalangeal* joint (MP), with *two* degrees of freedom.

— the *interphalangeal joint* (IP), with only **one** degree of freedom.

In sum, **five degrees of freedom** are necessary and adequate to achieve opposition of the thumb.

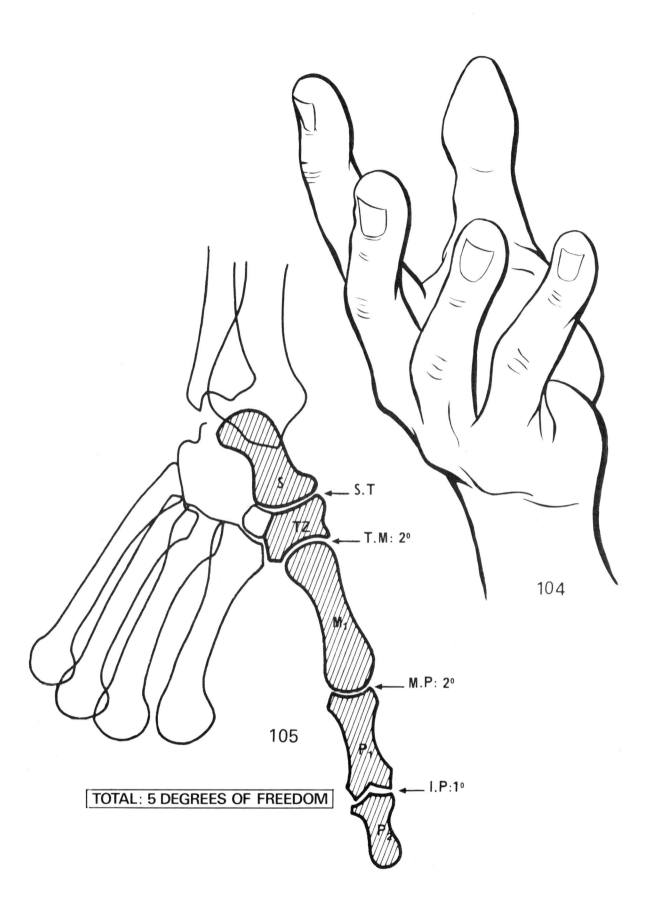

S.T

T.M: 2°

M.P: 2°

104

105

I.P: 1°

TOTAL: 5 DEGREES OF FREEDOM

209

THE GEOMETRY OF OPPOSITION OF THE THUMB

Geometrically speaking (Fig. 106), opposition of the thumb consists of bringing into contact the pulp of the thumb and that of another finger so that they touch at point A' (thumb) and A (finger). In other words, the tangential planes of the two pulps A and A' merge in space at a single point A + A'.

For two points to coincide in space (Fig. 107) *three degrees of freedom* are necessary in keeping with the three coordinates in space, x, y, z. *Two additional degrees of freedom* are needed for the planes of the pulps to coincide perfectly, i.e. two axes t and u are needed for rotation to occur. Since the pulps cannot come into contact 'back to back' a third degree of freedom about an axis v perpendicular to t and u is not necessary.

In sum, to achieve coincidence of these planes **five degrees of freedom** are necessary:

— three for coincidence of the points of contact.

— two for full coincidence of the planes of the pulps.

It can be easily demonstrated that each axis of a joint represents a degree of freedom and that these degrees of freedom can be added numerically. Thus the five degrees of freedom of the column of the thumb are both necessary and adequate to achieve opposition of the the thumb.

Let us consider only **in one plane** (Fig. 108) the movements of the three mobile segments (M_1, P_1 and P_2) of the column of the thumb about the three axes of flexion, i.e. YY' for the TM joint, f_1 for the MP joint and f_2 for the IP joint. It is clear that two degrees of freedom are necessary to place the tip of P_2 at a point H. If no movement is allowed about f_1 or f_2 then there is only one way of reaching the point H. But the use of a third degree of freedom allows H to be reached in many ways. The diagram contains two positions of the mobile segments. It is clear that *three degrees of freedom* are needed to get the tip of P_2 to lie on H in these two positions.

In space (Fig. 109) the addition of **a fourth degree of freedom** about the second axis XX' of the TM joint increases the range of orientation for the pulp of the thumb and allows a better *selection* of accurate positions for opposition with respect to each finger.

The addition of a **fifth degree of freedom** (Fig. 110), brought about by the second axis of the MP joint, allows the pulpar planes to rotate slightly with respect to each other at their point of contact and thus further improves the merging of these planes. It can be seen that the axis of flexion f_1 of the MP joint is strictly transverse only during direct flexion and is mostly *oblique* in one direction or another:

— with f_1' flexion is associated with *ulnar deviation and supination*.

— with f_1'', flexion is associated with *radial deviation and pronation*.

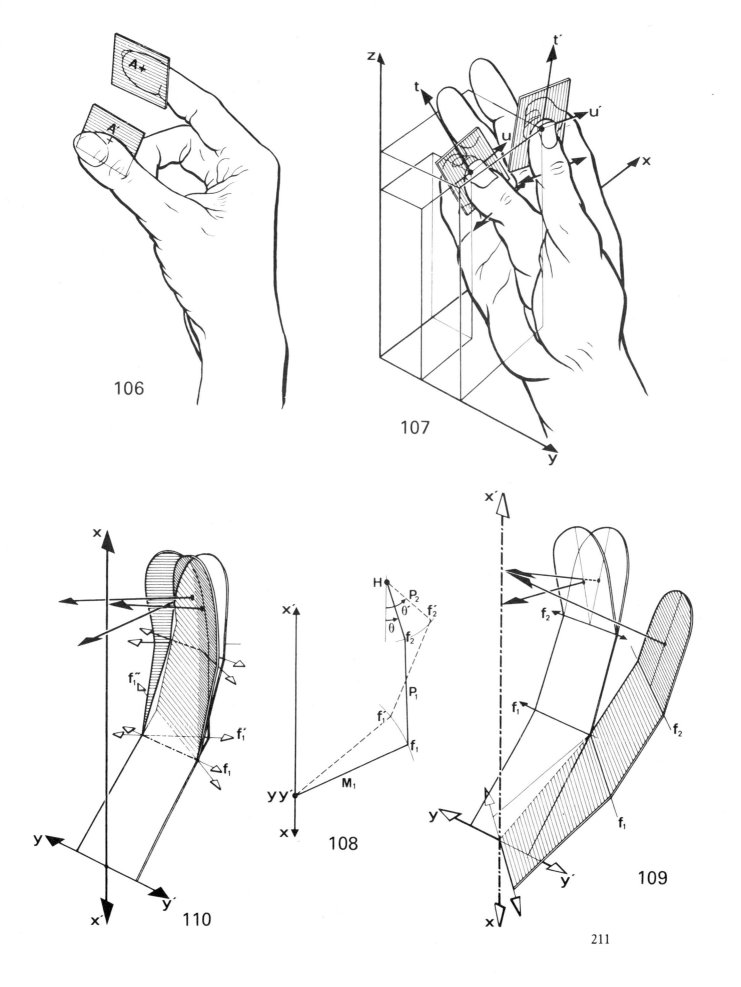

106

107

108

110

109

211

THE TRAPEZO-METACARPAL JOINT

The structure of the articular surfaces

The TM joint, lying at the base of the mobile column of the thumb, plays a vital role in movements of the thumb, especially opposition, by allowing the thumb to take up any position with respect to the hand.

It is a *saddle joint* (Fig. 111) with two saddle-shaped surfaces concave in one direction and convex in the other. These surfaces, one on the trapezium (TZ) and the other on the base of the first metacarpal (M_1), are congruent only after a 90° rotation when the convexity of one surface fits into the concavity of the other and vice versa.

The exact *contour* of these surfaces has been studied extensively but still remains controversial. The best account comes from Kuczynski (1974). When the TM joint is opened and the base of M_1 is tilted laterally (Fig. 112) the following observations can be made:

— The surface T of TZ bears a median ridge CD, which is slightly bent so that its concavity faces medially and anteriorly. The dorsal part of this ridge C is distinctly more pointed than that of the palmar part F, which is almost flat. This ridge is crossed transversely in its middle portion by a furrow AB, running from the postero-lateral border A to the anteromedial border B, where it is deeper. More importantly this furrow is curved with its convexity pointing anterolaterally. The posterolateral part E is almost flat.

— The surface of M_1 is inversely shaped with a ridge A'B' corresponding to the furrow AB of TZ and a furrow C'D' corresponding to the ridge CD on TZ.

When applied to TZ (Fig. 113) the metacarpal overhangs its borders at the ends a and b of the furrow. Also, on section (Fig. 114) it is clear that the correspondence of the surfaces is far from perfect. However, *when firmly pressed together*, the locking of the surfaces *prevents any longitudinal rotation of M_1* (Kuczynski).

Because the saddle is curved along its long axis, Kuczynski compares it to a (soft!) saddle placed on the back of a 'scoliotic horse' (Fig. 115). It can also be compared to a pass between two mountains traversed by a curved road (Fig. 116). Thus the path of a truck going uphill forms an angle r with that of the truck going downhill. According to Kuczynski this angle, which is equal to 90° between the points A and B of the furrow on TZ, accounts for the longitudinal rotation of M_1 during opposition. This could only be true if the base of M_1 traversed (as the truck on the mountain pass) the *entire length of the trapezial furrow*, which would produce total dislocation of the joint in either direction. This, of course, is not true. Hence we believe that another mechanism, to be discussed later, underlies this rotation.

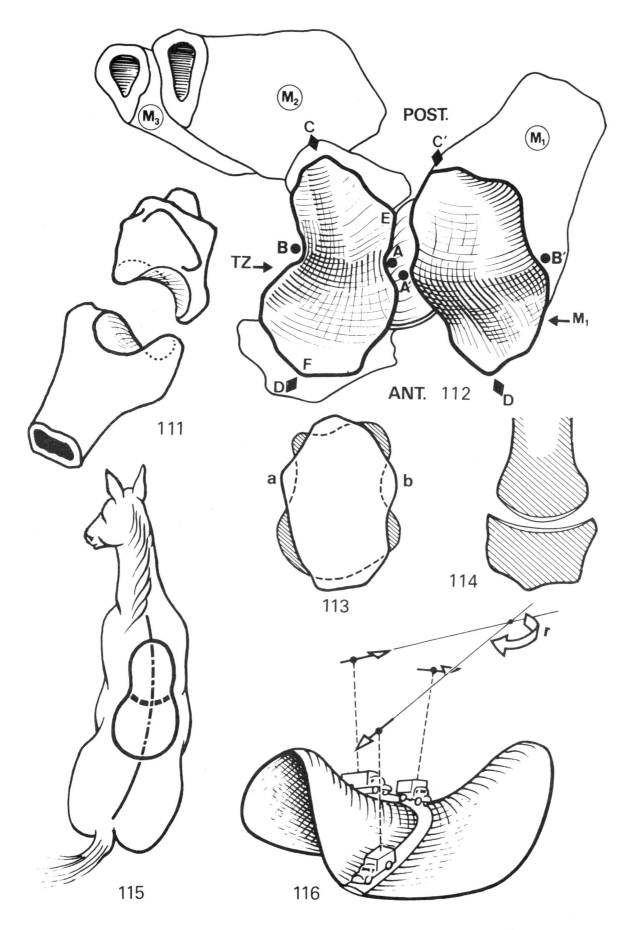

THE TRAPEZO-METACARPAL JOINT (continued)

Coaptation of articular surfaces

The capsule of the TM joint is considered to be lax with considerable play, thereby allowing M_1, according to many authors, to rotate about its long axis. This is incorrect, as will be shown later.

In fact, the laxity of the capsule only allows the articular surface of M_1 to move over that of TZ but the joint *works by axial compression*, i.e. one surface grinding on the other like a pivot (Fig. 117). Thus M_1 can assume any position in space, just like a *pylon* whose direction can be altered by shortening any one of its *stays*, which correspond here to the *thenar* muscles. These muscles therefore keep the articular surfaces together *in all positions*.

Likewise the *ligaments of the TM joint* help to keep these articular surfaces together, depending on their degree of stretching, and they also influence movements taking place at the joint. Their anatomy and functions have been recently defined by de la Caffinière (1970). Four components are recognised (Fig. 118: anterior aspect and Fig. 119: posterior aspect):

— the *intermetacarpal ligament* (IML), which is a short and thick band of fibres bridging the bases of M_1 and M_2 in the most proximal portion of the first interdigital cleft.

— the *oblique posteromedial ligament* (OPML), long recognised as a wide but thin band applied to the joint posteriorly and coursing anteriorly round the medial aspect of the base of M_1.

— the *oblique antero-medial ligament* (OAML), running from the distal tip of the ridge of TZ to the base of M_1. It crosses the anterior aspect of the joint after wrapping itself round the lateral aspect of the base of M_1.

— the *straight antero-lateral ligament* (SALL), stretching directly from TZ to the base of M_1 anterolaterally to the joint. Its medial border, well defined and sharp, bounds a small gap in the capsule, through which runs a synovial sheath for the tendon of the abductor pollicis longus (APL).

According to de la Caffinière these ligaments can be paired as follows:

— IML and SALL:

the widening and narrowing of the first interdigital cleft in the plane of the palm are checked by IML and SALL respectively.

— OPML and OAML:

they are stretched during axial rotation of M_1, with OPML limiting pronation and OAML supination.

214

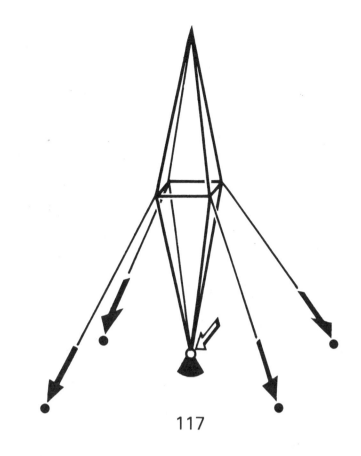

117

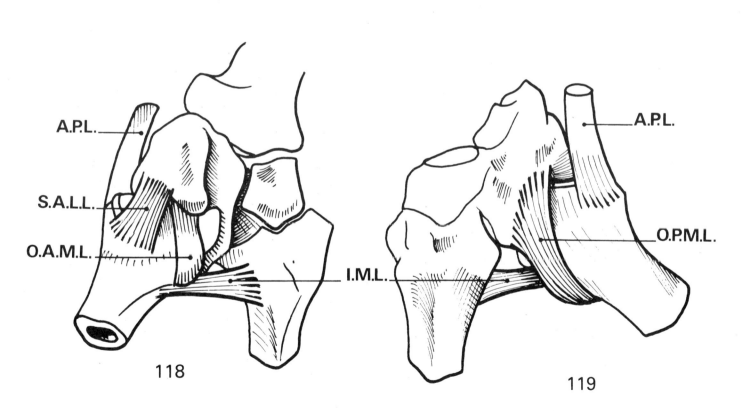

A.P.L.

S.A.L.L.

O.A.M.L.

I.M.L.

A.P.L.

O.P.M.L.

118

119

THE TRAPEZO-METACARPAL JOINT (continued)

The role of the ligaments

We feel the situation is more complex as one must also reckon with the action of the ligaments with regard to the movements of anteposition-retroposition and of flexion-extension of M_1, which will be further defined later.

During *movements of anteposition and retroposition:*

— in *anteposition* (Fig. 120: anterior view), OAML is stretched, SALL is slackened and OPML is stretched posteriorly (Fig. 121);

— in *retroposition* (Fig. 122: anterior view) SALL is stretched, OAML is slackened and OPML is slackened posteriorly (Fig. 123).

— IML (Fig. 124: anterior view) is tightened both in anteposition, when it pulls the base of M_1 towards M_2 and in retroposition, when it pulls back M_1 as it moves away on TZ. *It is relaxed only in the intermediate position.*

During *flexion and extension:*

— in *extension* (Fig. 125) the anterior ligaments SALL and OAML are stretched and OPML relaxes

— in *flexion* (Fig. 126): SALL and OAML are slackened and OPML is stretched.

Being wrapped around the base of M_1, in opposite directions (Fig. 127: an axial view of M_1 on TZ and M_2 and M_3), OPML and OAML control *longitudinal rotation* of M_1:

— OAML is stretched during pronation, so that its tension acting alone would tend to favour supination

— OPML is stretched during supination, so that its tendon acting alone would tend to favour pronation.

In *opposition*, which combines anteposition and flexion, *all the ligaments* are stretched except SALL, which runs parallel to the contracting muscles (abductor pollicis brevis, opponens pollicis, flexor pollicis brevis). It is noteworthy that the most stretched of the ligaments is OPML, which maintains joint stability posteriorly. Opposition thus corresponds to the *close-packed position*, as noted by Mac Conaill. It is the position in which the articular surfaces are most closely apposed, thus preventing, along with the two concurrently stretched oblique ligaments, any *axial rotation of M_1 that could result from any degree of 'play' within the joint. In the intermediate position*, as will be shown later, *all the ligaments are relaxed* and so 'play' within the joint is at a maximum, which, however, has no effect on axial rotation of M_1.

In *counter-opposition*, significant tension is developed only in OAML thus favouring some degree of axial rotation (supination) of M_1.

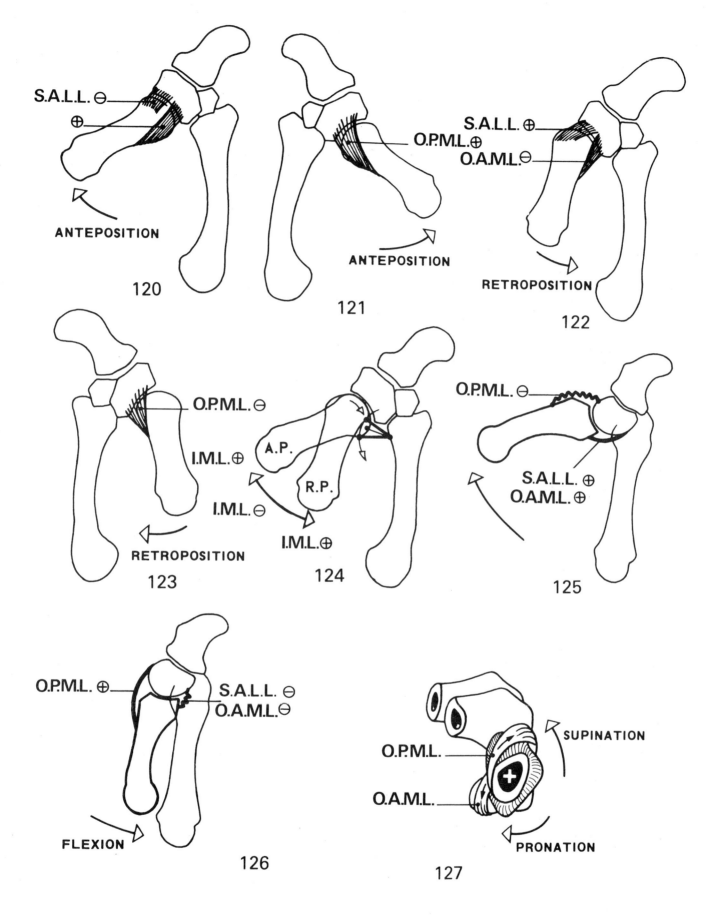

THE TRAPEZO-METACARPAL JOINT (continued)

Geometrical analysis of the articular surfaces

If free 'play' within the joint or the action of the ligaments cannot be invoked to explain axial rotation of M_1, the explanation can only rest with the structure of the articular surfaces, as with the hip joint. Mathematically speaking, *saddle-shaped surfaces* have a *negative curvature*, i.e. they are convex in one direction and concave in the other, so that they cannot be closed, unlike the sphere, which is the perfect example of positive curvature. These surfaces have been likened to a segment of a solid hyperbola (Fig. 128) (Bausenhart and Littler), or a segment of a parabolic hyperbola (Fig. 129: The hyperbola H rests on a parabola P) or to a segment of a double hyperbola (Fig. 130: the hyperbola H rests on another hyperbola H'). We feel it is more instructive to compare these saddle-shaped surfaces to an *axial segment of a torus* (annulus) (Fig. 131). The inner aspect of a tyre, which is a torus, has a concave surface with its centre lying on the axis of the wheel O and a convex surface with its centre lying on the axis of the tyre itself. (In reality there is a series of axes p, q, s etc. with q representing the mean). This surface or negative torus thus has two *main orthogonal axes* and *two degrees of freedom*. If Kuczynski's description, stressing the lateral curvature ('scoliotic horse'), is taken into account, then this axial segment must be demarcated *asymmetrically* (Fig. 132) on the surface of the torus, as if the saddle had slipped to one side on the back of a normal horse. The long axis (the ridge) of the saddle nm is bent to the side so that the radii u, v, w, passing through each point of the ridge, converge on a point O' located on the axis XX', which lies outside the plane of symmetry of the surface. However this saddle-shaped surface still remains a *negative torus* with two main orthogonal axes and two degrees of freedom. This of course is valid for a *small segment of the surface*, for otherwise the multiplicity of axes would make approximation unacceptable. In fact, as long as the surface involved is small, the successive axes (p, q, s . . .) are close enough to be viewed as identical. This applies to the articular surface of TZ and M_1 with their relatively small curvatures (less marked than shown in the diagrams).

Under these conditions, it is logical and permissible to *construct a theoretical model of the TM joint*, even as, in biomechanics, the model used for the hip-joint is that of a ball-and-socket model, although it is well known that the femoral head is not perfectly spherical.

The **mechanical model** of a biaxial joint is the **universal joint** (Fig. 133), with its two orthogonal axes XX' and YY' allowing movements in two planes AB and CD at right angles. In the same way, two saddle-shaped surfaces lying one on the other (Fig. 134) allow relative movements AB and CD to occur in two planes at right angles (Fig. 135).

But a study of the mechanics of the universal joint shows that biaxial joints have an accessory movement, i.e. *automatic rotation of the moving part on its long axis*.

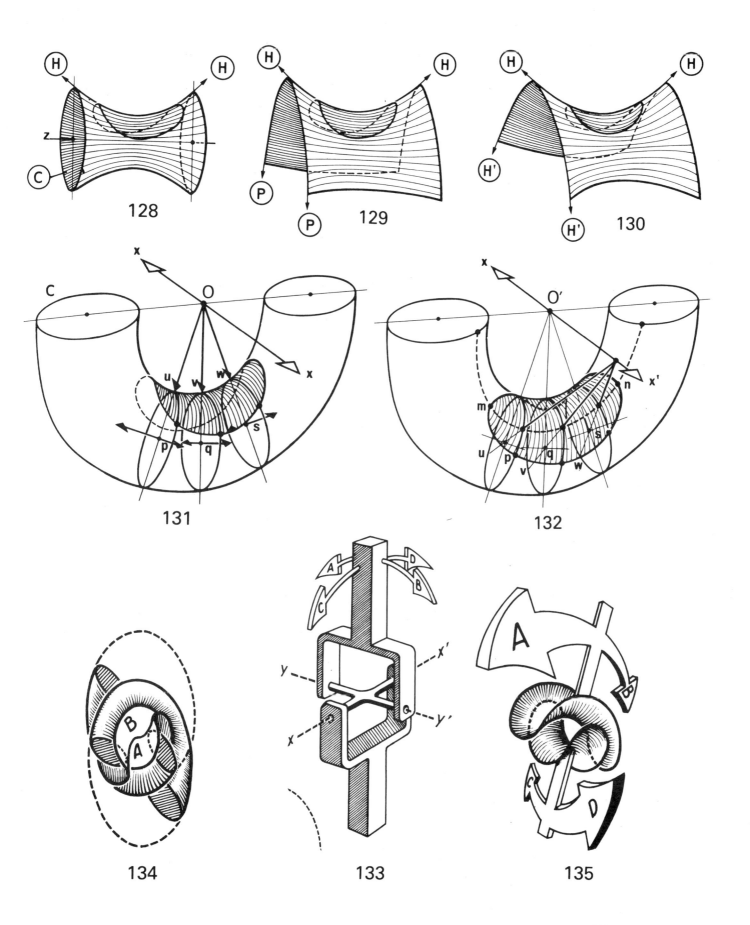

128

129

130

131

132

134

133

135

219

THE TRAPEZO-METACARPAL JOINT (continued)

Axial rotation of M_1

It is easy to construct a universal joint by cutting up pieces of cardboard and sticking them together (Fig. 136). To either side of the disc stick the semi-circular surfaces of the two strips b and c, folded at right angles along the lines 1–2 and 3–4. This *model of a universal joint* (you should try it!) will allow the physical demonstration of *automatic rotation of the moving part on its long axis.*

Let us note first (Fig. 137) that when one part is kept fixed the other can be moved about the two axes of the joint. When moving around the axis 1–2, the moving part (movement a) stays in the same plane, but as it moves about the axis 3–4 (movement b), it now forms a solid angle with its starting position.

If the part (Fig. 138) is moved again about the axis 1–2, without prior flexion or extension about the axis 3–4 which thus stays perpendicular to the moving part, it is clear that the moving part always 'faces' the same way, as shown by the arrows. It is thus a *pure rotation* in the same plane, as seen in hinge joints where the axis of movement is perpendicular to the moving part.

If the moving part (Fig. 139) is first 'flexed' through an angle b (less than 90°) about the axis 3–4, as shown by the small arrow, rotation about axis 1–2 leads to a change in the orientation of the moving part, demonstrated here by the large arrows pointing to a point P lying on the extended axis 1–2. This change of orientation of the moving part, as it goes through a *conical rotation*, underlies its *automatic axial rotation* (Mac Conaill's *conjunct rotation*). It is seen in hinge joints with one axis lying obliquely with respect to the moving part, when it is of *constant magnitude*. It can also vary in magnitude in relation to the degree of prior 'flexion'. Its value can be calculated using a simple trigonometrical formula.

A special case exists when prior flexion about axis 3–4 is exactly 90° (Fig. 140). Then the moving part goes through a *cylindrical rotation* about the axis 1–2, so that every degree of voluntary rotation is matched by an additional component of automatic rotation, which therefore is maximal.

Of course, between the two extreme values of automatic rotation associated with rotation in the same plane (nil) and cylindrical rotation (maximum), an infinite number of intermeidate values are possible.

It is also possible to demonstrate this cylindrical rotation (Fig. 141) if three hinged segments are attached to the universal joint at the axis 3–4, which is parallel to the other axes 5–6 and 7–8. Ninety degree flexion about the axis 3–4 is now distributed about the three axes so that the terminal segment lies parallel to the axis 1–2. It can be seen that the automatic rotation increases from the first to the third segment, reaching a maximum in the latter. This can be viewed as a model of the column of the thumb, which bears a universal joint at its base. Thus its second phalanx undergoes automatic rotation independently of a similar movement in the TM joint.

Thus axial rotation of the thumb depends on the coordinated function of the TM, MP and IP joints but the initiating movement occurs in the crucial joint, i.e. the TM joint.

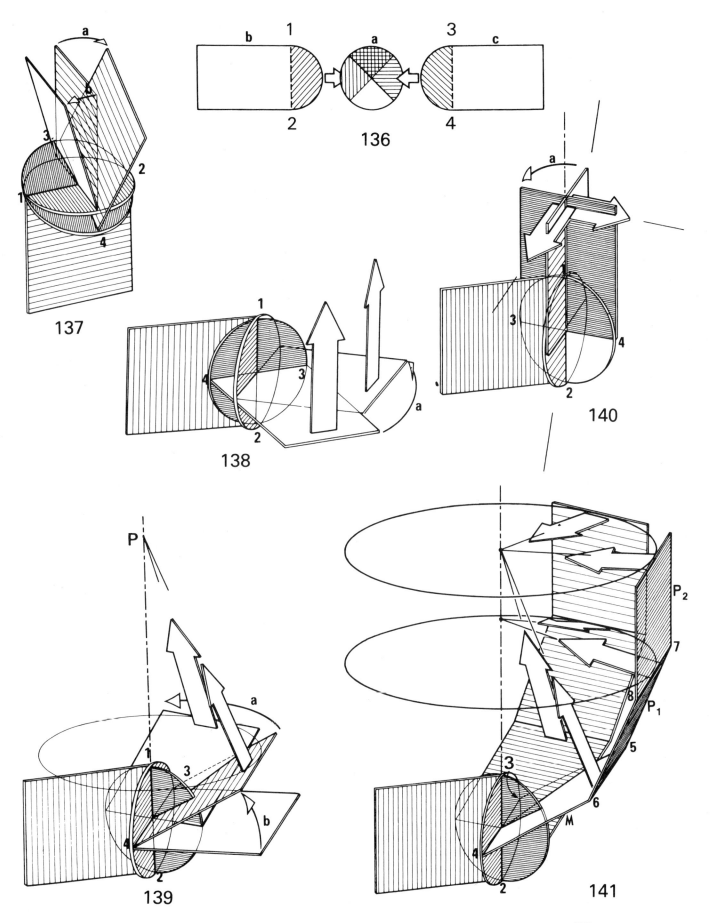

137

136

138

139

140

141

221

The movements of M_1

M_1 can move about its two orthogonal axes individually or simultaneously with a resulting automatic rotation about its long axis. The position in space of the main axes of the TM joint must now be defined.

If, on the skeleton (Fig. 142), a metallic pin is placed through the centre of mean curvature of the articular surfaces of the TZ and M_1, one can then recognise:

— the axis XX' at the base of M_1, corresponding to the concavity of TZ
— the axis YY' in TZ corresponding to the concavity of M_1.

Of course these axes are not fixed in life but *variable* during movements. (The pin only represents the mean position). However, to a first approximation, these axes can be considered as the two axes of the TM joint, with the realization that this *model is only a partial representation of reality*. Mechanically the joint is a *universal joint with two orthogonal axes*.

Two important points need to be stressed:

— on the one hand, the axis YY' is parallel to the axes of flexion-extension at the MP (f_1) and the IP (f_2) joints.
— on the other, the axis XX', perpendicular to YY' in space, is also perpendicular to f_1 and f_2, and thus lies in the plane of flexion-extension at the two IP joints, i.e. in the plane of flexion of the column of the thumb.

Finally it must be stressed that the two axes XX' and YY' of the TM joint are *oblique with respect to the three planes of reference*, frontal (F), sagittal (S) and transverse (T). Thus pure movements of M_1 take place in a plane which is *oblique to the three planes* of reference. Hence they cannot be described in terms of classical anatomy, at least at regards abduction taking placing in a frontal plane.

Thus **pure movements of M_1** (Fig. 143) *relative to TZ* can be defined as follows:

— *around the axis XX'*, which we call the *main* axis because it is the dominant axis during thumb opposition, occur *the movements of anteposition and retroposition*, during which the extended thumb moves in a plane AOR which contains the angle between the thumb and the palm. During *retroposition* (R) the thumb is displaced *posteriorly* to *reach the plane of the palm* while staying at an angle of 60° with M_2. During *anteposition* (A) the thumb moves anteriorly to a position *almost perpendicular to the plane of the palm*, rather confusingly called abduction by Anglo–Saxon authors.

— around axis YY', which we call *secondary*, occur the *movements of flexion and extension* in a plane FOE perpendicular to the axis YY' and the plane AOR. During *extension* (E) M_1 is displaced posteriorly and laterally and the range of this movement is increased by concurrent extension of P_1 and P_2. Thus the column of the thumb comes to lie almost in the plane of the palm. During *flexion* (F), P_1 is displaced distally, anteriorly and medially without crossing the sagittal plane through M_2. The range of this movement is increased by flexion of P_1 and P_2 so that the pulp of the thumb touches the palm at the base of the little finger.

Thus the concept of flexion and extension of P_1 is perfectly justified by the occurrence of similar movements at the other two joints of the column of the thumb.

Aside from these pure movements of anteposition-retroposition and flexion-extension, all the other movements of M_1 are *complex*, combined with varying degrees of successive or concurrent movement about the two axes and a component of *automatic or conjoint axial rotation*. The latter plays a vital role in opposition of the thumb, as will be shown later.

The movements of flexion and extension and anteposition and retroposition of M_1 start from *the neutral position* or *the position of rest of the thumb muscles* (Fig. 144). This corresponds to the *position of electromyographic silence* (Hamonet and Valentin), when the relaxed muscles give rise to no action potentials. This position N has been defined radiologically as the position when M_1 and M_2 lie at an angle of 30° frontally and at an angle of 40° sagittally.

This position N also corresponds to the position of relaxation of the ligaments and maximal congruence of the articular surfaces, which overspread each other precisely.

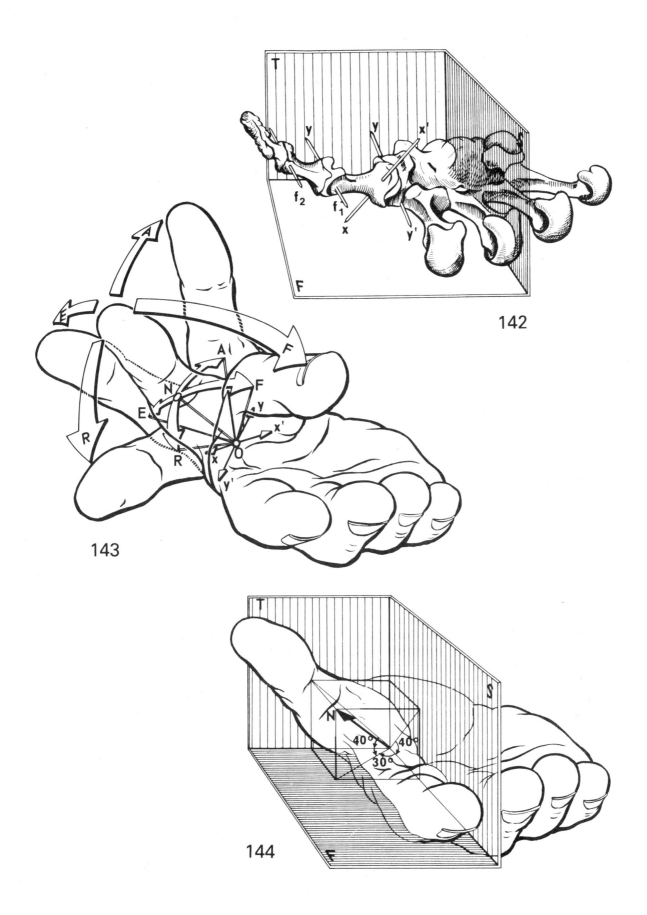

142

143

144

THE TRAPEZO-METACARPAL JOINT (continued)

Evaluation of the movements of M_1

The problem of evaluating movements of M_1 in practice is compounded by the current use of three methods.

In the *first method*, which could be called *classical* (Fig. 145), M_1 is made to move in a *rectangular solid of reference*: formed by three perpendicular planes, i.e. transverse (T), frontal (F) and sagittal (S). The latter two planes intersect along the long axis of M_2 and the plane of intersection of the three reference planes passes through the TM joint. The *reference position* is achieved when M_1 flanks M_2 in the plane of the palm, which is roughly the same as plane F. It should be noted that this position is not natural and also that M_1 cannot strictly be made to lie parallel to M_2.

Abduction (arrow 1) occurs when M_1 moves away from M_2 in the plane of the palm and the converse applies for *adduction*.

Flexion (arrow 2) of anterior displacement occurs when M_1 moves anteriorly and *extension* or posterior displacement when M_1 moves posteriorly.

The *position* of M_1 is also defined by two angles (inset): the angle a for abduction and the angle b for flexion.

This method has two disadvantages:

— the movements are projected on to abstract planes and are not related to real angles

— axial rotation is not evaluated.

The *second method* (Fig. 146), which could be called *modern* (Duparc, de la Caffinière and Pineau), determines not movements but rather *positions* of M_1 according to a system of polar coordinates. The position of M_1 is defined by its *position on a cone*, whose axis coincides with the long axis of M_2 and whose apex lies in the TM joint. The *angle formed by the plane of the thumb and the apex of the cone* (arrow 1) is the *angle of separation of the thumb* (a), which makes sense only when M_1 moves along the surface of the cone. The position of M_1 is established precisely by the angle b (arrow 2) between the plane passing through M_1 and M_2 and the frontal plane. This angle b is called by the above-mentioned authors '*the angle of rotation in space*', which is repetitious since rotation must take place in space. It would be more appropriate to call it the *angle of circumduction*, since the displacement of M_1 on the surface of the cone is analogous to circumduction.

The value of this method of assessment rests on the ease with which these two angles can be measured with a protractor.

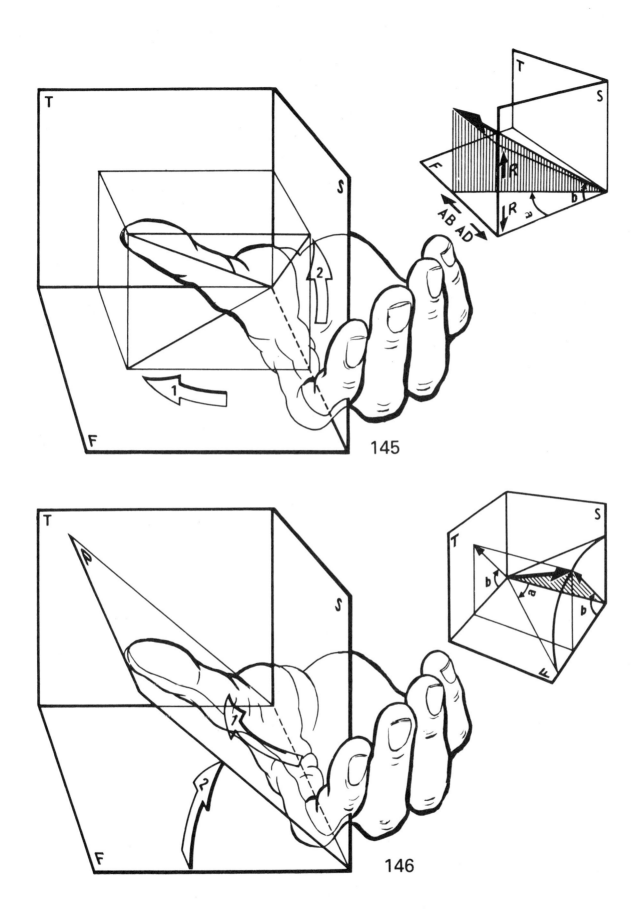

145

146

THE TRAPEZO-METACARPAL JOINT (continued)

The trapezium (TZ)

The major disadvantage of these two methods lies in the fact that they measure complex movements at the TM joint, *which must include a component of axial rotation*, generated by movements around the two axes of the joint.

The third method of assessment, which we put forward, *deals with movements of M_1 on TZ and* requires the use of special radiographic projections:

— when radiographs of the column of the thumb (Fig. 147) are taken *head on*, the concavity of TZ and the concavity of M_1 are seen only from the side. When such films are taken in anteposition and retroposition of the thumb, it is obvious that:

— during *retroposition* (15° to 25°) the axis of M_1 comes to lie almost parallel to that of M_2 while its base is displaced laterally past the surface of TZ;

— during *anteposition* (25° to 35°) the angle between M_1 and M_2 is widened to 65° while the base of M_1 slips medially towards that of M_2.

These displacements of M_1 over the saddle-shaped surface of TZ can easily be understood as resulting from rotation about the **centre of curvature of the concave surface of TZ**, which *lies on the main axis XX of the TM joint as its passes through the base of M_1*.

When radiographs of the column of the thumb are taken *from the side* (Fig. 148), the convexity of TZ and the concavity of M_1 are seen without any distortion due to perspective. Such lateral films taken with the thumb in full *flexion* and in *extension* will show:

— during *flexion* (20° to 25°) the axes of M_1 and M_2 come to lie almost parallel.

— during *extension* (30° to 45°) the axis of M_1 comes to lie at an angle of 65° with that of M_2. Here again the displacement of the concave surface of M_1 on TZ can be seen as due to rotation about the **centre of curvature of the convex surface of TZ**, which *lies on the secondary axis YY' of the TM joint as it passes through TZ*.

Thus the range of movements of the TM joint is definitely smaller than suggested by the great mobility of the column of the thumb:

— a range of 40° to 60° between extreme anteposition and retroposition

— a range of 50° to 60° between extreme flexion and extension.

Thus *special radiographs of the TM joint*, i.e. *taken with the column of the thumb seen head on and from the side,* are needed for the proper study of the functions and limitations of the TM joint (Kapandji 1980).

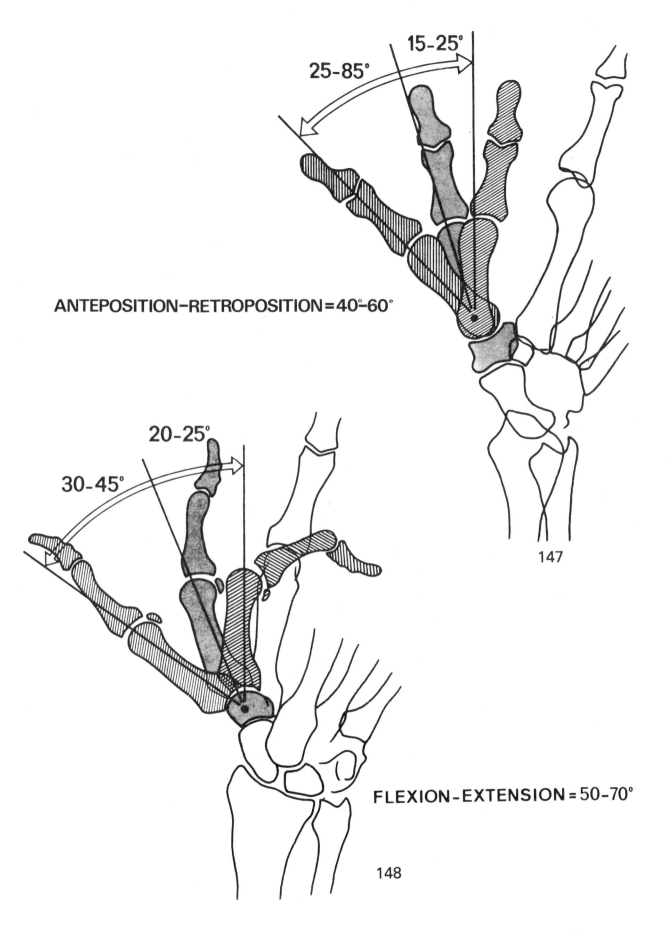

25-85°

15-25°

ANTEPOSITION-RETROPOSITION = 40°-60°

147

20-25°

30-45°

FLEXION-EXTENSION = 50-70°

148

227

THE METACARPO-PHALANGEAL JOINT OF THE THUMB

The MP joint is considered by anatomists to be of the *condyloid* variety, though Anglo-Saxon authors think of it as an ellipsoid (cotylic) joint. Thus, like every condyloid joint, it has *two degrees of freedom* allowing flexion and extension and side to side movements. In fact, as a result of its complex mechanics, there is also a *third degree of freedom* allowing axial rotation of P_1 (pronation and supination), which is both passive and *active* and essential for thumb opposition.

When the MP joint is opened *anteriorly* and P_1 is displaced posteriorly (Fig. 149), the *head of M_1* (1) appear biconvex, being longer than it is wide and expanded anteriorly by two asymmetrical swellings (the medial swelling **a** being more prominent than the lateral one **b**). To the cartilage-coated biconcave *base of P_1* (2) is attached the *fibrocartilaginous or palmar plate* (3), bearing near its distal edge two sesamoid bones (4 and 5), whose cartilage-covered surfaces are continuous with that of the plate. These bones lie respectively in the tendons of the medial sesamoid muscles (6), i.e. the adductor pollicis and the first anterior interosseous, and of the lateral sesamoid muscles (7), i.e. the flexor pollicis brevis and the abductor pollicis brevis. The capsule, seen sliced in the diagram (8), is thickened on both sides, medially (9) and laterally (10), by the ligaments bridging M_1 and the palmar plate. Also seen are the *anterior (11) and posterior (12) recesses of the capsule* and the *collateral ligaments*, the medial ligament (13) being shorter and more quickly stretched than the lateral (14). The arrows XX' and YY' represent respectively the axis of *flexion and extension* and that of *side-to-side movements*.

In Fig. 150 (*anterior view*) can also be seen more clearly: M_1 (15) below and P_1 (16) above, the palmar plate (3) and the sesamoid bones (4 and 5), linked by the intersesamoid ligament (17) and bound to the head of M_1 by the medial (18) and lateral (19) ligaments running between M_1 and the palmar plate and to the base of P_1 by the direct (20) and crossed (21) fibres of the phalango-sesamoid ligament. The medial sesamoid muscles (6) are inserted into the medial sesamoid bone and send an expansion (22) to the base of P_1, which partially masks the medial ligament (13). The phalangeal expansion (23) of the lateral sesamoid muscles (7) has been cut to display the lateral ligament (14).

In Figure 152 (*medial view*) and Figure 153 (*lateral view*) can also be seen the posterior (24) and anterior (25) recesses of the capsule, the tendon of insertion of the *extensor pollicis brevis* (26) and the clearly eccentric metacarpal attachment of the medial (13) and lateral (14) ligaments and of the ligaments joining the metacarpal to the palmar plate (18 and 19). It can be noted that the medial ligament (Fig. 152) is shorter and more readily tightened than the lateral (Fig. 153), so that the displacement of the base of P_1 is less marked on the medial than on the lateral aspect of the head of M_1. Figure 157 (proximal view) shows how the differential displacement of M_1 (striped), 1 medially and L laterally, produces an *axial rotation* (pronation) of the base of P_1, when the lateral sesamoid muscles (LSM) contract more vigorously than the medial sesamoid muscles (MSM).

This differential displacement is further enhanced by the asymmetry of the head of M_1 (Fig 51: seen head on), as the less prominent lateral swelling (b) extends further distally on its anterior aspect than the medial swelling (a). Thus laterally the base of P_1 moves further anteriorly and distally, giving rise to combined flexion, *pronation and lateral deviation* of P_1.

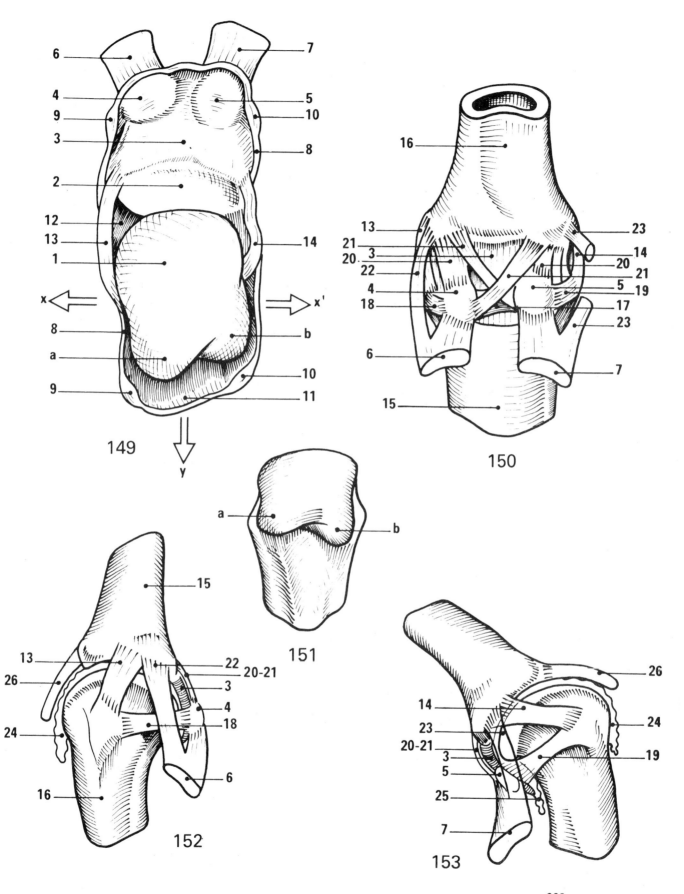

149

150

151

152

153

229

THE METACARPO-PHALANGEAL JOINT OF THE THUMB (continued)

The degree and nature of the side-to-side movements and of axial rotation of P_1 depend on the degree of flexion at the joint.

In *full extension* (Fig. 154) the collateral ligaments are slack while the ligament joining M_1 to the palmar plate and the plate itself are stretched, thus preventing axial rotation and side-to-side movements. It is thus the *locked position in extension*.

In *mid-flexion* (Fig. 155) the collateral ligaments are again slack, especially the lateral, while the palmar plate and the ligament binding it to M_1 are slackened as the sesamoid bones slip under the anterior swellings of the head of M_1. This is *the position of maximal mobility* when side-to-side movements and axial rotation can be produced by the muscles attached to the sesamoids. Thus contraction of the *medial* sesamoid muscles leads to medial displacement and supination (rotation) and that of the *lateral* sesamoid muscles produces lateral displacement and pronation (rotation).

In *full flexion* (Fig. 156) the palmar plate and the ligament binding it to M_1 are slackened while the collateral ligaments are maximally stretched so that the base of P_1 is *displaced laterally and pronated*. The joint is locked by the interaction of the maximally stretched collateral ligaments and of the posterior recess of the capsular ligaments and of the lateral thenar muscles in contraction. This is the *locked position* in **flexion** (Mac Conaill's close-packed position).

In sum, (Kapandji 1980) the MP joint of the thumb can undergo two types of movement starting from the position of full extension (Fig. 158: posterior view of the head of M_1 showing the axes of the various movements).

— *Pure flexion* (arrow 1) around a transverse axis F_1, produced by the balanced action of the medial and lateral sesamoid muscles up to the position of mid-flexion.

— the *complex movements of flexion, side-to-side displacement and axial rotation* (supination-pronation):

  * *flexion, medial displacement and supination* (arrow 2) about a moving oblique axis F_2 giving rise to a conical rotation.

    It is produced largely by the medial sesamoid muscles.

  * *flexion, lateral displacement and pronation* (arrow 3) about a moving oblique axis F_3, which is more oblique than F_2. Again the rotation takes place along the surface of a cone and is produced largely by the lateral sesamoid muscles.

Thus full flexion is always associated with lateral displacement and pronation because of the asymmetrical shape of the head of M_1 and the unequal tension in the collateral ligaments.

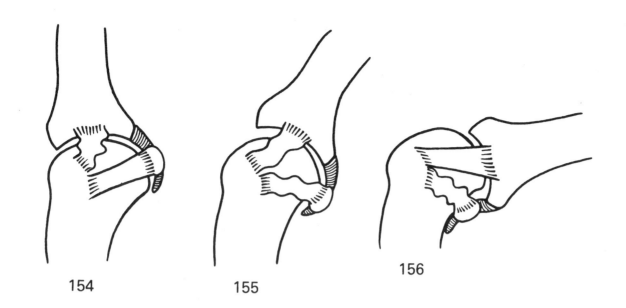

154   155   156

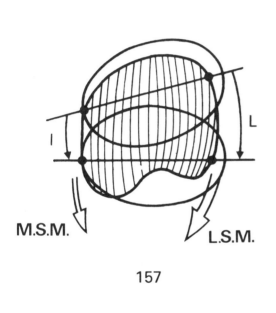

L

l

M.S.M.   L.S.M.

157

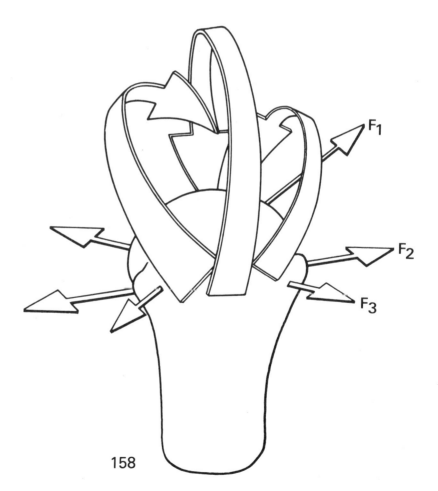

F_1

F_2

F_3

158

THE METACARPO-PHALANGEAL JOINT OF THE THUMB (continued)

The Movements

The *position of reference* of this joint coincides with that of *full extension* (Fig. 159), when the axes of P_1 and M_1 are collinear. Starting from this position no active or passive *extension* is possible normally. *Active flexion* (Fig. 160) reaches up to $60°-70°$, while *passive flexion* may attain 80° or even 90°. The ranges of the various components of movement at the MP joint can be studied as follows. Construct two *trihedral structures* with matches arranged orthogonally and place each of these structures on either side of the joint so that in the position of full extension they lie parallel (Fig. 161). In the position of mid-flexion either the medial or lateral sesamoid muscles can contract.

When *the former contract* (Fig. 162: seen distally with the thumb in anteposition; Fig. 163: seen proximally with the thumb lying in the plane of the palm), there is medial displacement of a few degrees and *supination* of 5° to 7°.

When *the latter contract* (Fig. 164: seen distally; Fig. 165: seen proximally) there is lateral displacement (well shown in Fig. 165) which is more marked than the medial displacement, and a *pronation* of 20°.

The significance of this combined movement of flexion-lateral displacement and pronation in opposition of the thumb will be discussed later.

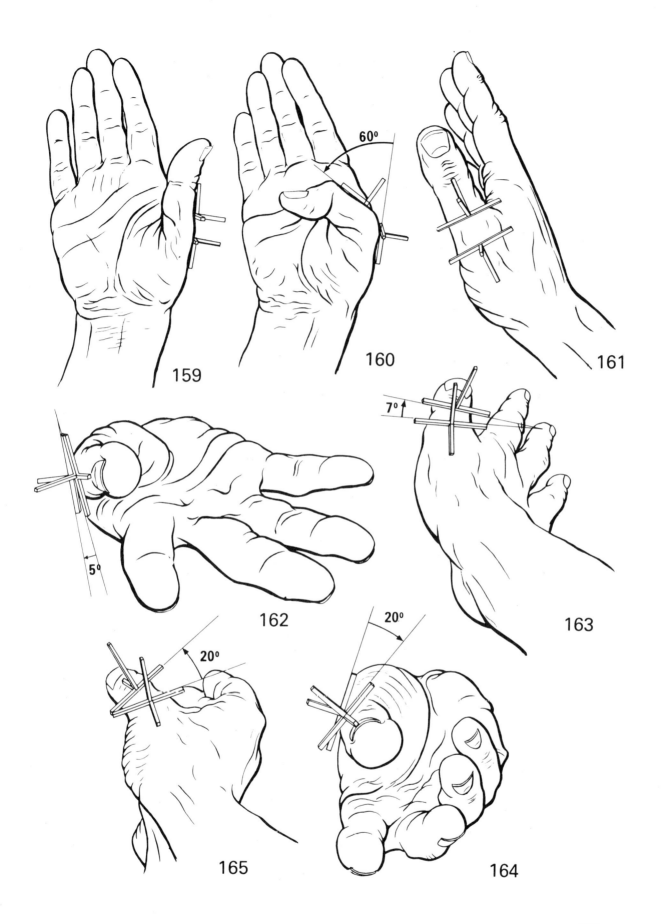

159

160

161

162

163

164

165

233

THE METACARPO-PHALANGEAL JOINT OF THE THUMB (continued)

When the *hand grips a cylinder with the whole palm*, the grip is *firmly locked* by the action of the lateral sesamoid muscles at the level of the MP joint. When the thumb is inactive (Fig. 166) and stays parallel to the axis of the cylinder, the grip is incompletely stabilised and the object can easily slip through the gap between the fingertips and the thenar eminence. If, on the other hand, the thumb moves towards the fingers (Fig. 167) the object cannot slip away. The medial displacement of P_1, seen clearly in the diagram, compounds the movement of anteposition of M_1. Thus the path taken by the thumb around the cylinder is circular and *the shortest possible* (f). Without medial displacement of P_1 the path would be elliptical and longer (d).

Thus *medial displacement is essential for the locking of the grip*, the more so as the ring formed by the thumb and the index is smaller and more completely closed (Fig. 168). In position a the thumb lies along the axis of the cylinder and the *ring of the grip* is broken. In positions b to e the ring closes progressively and finally in position f the thumb lies perpendicular to the axis of the cylinder and the ring is completely closed with locking of the grip.

Furthermore, *pronation of P_1* (Fig. 169), shown by the angle of 12° formed by the two transverse matchsticks, allows the thumb to *apply itself* to the object with the bulk of its palmar surface instead of its medial border. Thus by increasing the surface of contact, pronation of P_1 contributes to the *strengthening of the grip*.

If a smaller cylinder is being held (Fig. 170) the thumb comes to overlie the index partially so that the ring of the grip is narrower, the locking is more marked and the grip stronger.

Thus the function of the MP joint of the thumb and of its motor muscles is remarkably adapted to prehension.

The **stability of the MP joint of the thumb** depends not only on the articular surfaces but also on its *muscular cuff*. Normally, during opposition of the thumb (Fig. 171), the successive joints of the index and thumb are stabilised by the action of antagonistic muscles (shown by small black arrows). Under certain circumstances (Fig. 172, according to Bunnel) the MP joint goes into extension rather than flexion, i.e. 'inversion' of movement (white arrow). This occurs:

1. When paralysis of the abductor pollicis brevis and flexor pollicis brevis allows P_1 to be tilted posteriorly.

2. When shortening of the muscles of the first interosseous space draws M_1 nearer to M_2.

3. When paralysis of the abductor pollicis longus prevents abduction of the first MP joint.

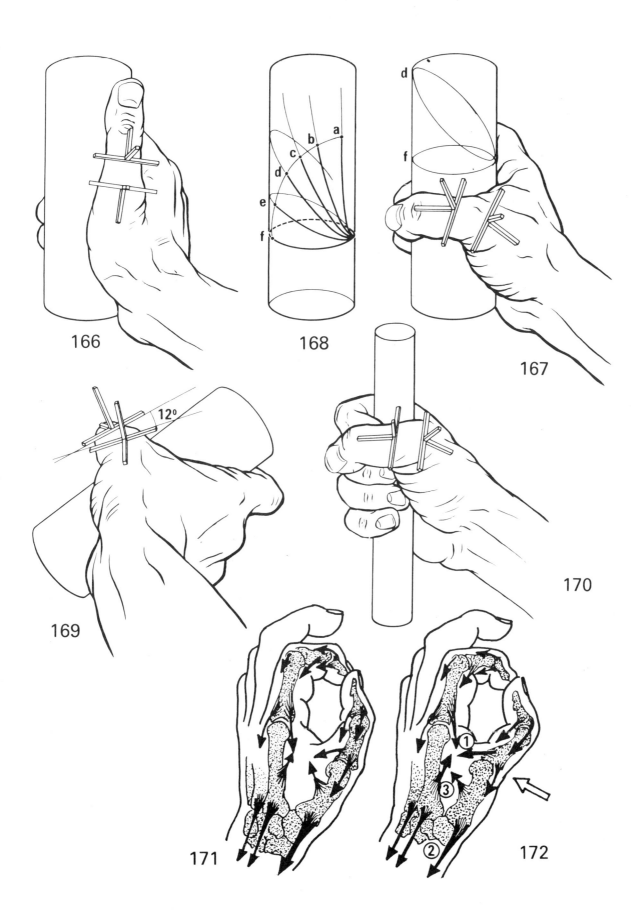

166

168

167

169

12°

170

171

172

235

THE INTERPHALANGEAL JOINT OF THE THUMB

At first sight the IP joint of the thumb is simple. It is a hinge joint with a fixed transverse axis, which runs through the centre of curvature of the condyles of the articular surface of P_1 and around which occur the movements of flexion and extension:

— *Flexion* (Fig. 173): active up to 75° to 80° and passive to 90°

— *Extension* (Fig. 174): active up to 5°–10° but *passive hyperextension* (Fig. 175) can be quite marked (30°) in certain people, e.g. sculptors who used their thumbs to press the clay.

In fact these movements are more complex since during flexion P_2 *is pronated (medially rotated)*.

In Fig. 176 two parallel pins have been inserted into the head of P_1 (a) and into the base of P_2 (b) in the position of full extension. During flexion at the IP joint the pins come to lie at an angle of 5° to 10°, concave medially, i.e. indicating medial rotation (pronation).

A similar experiment using matchsticks stuck to the posterior surfaces of P_1 and P_2 gives a similar result. P_2 is *pronated 5°–10°* during flexion.

This phenomenon can be explained by the anatomical structure of the articular surfaces. In Fig. 177 (the joint has been opened posteriorly) the medial condyle appears more prominent and larger anteriorly and medially than the lateral. The radius of curvature of the lateral condyle is shorter so that its anterior surface 'drops' more abruptly towards the anterior surface of P_1. Thus the medial ligament (ML) is stretched faster than the lateral (LL) during flexion, and thus brings the medial aspect of the base of P_2 to a halt while its lateral aspect goes on moving.

In other words (Fig. 178), the displacement of P_2 on the medial condyle (AA') is shorter than that on the lateral condyle (BB') so that P_2 is medially rotated. Thus it can be said that there is no single axis of flexion and extension but a *series of axes* between the initial position i and final position f. If a model of the IP joint is made with cardboard (Fig. 179), the strip must be folded along an axis, which is not perpendicular to that of the 'finger' but at an angle of 5°–10°. It can be seen that the phalanx is *rotated conically* during flexion secondary to a change in its direction, which is proportional to the degree of flexion.

This component of rotation at the IP joint contributes, as will be seen later, to the overall pronation (medial rotation) of the thumb during opposition.

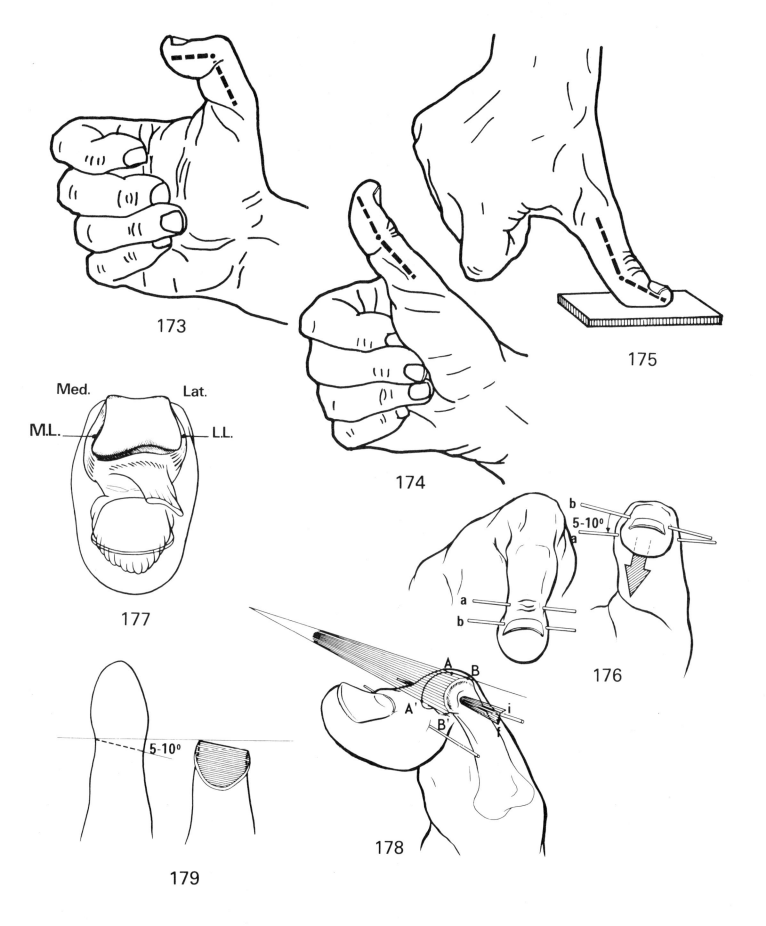

173

174

175

Med. Lat.

M.L. L.L.

177

176

5-10°

178

5-10°

179

237

THE MOTOR MUSCLES OF THE THUMB

The thumb has **nine motor muscles** and this abundance of muscles, as compared with the other fingers, determines its greater mobility and its essentiality.

These muscles fall into **two groups:**

a) the extrinsic or *long muscles*: four in all and lying mostly in the forearm. The three combined extensors and abductors release the grip while the fourth, a flexor, tightens and locks the grip.

b) the intrinsic muscles, *lying within the thenar eminence and the first interosseous space*. These five muscles allow the hand to achieve a variety of grips and the thumb to be opposed. Their main function is not to ensure strength but to *enhance precision and coordination*.

To understand the action of these muscles on the column of the thumb, their positions relative to the *two theoretical axes of the TM joint* must be known. These axes (Fig. 180), i.e. the axis YY' of flexion and extension, lying parallel to the axes of flexion of the MP joint (f_1) and IP joint (f_2), and the axis XX' of anteposition and retroposition, demarcate *four quadrants*:

— *quadrant X'Y'*, lying posterior to the axis YY' of flexion and extension of the TM joint and anterior to the axis XX' of anteposition and retroposition, and containing the tendon of a single muscle, the abductor pollicis longus (1). As the muscle lies close to the axis XX', it produces anteposition only weakly but powerfully extends the TM joint (Fig. 181: the wrist is seen 'running away' medially and distally).

— *quadrant X'Y*, lying posterior to the axes XX' and YY' and bearing the tendons of the extensor pollicis brevis (2) and the extensor pollicis longus (3)..

— *quadrant XY*, lying anterior to the axis YY' and posterior to the axis XX', containing two muscles, which run in the first interosseous space and cause retroposition combined with slight flexion at the TM joint:

   * the adductor pollicis with two bundles (8)

   * the first anterior interosseous (9), if present.

These two muscles adduct M_1 and narrow the first interdigital cleft by approximating M_1 and M_2 (Fig. 182).

— *quadrant XY'*, lying anterior to the axes XX' and YY' and bearing the muscles of opposition, which at once produce flexion and anteposition of M_1:

   * the opponens pollicis (6)

   * the abductor pollicis brevis (7)

   * the flexor pollicis longus (4)

   * the flexor pollicis brevis (5).

The last two muscles lie on the axis XX' and thus are pure flexors of the TM joint.

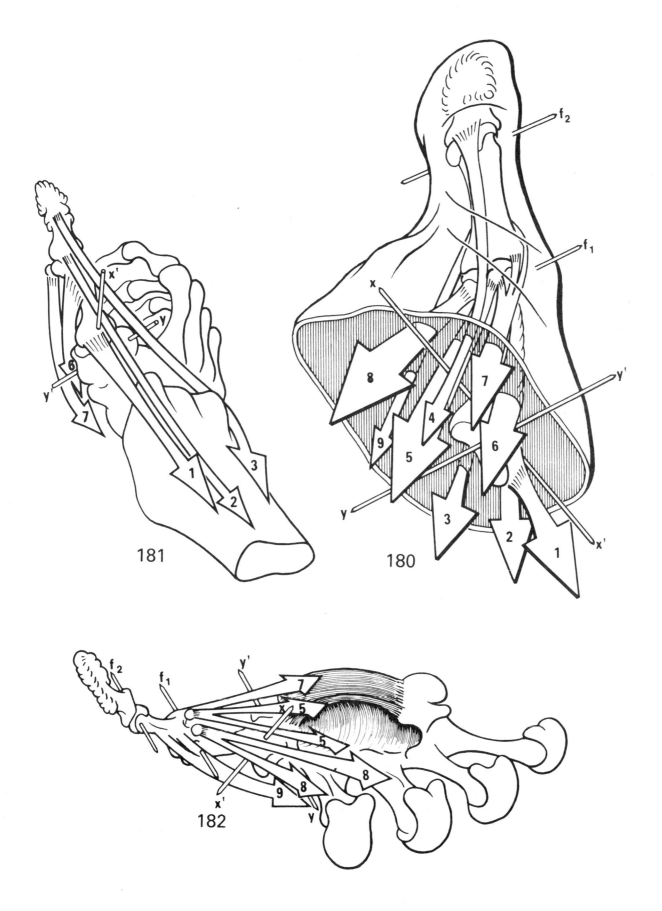

181

180

182

A brief account of their anatomy will shed considerable light on their physiology.

The **extrinsic muscles** are (Fig. 183: anterior view; Fig. 184: lateral view):

— the *abductor pollicis longus* (1), inserted into the antero-lateral aspect of the base of M_1

— the *extensor pollicis brevis* (2), which runs parallel to the latter

— *the extensor pollicis longus* (3) inserted posteriorly into the base of P_2.

Two points must be made regarding these three muscles:

(a) **anatomically speaking**, these three tendons, seen on the posterior and lateral aspects of the thumb, bound a triangular space with apex situated distally — the *'anatomical snuffbox'*. The floor of this space is formed by the tendons of the *extensor carpi radialis brevis* (10) *and extensor carpi radialis longus* (11);

(b) **physiologically speaking**, each muscle acts on a particular joint of the thumb and all three are extensors.

— *flexor pollicis longus* (4), which traverses the carpal tunnel, runs deep to the thenar eminence between the two heads of the flexor pollicis brevis and slips between the two sesamoid bones (Fig. 183) to be inserted into the anterior surface of the base of P_3.

The **intrinsic muscles** (Fig. 183 and 184) are further subdivided into *two groups*:

(a) The **lateral group** consists of three muscles, supplied by the median nerve, which are from deep to superficial:

— *flexor pollicis brevis* (5), which arises by two heads, one from the deep carpal surface of the carpal tunnel and the other from the lower border of the flexor retinaculum and the tubercle of the trapezium. Its single tendon is inserted into the outer sesamoid bone and the radial side of the base of P_1. Its general direction is oblique distally and laterally;

— *opponens pollicis* (6), arising from the flexor retinaculum and the crest of the trapezium, runs distally, laterally and posteriorly to be inserted into the lateral border of M_1;

— *abductor pollicis brevis* (7) arises from the flexor retinaculum and the crest of the scaphoid and lies superficial to the opponens, forming the superficial plane of the thenar eminence. It is inserted into the lateral aspect of the base of P_1, but some of its lateral fibres join the dorsal digital expansion of the thumb along with the first anterior interosseus (9). In functional terms it is important to realise that this muscle does not lie to the radial side of the metacarpal but *anteriorly and medially* and runs in the same direction as the opponens — i.e. distally, laterally and posteriorly.

These three muscles constitute the lateral group, *being inserted into the lateral aspects of M_1 and P_1*. The flexor pollicis brevis and the abductor pollicis brevis are called the *lateral sesamoid muscles*.

(b) The **medial group** consists of two muscles with tendons inserted into the medial side of the MP joint:

— *first anterior interosseus* (9), inserted by tendon into the medial side of the base of P_1 and into the dorsal expansion;

— *adductor pollicis* (8) with its transverse and oblique heads converging by a common tendon towards its insertion into the medial sesamoid bone and the medial aspect of the base of P_1.

These two muscles are the *medial sesamoid muscles* and are synergistic-antagonistic to the lateral sesamoid muscles.

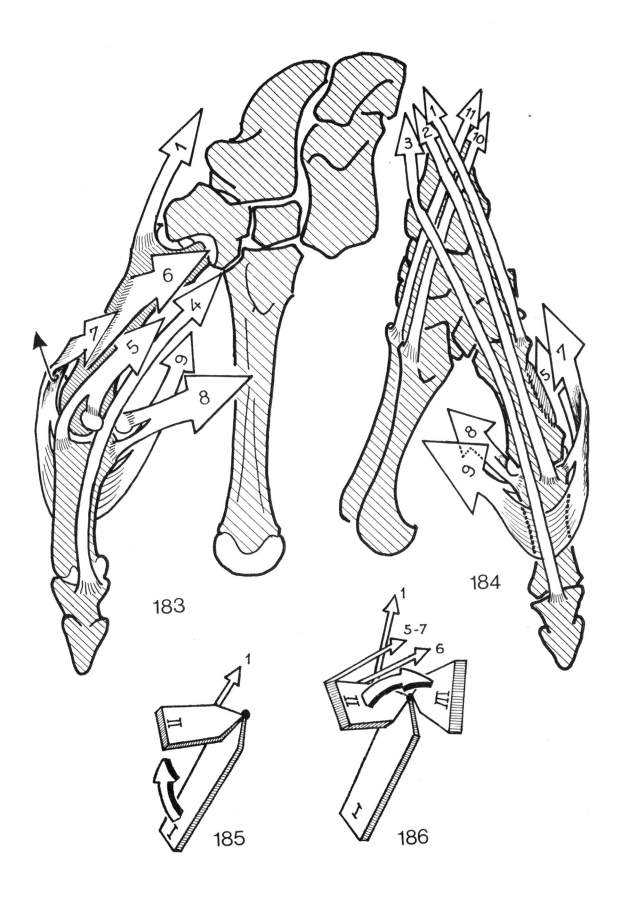

183

184

185

186

THE ACTIONS OF THE EXTRINSIC MUSCLES OF THE THUMB

The **abductor pollicis longus** (APL) moves M_1 (Fig. 187) *laterally and anteriorly*. Therefore it produces both *abduction* and *anteposition* at the TM joint. This latter movement is due to the fact that the abductor tendon runs anterior to the tendons of the muscles of the 'anatomical snuffbox' (cf. Fig. 184). When the wrist is not stabilised by the two radial extensors — especially the longus — the abductor pollicis longus *also flexes the wrist*. When the wrist is extended, APL extends the TM joint.

Functionally speaking, the couple formed by abductor pollicis longus and the lateral group of the intrinsic muscles plays a very important part in opposition. Before opposition can start M_1 must be raised directly above the plane of the palm so that the thenar eminence forms a *conical mass at the edge of the palm*. This is produced by this functional couple of muscles (Figs. 185 & 186: M_1 being represented diagrammatically):

— *First stage* (Fig. 185): abductor pollicis longus (1) moves M_1 anteriorly and laterally from position I to position II.
— *Second stage* (Fig. 186): from position II the muscles of the lateral group [flexor pollicis brevis and abductor pollicis brevis (5 & 7) and opponens (6)] tilt M_1 anteriorly and medially (position III), while producing a slight degree of axial rotation.

This movement has been divided into two successive stages for descriptive purposes. In fact, these stages occur simultaneously and position III — the final position of M_1 — represents the *resultant of the simultaneous forces exerted by the two sets of muscles*.

The **extensor pollicis brevis** (EPB) has two actions (Fig. 188):

(a) *It extends the MP joint*

(b) It moves M_1 and so the thumb laterally and thus produces *true abduction*, equivalent to extension and retroposition at the TM joint. For pure abduction to be produced, the wrist joint must be stabilised by the synergistic contraction of the flexor carpi ulnaris and especially the extensor carpi ulnaris *or else the extensor pollicis brevis also produces abduction at the wrist*.

The **extensor pollicis longus** (EPL) has three actions (Fig. 189):

(a) It *extends the PIP joint*

(b) It *extends the MP joint*

(c) It moves M_1 medially and posteriorly. By moving M_1 *medially* it 'closes' the first interosseous space and approximates M_1 and M_2. By moving the thumb *posteriorly* it extends the TM joint and so becomes an *antagonist of the opposition muscles*. It helps to flatten the palm and make the ball of the thumb face anteriorly.

The extensor pollicis longus *constitutes with the lateral group of thenar muscles a functional set of antagonistic and synergistic muscles*. In fact, when one wants to extend the IP joint without extending the thumb, these thenar muscles must act to stabilise the M_1 and P_1 and prevent their extension. The external thenar muscles therefore reduce the range of action of the EPL, and if they are paralysed the thumb is irresistibly adducted and extended. An accessory action of the extensor pollicis longus is *extension of the wrist*, when not cancelled by contraction of the flexor carpi radialis.

The **flexor pollicis longus** (FPL) flexes the IP joint (Fig. 190) and secondarily flexes the MP joint. For flexion of the IP joint to occur alone, the extensor pollicis brevis must contract and prevent flexion of the MP joint (synergistic action). The indispensable role of the flexor pollicis longus in prehension will be seen later (Figs. 211 & 212).

242

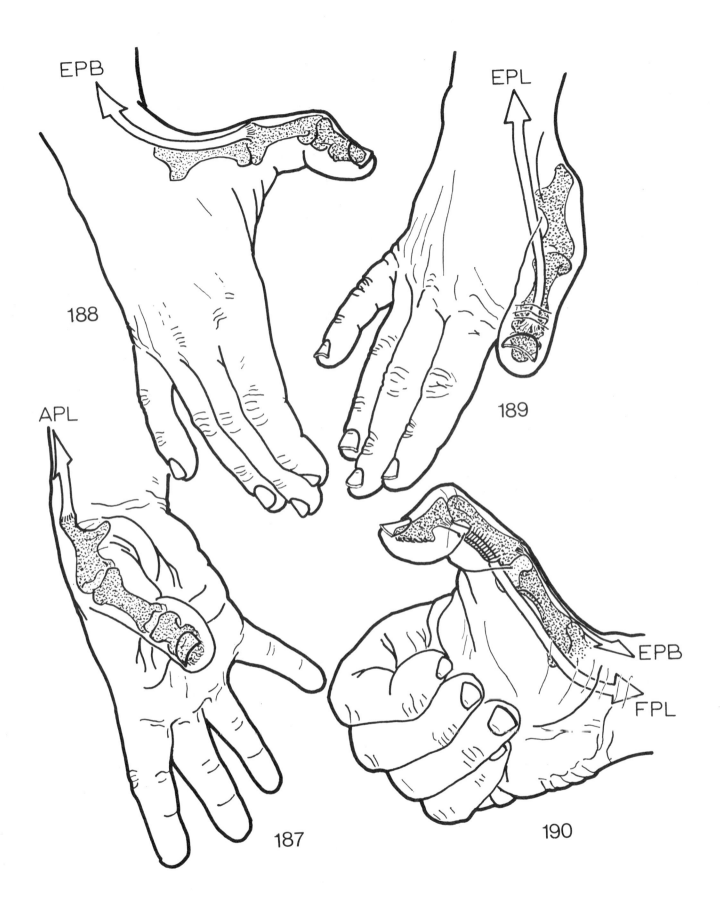

EPB

EPL

188

189

APL

EPB

FPL

187

190

THE ACTIONS OF THE INTRINSIC MUSCLES OF THE THUMB (continued)

Medial group of thenar muscles (or medial sesamoid muscles):

The **adductor pollicis** (Fig. 191), with its two heads of origin (1: transverse, 1': oblique), acts on the three bones of the thumb;

(a) on M_1 (diagram, Fig. 193): contraction of the adductor moves M_1 to a position of equilibrium, lying lateral and anterior to M_2 (position A). The type of movement produced by the muscle depends upon the starting point of M_1 (Duchenne de Boulogne):

1. the muscle is effectively adductor if M_1 starts from a position of maximal abduction (position 1);

2. it produces abduction if M_1 starts from a position of maximal adduction (position 2);

3. if M_1 is fully extended by the extensor pollicis longus (position 3), the adductor pollicis brings M_1 into anteposition;

4. it brings M_1 into retroposition if M_1 is already in anteposition as a result of contraction of the abductor pollicis brevis (position 4).

(R represents the position of rest of M_1).

Recent electromyographic studies have shown that the adductor pollicis is active not only during adduction but also during retroposition of the thumb, during full palmar prehension by subterminolateral opposition. During opposition of the thumb it becomes the more active as the thumb moves towards the more medial fingers. Hence it is maximally active during opposition of the thumb and the little finger.

The adductor is inactive during abduction, anteposition and termino-terminal grips.

It has also been confirmed electromyographically that it is particularly active when the thumb and M_2 are approximated during all phases of opposition, (Fig. 193: diagram showing action of adductor pollicis, according to Hamonet, de la Caffiniére and Opsomer).

(b) on P_1 (Fig. 191) it has a triple action: slight flexion, medial deviation and lateral rotation around its long axis (black arrow).

(c) on P_2: it acts as an extensor in so far as its insertion blends with that of the first interosseus.

— The first anterior interosseus has very similar actions:

— adduction (i.e. M_1 is drawn towards the axis of the hand).

— extension of the IP joint by means of the lateral extensor expansion.

The combined action of these two thenar muscles brings the pad of the thumb into contact with the radial aspect of P_1 of the index (Fig. 191). These muscles are essential for holding an object firmly between thumb and index.

244

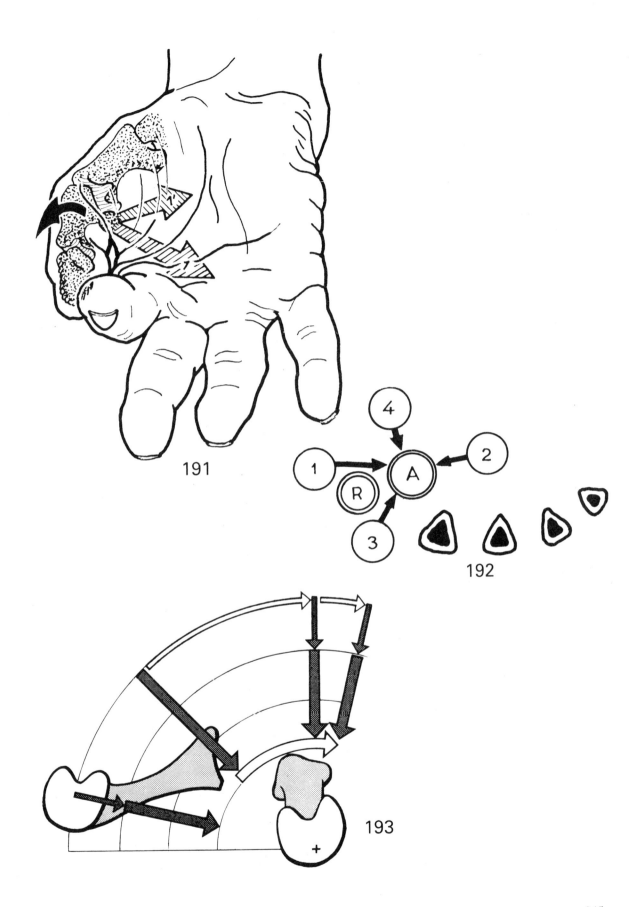

191

192

193

THE ACTIONS OF THE INTRINSIC MUSCLES OF THE THUMB (continued)

The **lateral group of thenar muscles** (Fig. 194):

— The **opponens pollicis** (2) has three actions, which correspond to those of the opponens digiti minimi (cf: Fig. 162). The electro-myographic diagram (Fig. 195) brings out its components:
— *anteposition* of M_1 with respect to the carpus
— *adduction*, i.e. M_1 and M_2 are approximated maximally
— *medial rotation*: **pronation**.

As these three simultaneous movements are essential for opposition, this muscle deserves its name.

Thus the opponens is active in every type of grip involving the thumb. Besides, electromyographs have shown that it is paradoxically recruited during abduction, when it *stabilises the column of the thumb*.

— The **abductor pollicis brevis** (3) further separates M_1 and M_2 at the end of opposition (Fig. 196: electromyographic diagram):
— it moves M_1 *anteriorly and medially*, especially when M_1 is furthest away from M_2
— it *flexes the MP joint* while causing P_1 to *tilt laterally* and *rotate medially* about its long axis i.e. **pronation** (black arrow).
— finally *it extends the IP joint*, as a result of its fibres which join the extensor pollicis longus.

When it contracts on its own, i.e. if electrically stimulated, it brings the pulp of the thumb into contact with the index and middle finger (Fig. 194). It is *thus an essential muscle for opposition*. As shown previously (cf. Fig. 185 & 186) it forms with the abductor pollicis longus a functional couple essential for opposition.

— The **flexor pollicis brevis** (4) takes part in the overall movements produced by the lateral group of thenar muscles (Fig. 197). However, when it is made to contract on its own (electrical studies by Duchenne de Boulogne), it is *primarily an adductor* and brings the ball of the thumb into opposition with the last two digits. On the other hand, its ability to *move M_1 into anteposition* is more restricted, because its deep head (4') antagonises its superficial head (4) in this movement. Thus it produces a very marked degree of medial rotation (*pronation*).

When action potentials are recorded from its superficial head (Fig. 198), it is clear that it has a similar action to the opponens and it is maximally active when the thumb moves into opposition with the small finger.

It also *flexes the MP joint* and is helped in this action by the abductor pollicis brevis and the first anterior interosseus, which form the extensor expansion of P_1.

The *combined action* of this group of muscles, along with the abductor pollicis longus, produces **opposition of the thumb.**

Extension of the IP joint can be produced (Duchenne de Boulogne) by *three muscles* or muscle groups which act under different circumstances:

1. *Extensor pollicis longus*: extension of the IP joint is accompanied by extension of the MP joint and flattening of the thenar eminence. These movements occur when one opens and flattens the hand.

2. The *internal group of thenar muscles* (first anterior interosseus): there is also adduction of the thumb. These movements take place when the ball of the thumb is opposed to the lateral aspect of P_1 of the index (cf. Fig. 214):

3. the *external group of thenar muscles* (especially abductor pollicis brevis): extension of the IP joint occurs during opposition of the thumb to other digits (cf. *Fig. 213*).

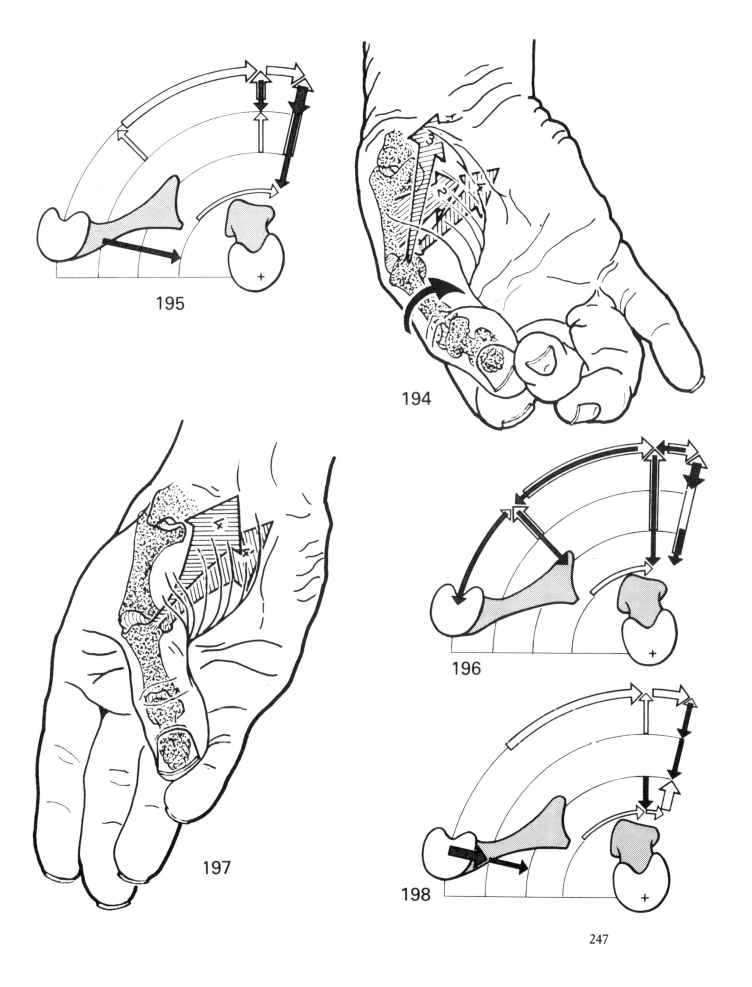

195

194

197

196

198

247

OPPOSITION OF THE THUMB

Opposition is the essential movement of the thumb and brings the pulp of the thumb into contact with that of any finger so as to form the *pollicidigital pincer*. There is thus not one movement of opposition but a series of movements of opposition, which underlie a wide variety of *static and dynnamic grips* depending on the number of fingers involved and the ways they are brought into action. Thus the full functional significance of the thumb is displayed when it is recruited in conjunction with the other fingers. Without the thumb the hand is virtually useless, so that complicated surgical techniques have been developed to reconstitute the thumb including 'pollicisation' of a finger and more recently transplantation.

The full spectrum of movements of opposition is contained within a conical sector of space, whose apex lies at the TM joint, i.e. the *cone of opposition*. This cone is markedly distorted as its base is cut short by the little finger and by the lateral border of the hand, when respectively the thumb moves towards the little finger, i.e. **in maximal opposition**, and when it moves into the plane of the palm to lie against the lateral border of the hand, i.e. **minimal opposition**. The movement of maximal opposition (Fig. 199) has been well illustrated by Sterling Bunnel's matchstick experiment (Fig. 203). The movement of minimal opposition (Fig. 200) is associated with almost linear displacement of M_1 so that its head comes progressively to lie anterior to M_2. This movement, occurring in the plane of the palm, is seldom used and of little functional value. It should not be classified as a movement of opposition, as it is not associated with a component of rotation, which is of fundamental importance in opposition. Also this creeping movement of the thumb is still seen when opposition is impaired as a result of damage to the median nerve.

248

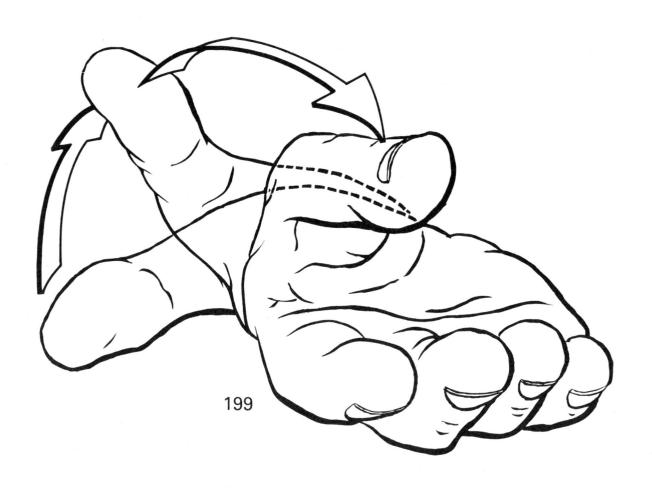

199

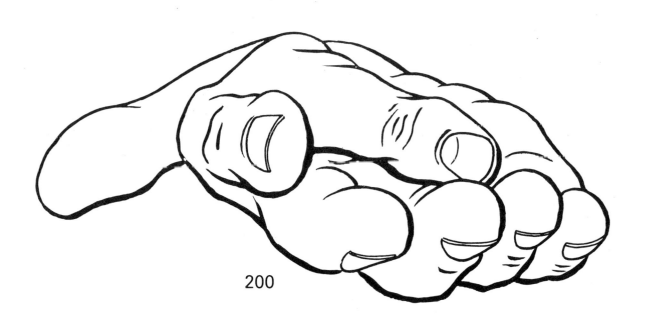

200

OPPOSITION OF THE THUMB (continued)

Mechanically speaking, thumb opposition is a complex movement variably made up of *three components*: anteposition, flexion and pronation of the osteoarticular column of the thumb.

— **anteposition** (Fig. 201) is the movement that brings the thumb to lie *anterior to the plane of the palm*, so that the thenar eminence looks like a cone in the proximo-lateral compartment of the hand. It occurs primarily at the *TM joint* and secondarily at the *MP joint*, where medial displacement of P_1 allows the thumb to rear itself up more readily. This movement of M_1 away from M_2 is called abduction by Anglo–Saxon authors, which is inappropriate as there is also an element of adduction in this movement. Thus abduction should only be used when M_1 moves away from M_2 strictly in the frontal plane.

— **flexion** (Fig. 202) moves the column of the thumb *medially* and is thus classically called adduction. All *three joints of the thumb* are involved:

— *the TM joint*, in particular, but movement at this joint cannot bring M_1 past the sagittal plane through the long axis of M_2. It is thus truly a movement of flexion as it merges with flexion at the MP joint.

— the *MP joint* allows flexion to proceed to a variable degree depending on the finger chosen for opposition.

— the *IP joint* allows flexion to reach completion by supplementing movement at the MP joint.

— **Pronation**, i.e. medial rotation (Fig. 203), is essential for opposition of the thumb as it allows the pulps of the thumb and of the fingers to achieve full contact. It can be defined as the change in the spatial orientation of P_2 so that it 'looks' in different directions depending on the degree of axial rotation. The term pronation is used *by analogy with the movement of the forearm and has a similar meaning*. This medial rotation of P_2 is produced by the summation of movements occurring to a variable degree at the joints of the column of the thumb. It is well demonstrated by the **matchstick experiment** of Sterling Bunnel (Fig. 203). A matchstick is glued across the base of the nail of the thumb and the hand is viewed head on. The angle between the initial position of the thumb (with the hand flat) and its final position in maximal opposition (with the thumb touching the little finger) is 90° to 120°. It was first thought that this rotation of the column of the thumb was the result of the laxity of the capsule of the TM joint. But recent studies have shown that it is precisely in full opposition that the TM joint assumes the close-packed position with little free 'play'. It is now recognised that the rotation, occurring essentially at the TM joint, is due to the mechanical properties of this biaxial joint. Thus a biaxial prosthesis of the TM joint allows opposition to occur normally.

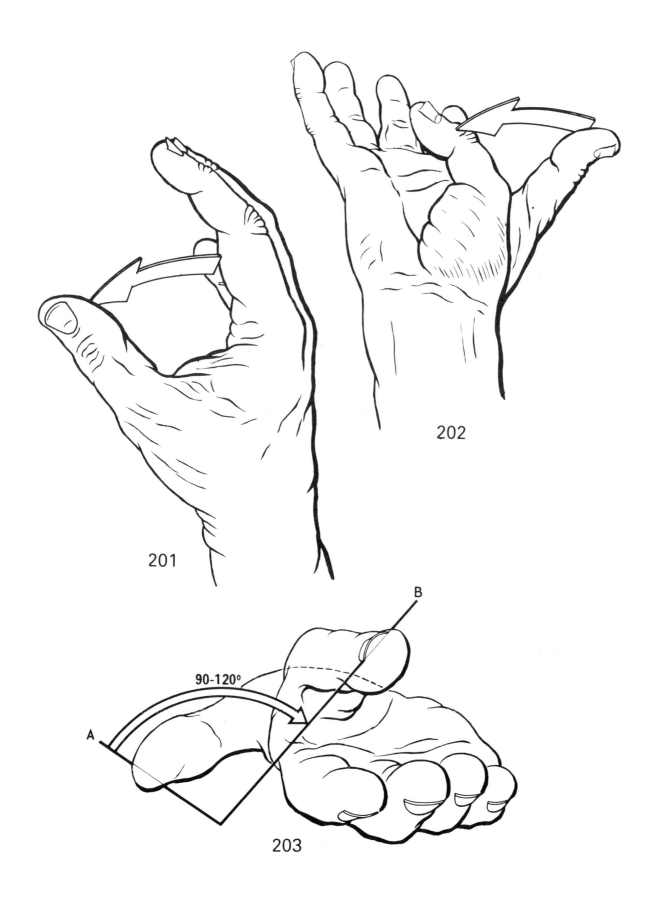

201

202

90-120°

A

B

203

251

OPPOSITION OF THE THUMB (continued)

The Component of Pronation

Pronation of the column of the thumb consists of *two components of rotation*:

— **automatic (conjunct) rotation** due to the mechanical properties of the TM joint (p. 220). The MP and IP joints contribute to this rotation by adding their movements of flexion to that of the TM joint. Thus the long axis of P_2 becomes almost parallel to the axis XX' of anteposition and retroposition, so that P_2 is rotated to the same degree as P_1 at the TM joint.

From the *initial* (Fig. 204) to the *final* (Fig. 205) position during opposition to the little finger, the successive changes in the orientation of P_2 have occurred about the four axes XX', YY', f_1 and f_2, without any distortion of the cardboard which would signify free 'play' at one of the joints.

When this movement is examined in detail (Fig. 206), it is found to consist of four successive (or simultaneous) movements, as follows:

1. At the TM joint, (about the axis XX') rotation of M_1 from position 1 to position 2 (arrow 1), i.e. in the direction of anteposition, so that the axis Y_1Y_1' comes to lie at Y_2Y_2'.

2. At the TM joint, rotation of M_1 (arrow 2) from position 2 to position 3 due to flexion around the axis Y_2Y_2'.

3. At the MP joint, flexion of P_1 around the axis f_1.

4. At the IP joint, flexion of P_2 around the axis f_2.

Hence we have shown, not by theoretical arguments but by practical demonstration, that the TM joint plays an essential role in axial rotation of the thumb.

— **Voluntary or 'adjunct' rotation** (Fig. 207), which is well brought out by fixing matchsticks transversely along the three mobile segments of the thumb. When the thumb is maximally opposed, it can be seen that this pronation of nearly 30° takes place at two joints:

— *at the MP joint*, where pronation of 24° is produced by the abductor pollicis brevis and the flexor pollicis brevis. It is *active* rotation.

— *at the IP joint*, where pronation of 7°, purely *automatic*, is due to the phenomenon of conical rotation (cf. Fig. 176).

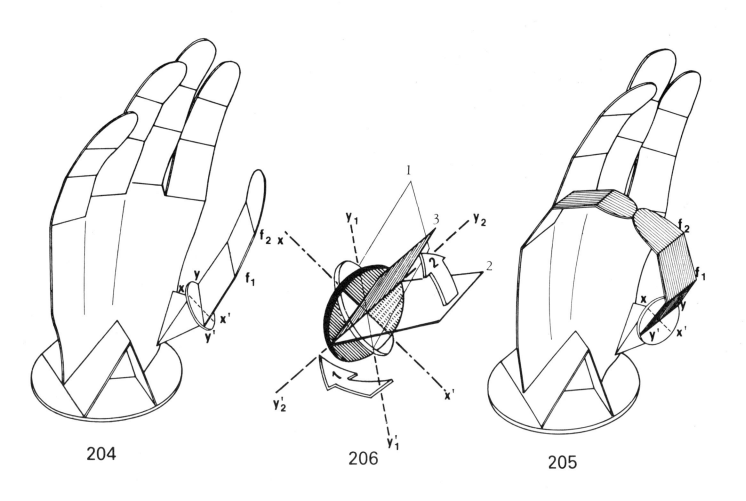

204

206

205

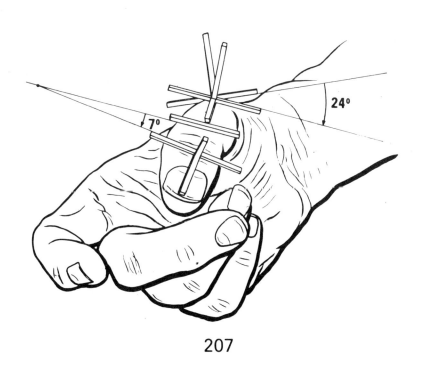

207

253

OPPOSITION AND COUNTEROPPOSITION

We have seen the crucial role played by the TM joint during opposition of the thumb but the MP and the IP joints are important in determining which finger will participate in opposition with the thumb. In fact, it is the occurrence of variable degrees of flexion at these joints that permits the thumb to select a finger for opposition.

When the thumb and index are opposed with close contact of their pulps (Fig. 208), there is very little flexion at the MP joint with no medial rotation (pronation) or medial displacement of P_1, which is prevented by the medial ligament. The IP joint is extended. There are other modes of opposition between the thumb and the index, e.g. termino-terminal where the MP joint is in full extension and the IP joint flexed.

When the thumb and little finger are opposed termino-terminally (Fig. 208a), the MP joint is flexed and there is concurrent medial displacement and pronation of P_1, while the IP joint is flexed. When there is opposition with contact of the pads, the IP joint is extended.

Opposition with the ring finger and the middle finger occurs as a result of an intermediate degree of flexion at the MP joint and medial displacement and pronation of P_1.

Thus it can be said that during opposition, *after the thumb has come to lie anterior to the plane of the palm, it is the MP joint that allows the thumb to choose a finger for contact.*

Opposition, which is essential to grasp an object, would be useless without *counteropposition*, which allows the hand to release its grip or makes it capable of grasping very large objects. This movement, starting from the position of opposition, is comprised of three components:

— Extension

— Retroposition

— Supination (lateral rotation) of the column of the thumb.

The motor muscles of counteropposition are:

— the abductor pollicis longus

— the extensor pollicis brevis

— especially, the extensor pollicis longus, which alone can bring it into the position of extreme retroposition, i.e. in the plane of the palm.

The *motor nerves of the muscles of the thumb* are (Fig. 210):

— the radial nerve for counteropposition

— the ulnar nerve and particularly the median nerve for opposition.

The *movements used to test integrity of the nerve supply* are:

— extension of the wrist and of the MP joints of the four fingers, extension and counteropposition of the thumb for the radial nerve

— extension of the two distal phalanges of the fingers and the approximation or separation of the fingers for the ulnar nerve

— 'making at fist' and opposition of the thumb for the median nerve.

254

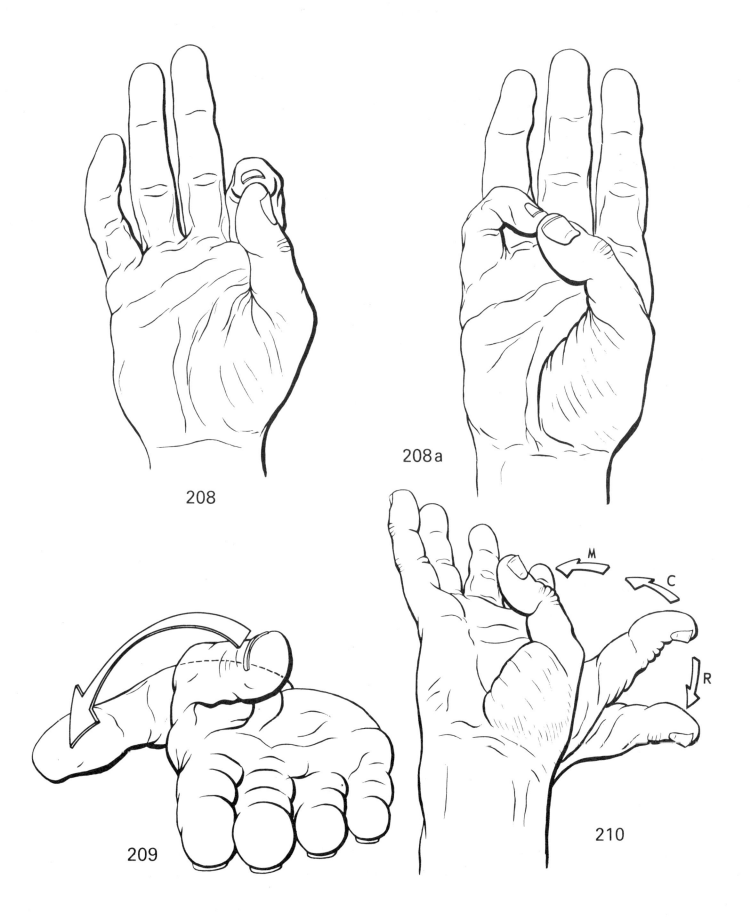

208

208a

209

210

M

C

R

THE MODES OF PREHENSION

The complex anatomical and physiological organization of the hand contributes to prehension. There are many modes of prehension which fall into three broad categories: static grips, grips associated with gravity and dynamic grips (associated with actions). In addition to prehension, the hand can act as an instrument of percussion, as a means of contact and in the performance of gestures. These will be discussed sequentially.

PREHENSION

Static grips can be classified into three groups: digital, palmar and symmetrical. They share one property: they do not require the help of gravity, unlike the other forms of grip.

A) The **digital grips** can be further subdivided into: bi-digital and pluri-digital.

(a) *Bi-digital grips* give rise to the classical *pollici-digital pincer* (usually between the thumb and the index) and fall into three types depending on whether opposition occurs by terminal, subterminal or subtermino-lateral contact.

1. **Prehension by terminal opposition** (Figs. 211 & 212) is the finest and most precise. It allows one to hold a *thin object* (Fig. 211) or to pick up a very fine object like a matchstick or a pin (Fig. 212). The thumb and the index (or the middle finger) come into contact during opposition at the tips of their pulps or even the edges of the nails, when fine objects (e.g. a hair) are being grasped. This requires that the pulp be elastic and properly supported by the nail which plays an all-important part in this mode of prehension. This mode of prehension is most easily upset by any disease of the hand, as it requires the whole range of movements of the joints (flexion reaches its maximum) and especially the intactness of the muscles and tendons, in particular the following:

— *flexor digitorum profundus* (for the index) which stabilises the flexed phalanx; hence the prime importance of repair of this tendon
— *flexor pollicis longus* which has a similar action on the thumb.

2. **Prehension by subterminal opposition** (Fig. 213) is the commonest. It allows one to hold relatively large objects like a pencil or a sheet of paper. The **efficiency of this mode of prehension can be tested** by attempting to pull out a sheet of paper from between the thumb and index. If it is efficient the sheet cannot be pulled out. This test, known as Froment's sign, assesses the strength of the adductor pollicis and thus the integrity of its motor nerve, the ulnar nerve.

In this mode of prehension the thumb and index (or any other finger) are in contact on the palmar surfaces of their pulps. The state of the pulp is of course important but the distal IP joint can be extended or even frozen in mid-flexion by an arthrodesis. The important muscles for this mode of prehension are:

— *flexor digitorum sublimis* (for the index) which stabilises the flexed distal IP joint
— the *thenar muscles which flex the MP joint of the thumb*: flexor pollicis brevis, first anterior interosseus, abductor pollicis brevis and adductor pollicis especially.

3. **Prehension by subtermino-lateral opposition** (Fig. 214). This occurs when one holds a coin. It can replace the first two types when the two distal phalanges of the index have been amputated. The grip is less fine but nevertheless strong. The palmar aspect of the pulp of the thumb presses on the radial surface of the first phalanx of the index. This requires the following muscles:

— *first posterior interosseus* to stabilise the index on the radial side (the index is medially supported by the other fingers)
— *flexor pollicis brevis, first anterior interosseus* and especially *adductor pollicis*.

The involvement of this last muscle has been confirmed electromyographically.

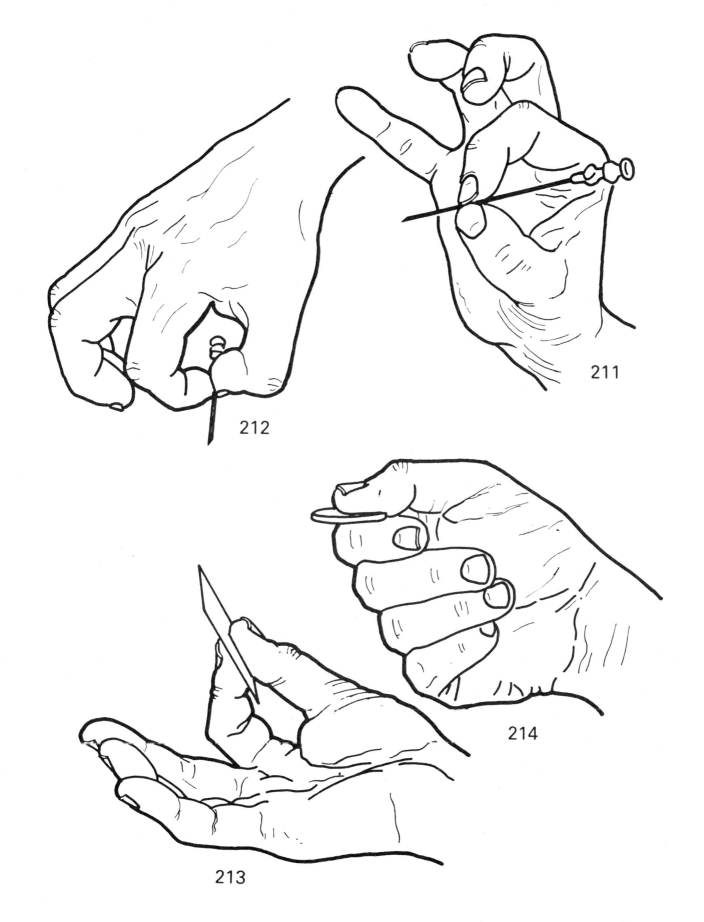

211

212

213

214

THE MODES OF PREHENSION (continued)

4. **Interdigital latero-lateral prehension,** i.e. between the two sides of the fingers (Fig. 215) is the only type of bidigital grip where the thumb is not involved. It is an accessory mode of prehension (e.g. holding a cigarette) and usually occurs between the index and the middle finger. The muscles concerned are *the interossei* (second interossei, anterior and posterior). The grip is weak and has little precision but thumb amputees can develop this grip to an astonishing degree.

(b) *Pluri-digital grips* involve the thumb and any number of fingers and are much stronger than the bi-digital grips, which are essentially precise.

1. **Tridigital grips,** most commonly used, involve the thumb, index and middle finger. The greater part of the world population does not use the fork, and uses this grip to bring food to the mouth. It is a form of *subterminal tridigital prehension* (Fig. 216) and is used when holding a small ball, when the pulp of the thumb presses against the object supported by the pulps of the index and middle finger. It is also used when writing with a pencil (Fig. 217), which is held between *the pulps of the thumb and index and the lateral aspect of the middle finger*. Support is provided by the latter and by the first interdigital cleft. In this sense this grip is directional and resembles symmetrical grips and dynamic grips, since writing results from movements of the shoulder and hand, which slips on the table on its ulnar border and on the little finger, and also of the three fingers. The to and fro movements of the pencil are produced by the flexor pollicis longus and the flexor indicis sublimis, while the lateral sesamoid muscles and the second posterior interosseus keep the pencil in position.

When the cap of a flask is unscrewed (Fig. 218) the grip is tridigital, *with the lateral aspects of the thumb and of P_2 of the middle finger* holding the cap across and *the pulp of the index* helping to stabilize it on the other side. The thumb presses the cap strongly against the middle finger as a result of contraction of the thenar muscles. Tightening of the grip is secured by the flexor pollicis longus and by the flexor indicis sublimis. After the cap has been loosened, it is unscrewed without the help of the index and simply by unwinding of the thumb and middle finger.

If from the start the cap is loose, the unscrewing can be done by a tridigital grip so that the thumb is flexed, the middle finger extended and the index abducted by the first posterior interosseus. This is a grip associated with movement (a dynamic grip).

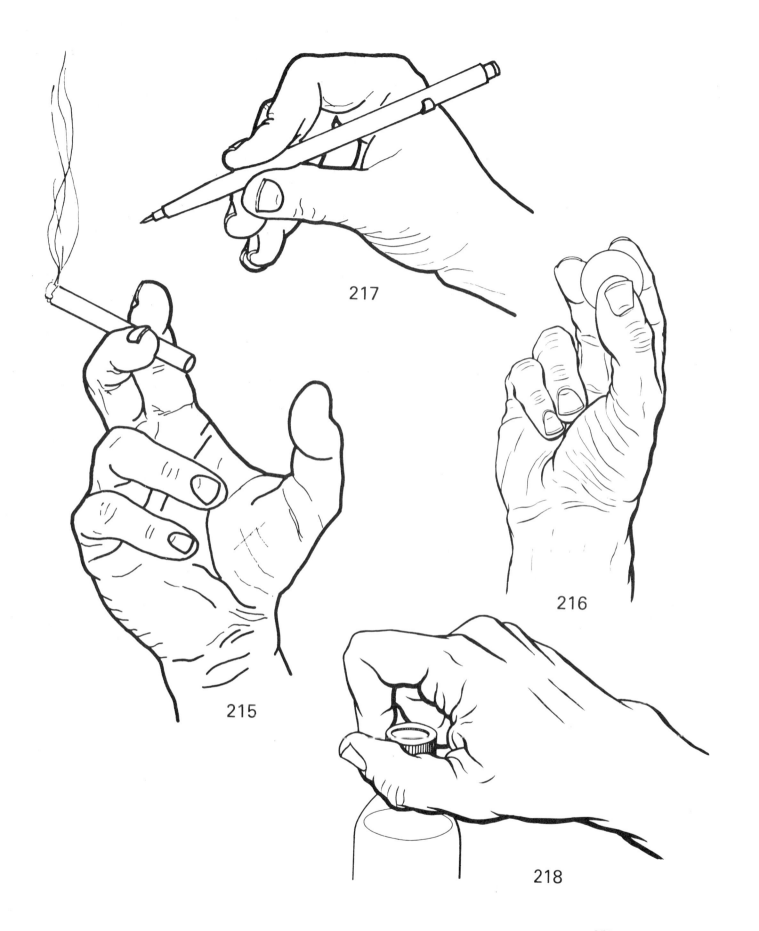

217

215

216

218

259

THE MODES OF PREHENSION (continued)

2. **Tetradigital grips** are used when the object is larger and must be more firmly grasped. They can occur as follows:

— *tetradigital grip with pulp contact* (Fig. 219), when the hand takes hold of a spherical object like a ping-pong ball. The thumb, the index and the middle finger show pulp contact while the ball presses against the side of the ring finger, whose function is to stop the ball from slipping away medially.

— *Tetradigital grip with pulp to side contact* (Fig. 220), as when a lid is unscrewed. The area of contact is extensive, involving the pulps and the palmar surfaces of the first phalanges of the thumb, index and middle finger, and the pulp and lateral aspect of the second phalanx of the ring finger, which stops the lid from slipping medially. As the thumb and fingers surround the lid, the fingers move spirally and it can be shown that the resultant of forces is nil at the centre of the lid, which is displaced in the direction of the MP joint of the index.

— *Tetradigital grip by pulp contact* (pollici-tridigital), as when one holds a charcoal pencil, a brush or a pencil. The pulp of the thumb presses the object firmly agains the pulps of the index, middle and ring fingers, which are almost completely extended. This is also how the violinist or the cellist holds his bow.

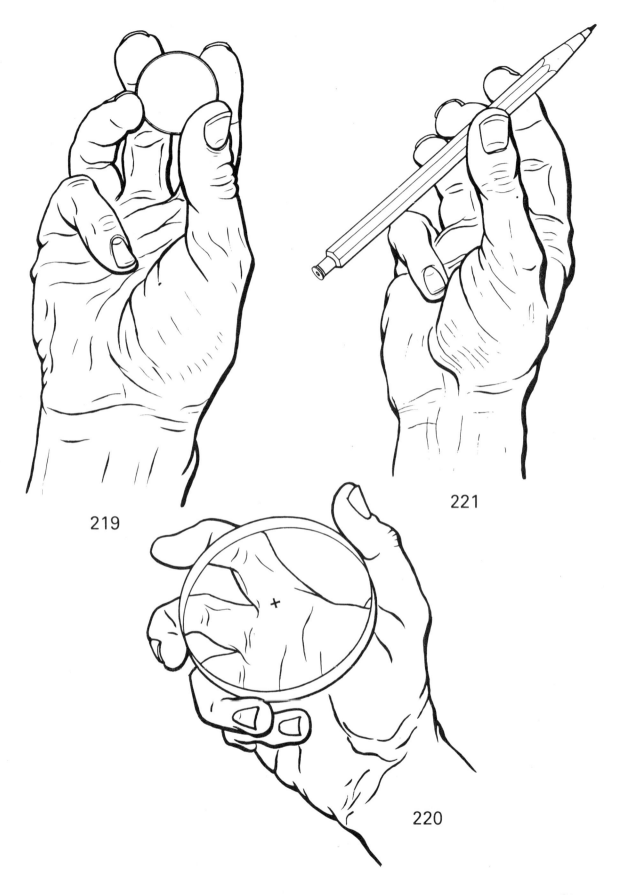

219

221

220

THE MODES OF PREHENSION (continued)

3. **Pentadigital grips** utilise all the fingers with the thumb in variable positions of opposition. They are used, as a rule, to grasp large objects. However even small objects can be held in a penta-digital grip with pulp contact (Fig. 222), with only the little finger showing lateral contact. As the object gets bigger, as for example a tennis ball, the *pentadigital grip is by pulp and side contact* (Fig. 223). The palmar surfaces of the thumb, index, middle and ring fingers are in contact with the ball and surround it almost completely. The thumb lies in opposition to these three fingers. The little finger is in contact on its lateral surface and prevents the ball from slipping medially and proximally. Though not a palmar grip, as the ball is held by the fingers above the palm, it is very strong.

Another pentadigital grip involves holding a large hemispherical object (e.g. a bowl) in the first interdigital cleft (Fig. 224). The thumb and index, widely extended and separated from each other, touch the object along their entire palmar surfaces. This can only occur if the first interdigital cleft can be widened normally, which is not the case when fractures of M_1 or traumatic lesions of the cleft cause its retraction. The bowl is also supported (Fig. 225) by the middle, ring and little fingers, which make contact with their two distal phalanges. It is thus a truly digital grip.

The *'panoramic' pentadigital grip* (Fig. 226) allows one to take hold of large flat objects, e.g. a saucer. It depends on wide separation of the fingers with the thumb in maximal counteropposition, i.e. retroposition and extension. It lies diametrically opposite to the little finger (white arrows), with which it forms an angle of 180°. In between lie the index and middle finger. The little finger lies on the other semicircle and forms an angle of 215° with the thumb. These two fingers are maximally separated, as when spanning an octave on the piano, and constitute a 'triangular' grip with the index and a 'spider' grip with the others, so that the object cannot escape. Note that the efficiency of this grip depends of the integrity of the DIP joints and on the action of the deep flexors.

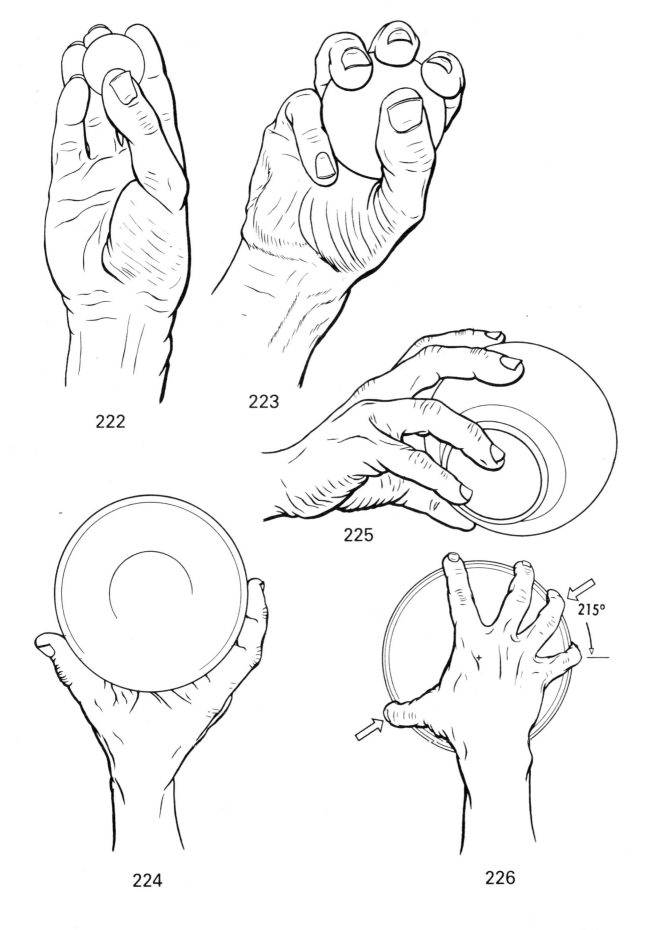

222

223

225

224

226

215°

THE MODES OF PREHENSION (continued)

B) **Palmar grips** involve both the fingers and the palm. They are of two types depending on whether or not the thumb is included.

(a) **Digito-palmar prehension** (Fig. 227) is an accessory mode of prehension but it is fairly commonly used, e.g. to manipulate a handle or hold a steering wheel. The object of *small diameter* (3–4 cm) is held between the flexed fingers and the palm, and the thumb is not involved. The grip is strong up to a certain point in the disto-proximal direction. When held near the wrist the object can easily slip away as the grip is not locked. The axis of the grip is perpendicular to the axis of the hand and does not follow the oblique direction of the palmar gutter. This digito-palmar grip can also be used when holding a larger object, such as a glass (Fig. 228) but the greater the diameter of the object the weaker the grip.

(b) **Full palmar prehension**, i.e. with the whole palm or the whole hand (Fig. 229 & Fig. 230), allows one to grasp powerfully *heavy and relatively large objects*. The hand wraps itself round cylindrical objects (Fig. 229) and the axis of the object coincides with that of the palmar gutter i.e. *it runs obliquely from the hypothenar eminence to the base of the index*. The obliquity of this axis with respect to the axis of the hand and that of the forearm corresponds to the obliquity of the handle of a tool (Fig. 230), which forms an angle of 100° to 110° with the body of the tool. It is easy to note that one can compensate more easily for a wider (120°–130°) than for a narrower (90°) angle, because ulnar deviation of the wrist is greater than its radial deviation.

The *volume* of the object grasped determines the strength of the grip, which is maximal when the thumb can still touch (or nearly so) the index. The thumb in fact forms the only buttress against the force of the other four fingers and its efficiency is greater the more flexed it is. This determines the size of the diameter of the handles of the tools.

The *shape* of the object grasped is also important and nowadays handles are made bearing the imprints appropriate for the fingers.

The important muscles for this mode of prehension are:

— The *digital flexors* and especially *the interossei* to flex the MP joints of the fingers powerfully

— *All the muscles of the thenar eminence* (especially adductor pollicis) and the flexor pollicis longus to lock the grip thanks to flexion of the IP joint of the thumb.

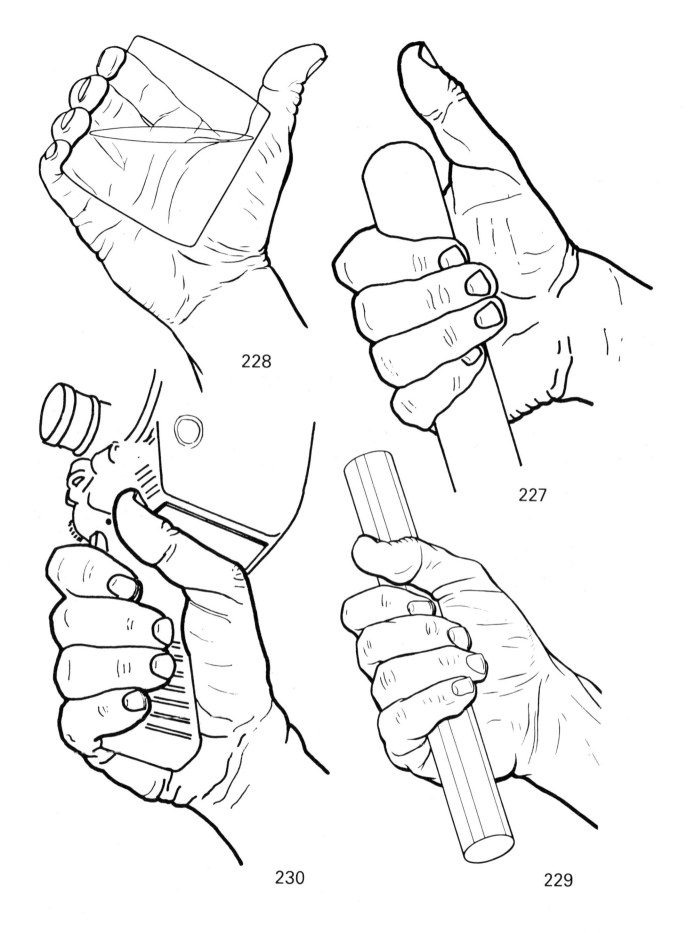

228

227

230

229

THE MODES OF PREHENSION (continued)

1) During **cylindrical palmar prehension** large objects are less firmly gripped the larger they are (Figs. 231 & 232). The grip is locked because medial displacement of P_1 at the MP joint of the thumb allows the thumb to hold the object along the shortest path and thus to surround it (see p. 234). On the other hand, because of the size of the object, the first interdigital cleft must be opened at its widest.

2) **Spherical palmar prehension** may concern three, four or five fingers. When *three* (Fig. 233) or *four* (Fig. 234) fingers are involved, the most medial finger, i.e. the middle finger or the ring finger respectively, is in contact with the object on its lateral aspect and, helped by the uninvolved fingers (the little finger alone or the little and ring fingers), it prevents it from escaping medially. As the object is also held by the thumb laterally, it is locked distally by the palmar surfaces of the fingers involved.

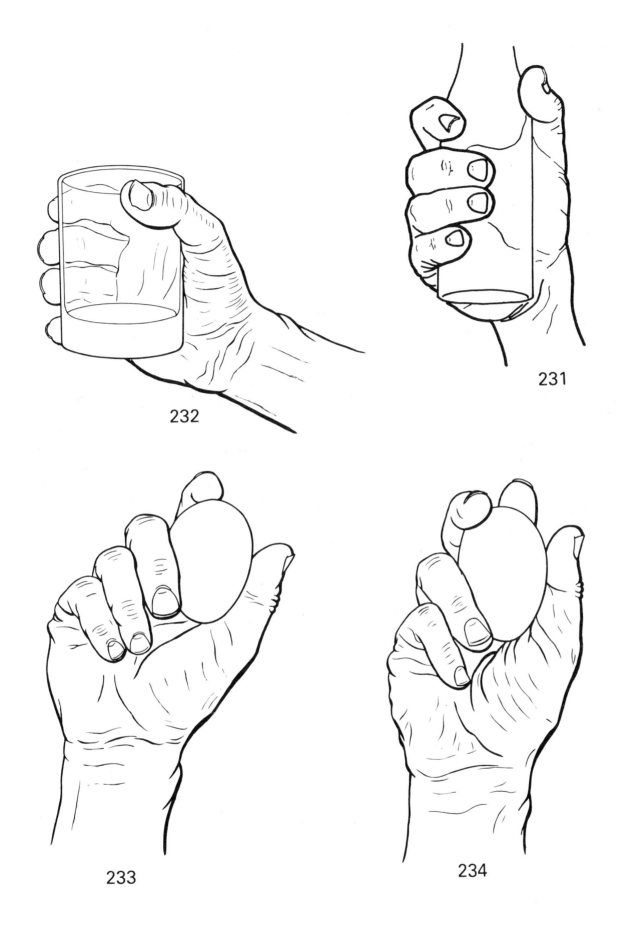

232

231

233

234

THE MODES OF PREHENSION (continued)

During **spherical pentadigital palmar prehension** (Fig. 235), all the fingers have palmar contact with the object. The thumb is directly opposite the little finger and they are the most widely separated. The grip is locked distally by the index and the middle finger and proximally by the thenar eminence and the little finger. The object in contact with the palm is firmly hooked by the flexed fingers and this is possible only if the interdigital clefts can be maximally widened and if the superficial and deep flexors of the fingers are working efficiently. This grip is much more symmetrical than the last two and thus is closer to the following types.

C) **Centralised grips** are in fact symmetrical about a longitudinal axis, which generally coincides with the axis of the forearm. This is seen when the conductor holds his baton (Fig. 236), which is in line with the axis of the forearm and presents an extension of the index in its role of indicator. This coincidence of axes is mechanically essential when *one holds a screwdriver* (Fig. 237), i.e. its axis coincides with the axis of pronation-supination during screwing or unscrewing. This is also the case when *one holds a fork* (Fig. 238) or a knife, which essentially elongates the hand distally. In every case the long object is firmly grasped in a palmar grip using the thumb and the three fingers while *the index orientates the tool*.

Centralised or directional grips are in common use and can be achieved only when the three fingers can be flexed, the index completely extended with its flexors in good trim and the thumb can be minimally opposed, even though flexion at the IP joint is prevented.

268

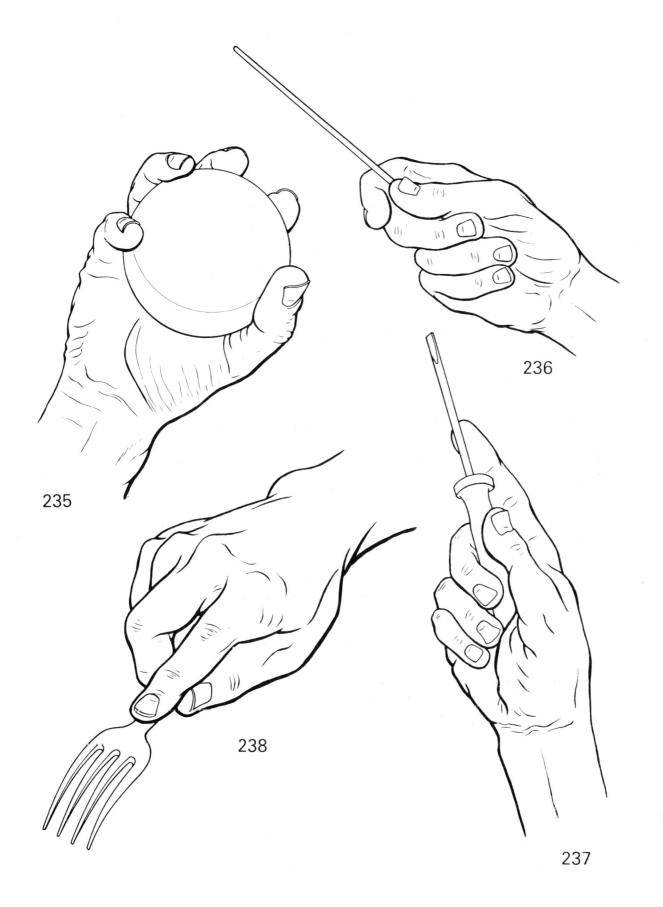

235

236

238

237

THE MODES OF PREHENSION (continued)

So far only grips where gravity is not involved have been discussed, but there are others which depend critically on the action of gravity and cannot operate under conditions of weightlessness, e.g. in a space cabin.

In these **gravity-dependent grips** the hand acts as a *supportive* platform, e.g. when it supports a tray (Fig. 239). This can only be done when the hand can be flattened with the palm facing superiorly or can form a tripod under the object.

Under the force of gravity, the hand can act as a *spoon*, as when it contains grains (Fig. 240) or a liquid. The hollow of the hand is extended by that of the fingers as they are closely approximated by the anterior interossei to prevent any leaks. The thumb is very important as it closes the palmar gutter laterally. Half flexed, it is pulled against M_2 and P_1 of the index by its adductor. A larger shell can be made by hollowing both hands (Fig. 241), and bringing them together along their ulnar borders.

All these gravity-dependent modes of prehension depend on the *integrity of supination*. Without it, the palm, which is the only part able to form a concave surface, cannot be oriented anteriorly. Thus the tray test allows one to assess recovery of supination, which cannot be compensated for by shoulder movements.

Grasping a bowl with three fingers (Fig. 242) needs the effect of gravity, as its edge is held between two prongs, formed by the thumb and the middle finger and a hook, i.e. the index. This grip depends on the stability of the thumb and the middle finger and the integrity of the flexor profundus indicis, which helps P_3 of the index to hold the sickle-shaped fold of the bowl. The adductor pollicis is also indispensable.

Grips with one or more fingers in the claw position, as when carrying a pail or a suitcase or trying to cling to a rocky surface, also depend on gravity.

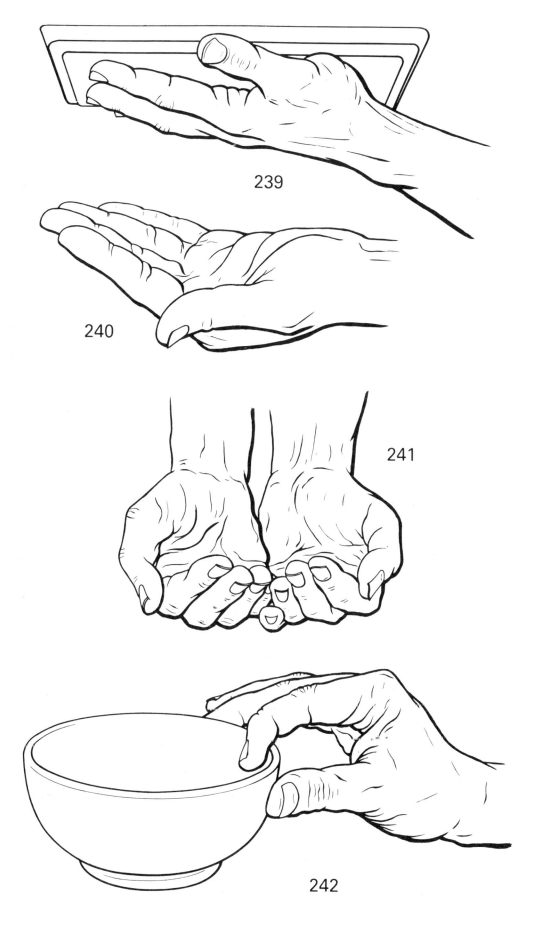

239

240

241

242

271

THE MODES OF PREHENSION (continued)

These static grips, discussed so far, do not include all the possible grips of the hand. The hand can also act while grasping. We call these **dynamic grips.**

Some of these actions are simple. For example, when *one sets a top turning* (Fig. 243), it is held *tangentially* between the thumb and index; when a *marble is shot* by a sudden flick of P_2 of the thumb, produced by the extensor pollicis longus, the marble is first of all held in the hollow of the index, fully flexed by the deep flexor.

Other actions are more *complex* with the hand bending back on itself. In this case the object held by one part of the hand is acted upon by another part. These types of dynamic grips are innumerable and the following examples are given:

— the *lighting of a cigarette lighter* (Fig. 245), which resembles fairly closely the shooting of the marble. The lighter is held in the hollow of the index and of the other fingers, while the flexed thumb presses on the top (action of the flexor pollicis longus and the thenar muscles).

— *squeezing the top of a spray can* (Fig. 246): this time the object is held by a palmar grip and it is the flexed index that presses on the top (action of the flexor indicis profundus).

— *cutting with scissors* (Fig. 247): the handles are threaded on to the thumb and the middle or ring finger. The thumb muscles provide the force needed to open (thenar muscles) or close (extensor pollicis longus) the scissors. The opening of the scissors, when excessively repeated professionally, may lead to rupture of the extensor longus. The index orients the scissors, thus providing an example of a directional dynamic grip.

— *eating with chopsticks* (Fig. 248): one stick, jammed in the first interdigital cleft by the ring finger, stays put while the other, held in a tridigital grip with the thumb, index and middle finger, forms a pincer with the former. This is certainly a good test of manual dexterity for Europeans while Asiatics use chopsticks almost unconsciously.

— *tying knots with one hand* (Fig. 249): this also is a test of manual dexterity based on the independent and coordinated action of two bidigital pincers, i.e. the one formed by the index and middle finger laterally apposed and the other by the thumb and the ring finger, a rarely used pollici-digital grip. Surgeons use a closely related grip to tie knots with one hand. Such complex actions involving one hand are very commonly used by jugglers and conjurers, whose above-average manual dexterity is maintained by daily exercises.

— *the left hand of the violinist* (Fig. 250) or of the guitarist achieves a *very flexible dynamic grip.* The thumb supports the neck of the violin and, while moving up and down, 'opposes' the pressure applied by the other four fingers. This pressure must be at once precise, firm and modulated to produce the vibrato. These complex actions can only be performed after many years of training and require daily exercises.

Each reader can find for himself the *infinite variety of dynamic grips* which represent the most elaborate activity of the hand when endowed with its full functional capacity.

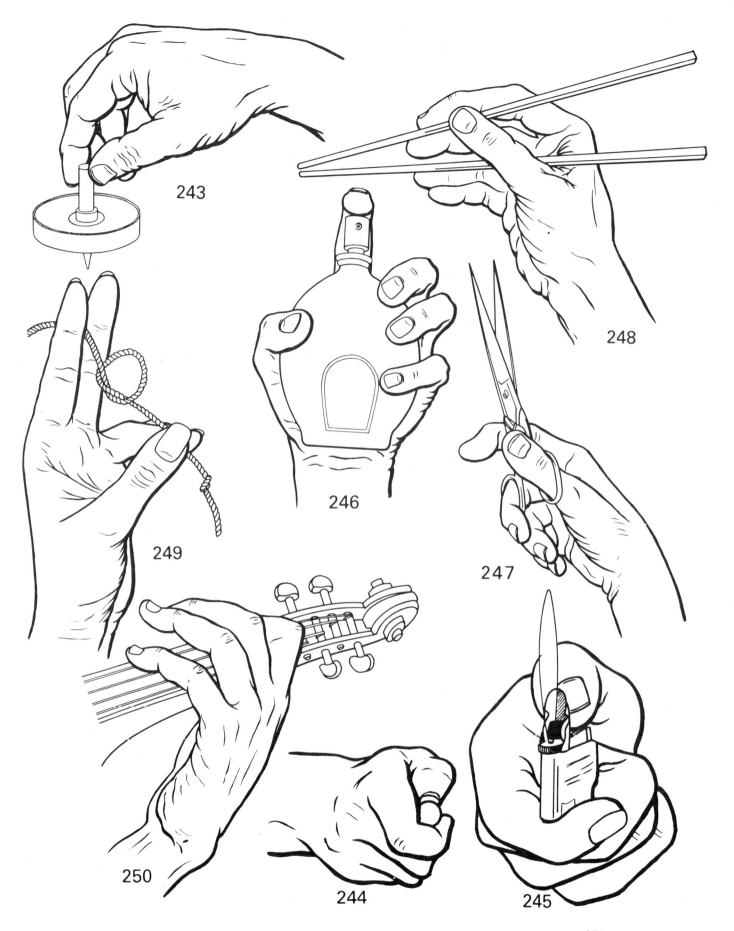

273

PERCUSSION — CONTACT — GESTURES

The human hand can also be used as an **instrument of percussion:**

— when, for instance, one uses a calculating or a typewriting machine (Fig. 251) or plays the piano. Each finger behaves as a little hammer hitting the keyboard as a result of the coordinated action of the interossei and the flexors, especially the profundus. The difficulty lies in acquiring functional independence among the fingers and between the two hands. This requires special training of brain and muscles and constant practice.

— when blows are dealt by the fist (Fig. 252) in boxing, by the ulnar border or tip of the hand in karate or by the outspread hand when a slap is given.

Contact achieved by the hand is softer when it *caresses* (Fig. 253), an action of fundamental importance in social and particularly affective interaction. Note that intact cutaneous sensitivity is essential for the hand that caresses and the hand being caressed. In some cases contact with two hands may heal as in the laying on of hands, which may be effective even at a distance. Finally the most banal gesture of everyday life in the West, the handshake, (Fig. 254), represents a social contact charged with symbolic meaning.

This brings us to the irreplaceable role of the hands in the *performance of gestures*. In fact gestures are performed as a result of close cooperation between the face and the hand. They are under subcortical control, as they disappear in Parkinsonism. This language of the face and hands is codified in the language of the deaf and mute but *the gamut of instinctive gestures constitutes a second language*, which, unlike spoken language, is *universally understood*. This mode of expression consists of innumerable gestures, which may show geographical variations but are generally understood all over the world, as, for example, the wrist raised in threat (Fig. 252), the peace greeting with the hand wide open, the finger pointed accusingly (Fig. 255) or applause expressing approval. This instinctive language is developed professionally by actors but it is also an integral part of every man's behaviour. Its goal is to underline and stress a particular facial expression but often it does so without any words and is enough by itself to express sentiments and situations. Hence the extensive use of the 'posturing hand' in painting and sculpture. This role of the hand is as important as its role in grasping and feeling. In certain jobs, as in *pottery* (Fig. 256), the hand is multi-functional. It is the effector organ that models the object, it is the sensory organ that recognises and modifies its shape constantly and finally it is the organ of symbolic expression, as it offers the object of its creation to mankind. It is the *completeness of the creative gesture* that makes it so valuable.

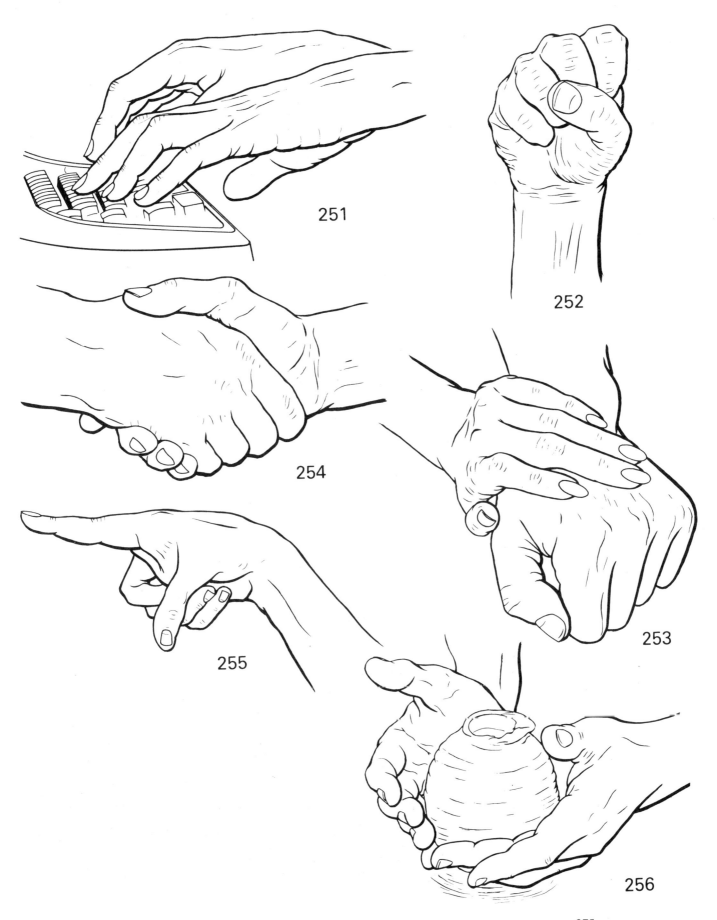

251

252

254

253

255

256

275

THE POSITIONS OF FUNCTION AND IMMOBILISATION

The position of function of the hand, initially described by Bunnel (1948) as the position of the hand at rest, is quite different from that observed during sleep (Fig. 257, according to Michelangelo). The latter position, called **the position of relaxation**, is also that assumed by the wounded arm so as to reduce pain and consists of: forearm in pronation, wrist flexed, thumb in adduction and retroposition, the first interdigital cleft closed, fingers relatively extended particularly at the level of the MP joints.

The **position of function** (Figs. 28 & 29) was redefined by Littler (1951) as follows: forearm in semi-pronation, wrist *in 30° extension* and adduction, the thumb in a straight line with the radius and forming an angle of 45° with M_2, the MP and IP joints of the thumb almost fully extended, fingers slightly flexed and the MP joints of the fingers flexed, the degree of flexion increasing towards the little finger. As a whole this position of function corresponds with that in which prehension could take place with minimal articular mobility, if one or more of the joints of the fingers and thumb were ankylosed, or with that in which the recovery of useful movements could be relatively easy, since opposition is already almost full and could be completed by a few degrees of flexion in any one of the still active joints.

There are, however, in practice *three positions of immobilisation* (Tubiana 1951):
— **The temporary or protective position of immobilisation** (Fig. 260), which aims at preserving the eventual mobility of the hand:
  — forearm in mid-flexion and pronation with the elbow flexed to 100°
  — wrist in extension to 20° and slight adduction
  — fingers flexed, the more so as they are more medial
  — the MP joint flexed between 50° and 80°, the more so the less flexed are the PIP joints
  — the IP joints moderately flexed to reduce tension and possible ischaemia:
    • the PIP joints between 10° and 40°
    • the DIP joints between 10° and 20°
  — the thumb in the initial stage of opposition:
    • M_1 in slight adduction but also in anteposition keeping the interdigital cleft open;
    • MP and IP joints in very slight extension so that the pulp of the thumb points towards those of the index and middle finger.
— The **positions of definitive immobilisation or functional fixation,** which depend on the individual case:
  — as regards the **wrist:**
    • when the fingers are still able to grip, the wrist should fused in 25° extension so as to place the hand in a gripping position.
    • when the fingers are unable to grip, it is better to fix the wrist in flexion
    • if both wrists are fused then it is imperative to keep one in flexion to facilitate personal hygiene
    • if a cane is to be used it is necessary to fix the wrist in full extension. If two canes are to be used the wrist of the dominant hand should be fixed in 10° extension and the other in 10° flexion.
  — the *forearm* is immobilised in more or less full pronation
  — the *MP joints* are fixed in flexion varying from 35° for the index to 50° for the little finger
  — the *PIP joints* are fixed in flexion varying from 40° to 60°
  — the *TM joint* is arthrodesed in a position that suits each case but, every time one of the elements of the pollici-digital pincer is put out of action, the functional capabilities of the other elements must be considered.
— **The non-functional positions of 'temporary immobilisation' or of partial relaxation.**
These should only be used for a very short time to achieve stability at the level of a fracture or a dehiscence in sutures applied to a tendon or a nerve.
There is a serious risk of developing stiffness as a result of venous and lymphatic stasis. It is considerably reduced if the joints near those immobilised are actively exercised.
  — when the median or ulnar nerve or the flexor tendons have been sutured, the wrist can be safely kept in flexion at 40° for *three weeks* but it is crucial to immobilise the MP joints in approximately 80° flexion, while keeping the IP joints in their state of natural extension, since recovery of extension is difficult to achieve after forced flexion.
  — when the dorsal structures have been repaired, the joints must be immobilised in extension but the MP joints must be kept in at least 10° flexion. The IP joints should be flexed at 20°, if the damage occurred proximal to the MP joints but they should be in the neutral position if the damage was at the level of P_1;
  — when 'buttonhole' lesions are being repaired, the PIP joint is immobilised in extension and the DIP joint in flexion so as to pull the extensor tendons distally.
  — conversely, when the lesion is near the DIP joint, it is immobilised in extension and the PIP joint in flexion so as to relax the lateral **fibres** of the extensors.

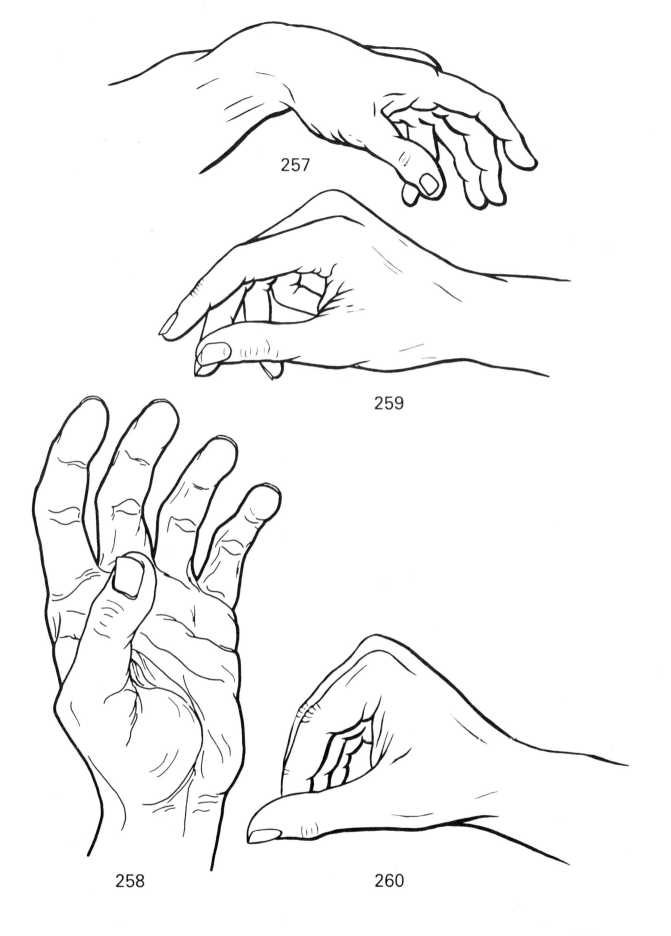

257

259

258

260

FICTIONAL HANDS

The study of fictional hands is not simply an exercise of the imagination: it allows a better understanding of the structural rationale of the human hand. The types of hand that can be imagined fall into two categories: asymmetrical and symmetrical.

The **asymmetrical hands** can be derived from the normal hand by reducing or increasing the number of fingers or by inverting its symmetry.

An *increase in the number of fingers*, a sixth or seventh finger added beyond the little finger on the ulnar border of the hand, would certainly strengthen the full palmar grip but it would give rise to unacceptable functional complications.

A *decrease in the number of fingers* to four or three would reduce the capabilities of the hand. In some monkeys of Central America the upper limb is a hand with four fingers and no thumb, which can only cling to tree branches, while the lower limb is a hand with five fingers and a thumb capable of opposition. The *hand with three fingers* (Fig. 261), as seen after certain amputations, retains the tridigital and bidigital grips, which are the most commonly used and the most precise but has lost the full palmar grip needed to grasp the handles of tools etc. In the *hand with two fingers* (Fig. 262), the thumb and index can still form a hook and a bidigital pincer to grasp small objects but tridigital and full palmar grips are impossible. Yet unexpected results are obtained when such a hand is retained or reconstructed in some patients. Note also that this hand is symmetrical with all the inherent defects of a symmetrical hand.

The *symmetrically inverted hand*, i.e. the hand with the thumb located medially, would have a palmar gutter running obliquely in the opposite direction. Thus in the neutral position of pronation-supination the head of the hammer, instead of looking distally and superiorly would look distally and inferiorly and this change of orientation would prevent one from hitting a nail on the head, unless the neutral position of pronation-supination were reversed +180°, i.e. with the palm pointing laterally! The ulna would override the radius and the insertion of the biceps on the radius would reduce the efficiency of the muscle. In sum the entire architecture of the upper limb would have to be altered without any evident functional advantage.

Symmetrical hands would have *two thumbs*, one medial and one lateral, with two or three fingers lying in between. In *the symmetrical hand with three fingers* (Fig. 263), the simplest type, the following grips would be possible: pollici-digital, bipollical (between the two thumbs) and a tridigital grip (Fig. 264) with the thumbs opposing the index. Thus four precision grips would be possible. A full palmar grip (Fig. 265) would be achieved between the thumbs on the one hand and the palm and the index on the other. Though fairly strong, this grip would suffer from a serious disadvantage, i.e because of its symmetry, the handle of a tool would lie *perpendicular to the axis of the forearm*. Now we have seen that the tool can only be properly oriented for use when the handle runs obliquely with respect to the axis of pronation-supination. The same would apply to symmetrical hands with two or three intermediate fingers (Fig. 266), i.e. with five fingers. Parrots have two fingers posteriorly forming a symmetrical claw, which allows them to stand firmly on a branch.

An unfortunate consequence of the symmetrical hand with two thumbs would be the need for a symmetrical disposition of the forearm, which would exclude pronation-supination.

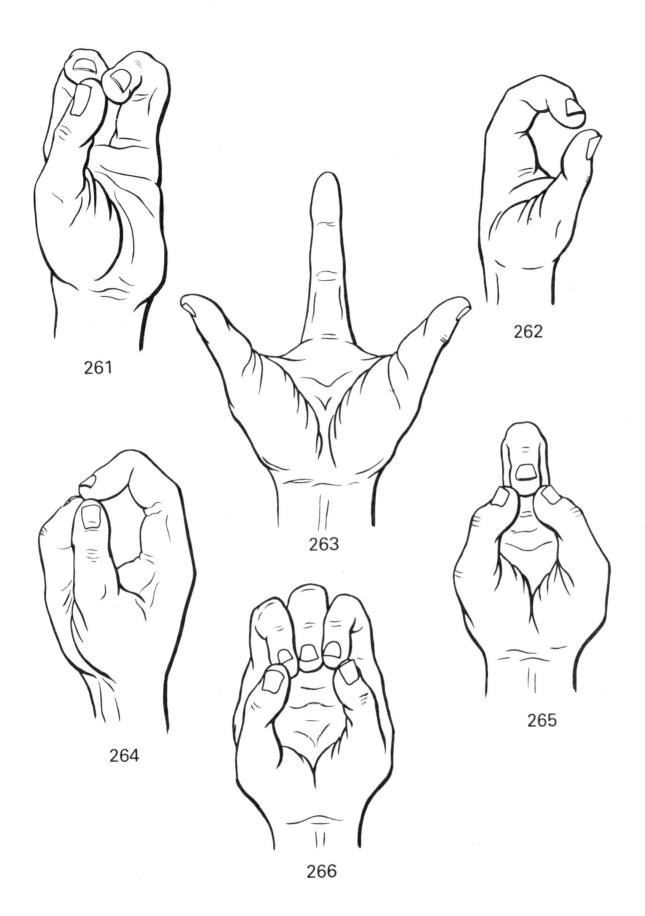

261

262

263

264

266

265

279

THE HUMAN HAND

The human hand, despite its complexity, turns out to be a perfectly logical structure, fully adapted to its multiple functions. Its architecture reflects Occam's principle of universal economy. It is one of the most beautiful achievements of nature.

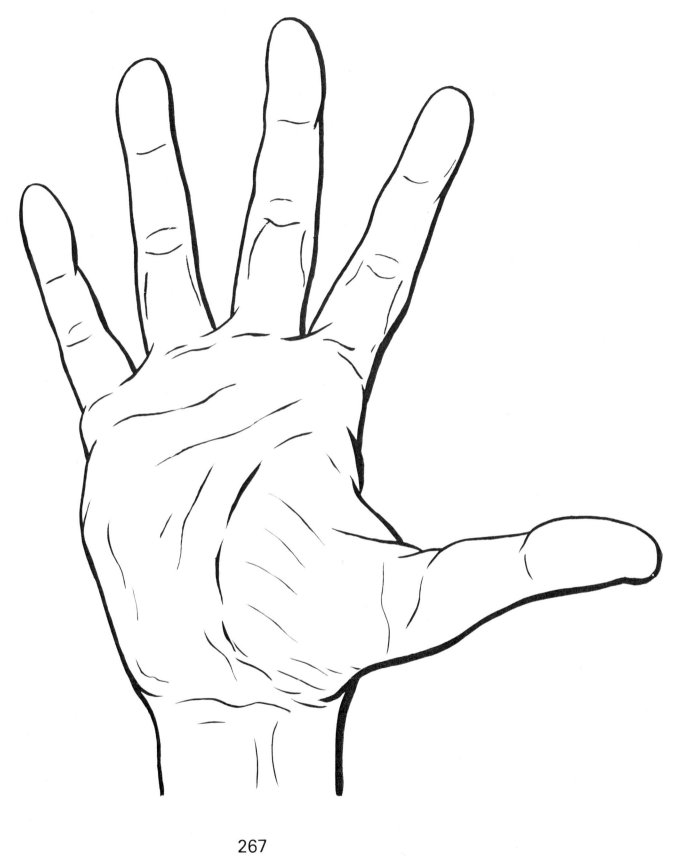

267

281

REFERENCES

BARNETT C.H., DAVIES D.V. & MAC CON-AILL M.A. — Synovial Joints. Their structure and mechanics. 1961, C.C. Thomas, Springfield U.S.A.

BARNIER L. — L'analyse des mouvements, 1950, P.U.F., Ed. Paris.

BAUSENHARDT D. — Uber das carpo-metacarpalgelenk des Daumens, 1949, Zeitschr. Anat. Entw. Gesch. Bd, 114–251.

COMTET J.J. & AUFFRAY Y. — Physiologie des muscles élévateurs de l'épaule. Rev. Chir. Ortho., 1970, *56*, 3, 105–117.

DAUTRY P. & GOSSET J. — A propos de la rupture de la coiffe des rotateurs de l'épaule. Rev. Chir. Ortho., 1969, *55*, 2, 157.

DBJAY H.C. — L'humérus dans la prono-supination. Rev. Méd. Limoges, 1972, *3*, 3, 147–150.

DE LA CAFFINIERE J.Y. — L'articulation trapézo-métacarpienne, approche biomécanique et appareil ligamentaire. Arch. Anat. Path., 1970, *18*, 4, 277–284.

DE LA CAFFINIERE J.Y., MAZAS F., MAZAS Y., PELISSE F. & PRESENT D. — Prothèse totale d'épaule, bases expérimentales et premiers résultats cliniques. Vol. IV, N° 5, 1975, Editions INSERM (Paris).

DESCAMPS Louis — Le jeu de la hanche. Thèse, Paris 1950.

DUBOUSSET J. — Les phénomènes de rotation lors de la préhension au niveau des doigts (sauf le pouce). Ann. Chir., 1971, *25*, (19–20), C. 935–944.

DUCHENNE G.B.A. (DE BOULOGNE) — Physiologie des mouvements. 1867: Réédition en fac-similé, Ann. Med. Physique, Lille. 1959: Ed. Américaine translated by E.B. KAPLAN (1949). W.B. Saunders Co, Philadelphia and London.

DUPARC J., DE LA CAFFINIERE J.Y. & PINEAU H. — Approche biomécanique et cotation des mouvements du premier métacarpien. Rev. Chir. Orthop., 1971, *57*, 1, 3–12.

FICK R. — Handbuch der Anatomie und mechanik Gelenke. 1911, Gustav Fischer, Iéna, Allemagne.

FISCHER L.P., NOIRCLERC J.A., NEIDART J.M., SPAY G. COMTET J.J. — Etude anatomoradiologique de l'importance des différents ligaments dans la contention verticale de la tête de l'humérus. Lyon, Méd., 1970, *223*, 11, 629–633.

FISCHER L.P., CARRET J.P., GONON G.P. & DIMMET J. — Etude cinématique des mouvements de l'articulation scapulo-humérale. Rev. Chir. Orth., 1977, Suppl. 11, *63*, 108–112.

HAMONET C., DE LA CAFFINIERE J.Y., OPSOMER G. — Mouvements du pouce. Détermination électromyographique des secteurs d'activité des muscles thénariens. Arch. Anat. Path., 1972, *20*, 4, 363–367.

HAMONET C., DE LA CAFFINIERE J.Y. & tromyographique du rôle de l'opposant du pouce (opponens pollicis) et de l'adducteur du pouce (adductor pollocis). Rev. Chir. Ortho., 1970, *56*, 2, 165–176.

HENKE W. — Handbuch der anatomie und mechanik der gelenke, 1863. C.F. Wintersche Verlashandlung, Heidelberg.

INMAN-VERNET T. et al — Observations on the function of the shoulder joint. 1944, J. Bone Joint Surg., 26, 1, 30.

KAPANDJI I.A. — La flexion-pronation de l'interphalangienne du pouce. Ann. Chir., 1976, *30*, 11–12, 855–857.

KAPANDJI I.A. — Pourquoi l'avant-bras comporte-til deux os? Ann. Chir., 1975, *29*, 5, 463–470.

KAPANDJI I.A. — Le membre supérieur, support logistique de la main. Ann. Chir., 1977, *31*, 12, 1021–1030.

KAPANDJI I.A. — La radio-cubitale inférieure vue sous l'angle de la prono-supination. Ann. Chir., 1977, *31*, 12, 1031–1039.

KAPANDJI I.A. — La rotation du pouce sur son axe longitudinal lors de l'opposition. Etude géométrique et mécanique de la trapézo-métacarpienne. Modèle mècanique de la main. Rev. Chir. Orthop., 1972, *58*, 4, 273–289.

KAPANDJI I.A. — Anatomie fonctionnelle de la métacarpo-phalangienne du pouce. Ann. Chir. 1980.

KAPANDJI I.A. & MOATTI E. — La radiographie spécifique de la trapézo-métacarpienne, sa technique, son intérêt. Ann. Chir. 1980.

KUCZYNSKI K. — Carpometacarpal joint of the human thumb. J. Anat., 1974, *118*, 1, 119–126.

KUHLMANN N., GALLAIRE M. & PINEAU H. — Déplacements du scaphoïde et du semi-lunaire au cours des mouvements du poignet. Ann. Chir., 1978, *32*, 9, 543–553.

LANDSMEER J.M.F. — A report on the coordination of the interphalangeal joints of the human finger and its disturbances. Acta morph. neerl. scand., 1953, 2, 59–84.

LANDSMEER J.M.F. — Anatomical and functional investigations on the articulation of the human finger. Acta anat. (supp. 24), 1955, 25, 1, 69.

LANDSMEER J.M.F. — Studies in the anatomy of articulations. 1) The equilibrium of the intercalated bone; 2) Patterns of movements of bimuscular, biarticular systems. Acta morph. neerl Scand, 1961, 3, 3–4, 287–321.

LANDSMEER J.M.F. — Atlas of anatomy of the hand. Churchill Livingstone. Edinburgh London and New York, 1976.

LITTLER J.W. — Les principes architecturaux et fonctionnels de l'anatomie de la main. Rev. Chir. Orthop., 1960, 46, 2, 131–139.

LUNDBORD G., MYRHAGE E. & RYDEVIK B. — Vascularisation des tendons fléchisseurs dans la gaine digitale. J. Hand Surg., 1977, 2, 6, 417–427.

LONG C., BROWN M.E. — Electromyographic-Kinesiology of the hand: muscles moving the long finger. J. Bone & Joint Surg., 1964, 46 A, 1638–1706.

LONG C. & BROWN M.E. — Electromyographic kinesiology of the hand. Part III. Lumbricalis and flexor digitonum profundus to the long finger. Arch. Phys. Med., 1962, 43, 450–460.

LONG C., BROWN M.E. & WEISS G. — Electromyographic study of the extrinsic-intrinsic kinesiology of the hand. Preliminary report. Arch. Phys. Med., 1960, 41, 175–181.

MAC CONAILL M.A. — Studies on the anatomy and function of Bone and Joints. 1966, F. Gaynor Evans Ed. New York.

MAC CONAILL M.A. — Studies in mechanics of synovial joints. Displacements of articular surfaces and significance of saddle joints. Irish J.M. Sc. Med. Sci, 1946, July, 223–235.

MAC CONAILL M.A. — Studies in mechanics of synovial joints; hinge joints and nature of intra-articular displacements. Irish J.M., Sci, 1946, Sept., 620.

MAC CONAILL M.A. — Movements of bones and joints. Significance of shape. J. Bone and Joint Surg., 1953, May, 35 B, 290.

MAC CONAILL M.A. — The geometry and algebra of articular kinematics. Bio. Med. Eng., 1966, 1, 205–212.

MAC CONAILL M.A. & BASMAJIAN J.V. — Muscles and movements: a basis for human kinesiology. Williams & Wilkins Co, Baltimore, 1969.

PIERON A.P. — The mechanism of the first carpometacarpal joint. An anatomic and mechanical analysis. Acta Orthop. Scand., 1973 supplementum, 148.

POIRIER P. & CHARPY A. — Traité d'Anatomie Humaine, 1926 (4e édition), Masson Ed. Paris.

RASCH P.J. & BURKE R.K. — Kinesiology and applied anatomy. 1971, Leax Febiger (4e ed.), Philadelphia, U.S.A.

ROCHER C.H. & RIGAUD A. — Fonctions et bilans articulares. Kinésithérapie et rééducation a 1964, Masson Ed., Paris.

ROUD A. — Mécanique des articulations et des muscles de l'homme. 1913, Librairie de l'Université, Lausanne, F. ROUGE & Cie.

ROUVIERE H. — Anatomie humaine descriptive et topographique. 1948 (4e éd.), Masson Ed., Paris.

STEINDLER A. — Kinesiology of the human body. 1955, Charles C. Thomas, Springfield, Illinois, U.S.A.

STRASSER H. — Lehrbuch der Muskel und gelenk-mechanik. 1917, J. Springer, Berlin.

TESTUT L. — Traité d'anatomie humaine. 1921, Doin Ed., Paris.

TUBIANA R. — Les positions d'immobilisation de la main. Ann. Chir., 1973, 27, 5, pp. C. 459–466.

TUBIANA R., HAKSTIAN R. — Les déviations cubitales normales et pathologiques des doigts. Etude de l'architecture des articulations métacarpo-phalangiennes des doigts. La main rhumatoïde. Monographie du GEM, 1969. L'expansion scientifique francaise Ed.

TUBIANA R., VALENTIN P. — L'extension des doigts. Rev. Chir. Orthop., 1963, T 49, 543–562.

VANDERVAEL F. — Analyse des mouvements du corps humain. 1956, Maloine Ed., Paris.

VAN LINGE B. & MULDER J.D. — Fonction du muscle sus-épineux et sa relation avec le syndrome sus-épineux. Etude expérimentale chez l'homme. J. Bone & Joint Surg., 1963, 45 B, 4, 750–754.